Cardiac Emergencies

Edited by
Robert S. Eliot, M.D.

Professor Medicine
University of Nebraska College of Medicine
Director, Cardiovascular Center
Head, Division of Cardiovascular Medicine
University of Nebraska Medical Center

Associate Editors
Gerald L. Wolf, Ph.D., M.D.

Associate Professor of Pharmacology and Radiology
University of Nebraska College of Medicine
Director of Cardiovascular Radiology Research
Cardiovascular Center
University of Nebraska Medical Center

and
Alan D. Forker, M.D.

Associate Professor of Medicine
University of Nebraska College of Medicine
Director of Medical Education
Cardiovascular Center
University of Nebraska Medical Center

 FUTURA PUBLISHING COMPANY, INC.
Mount Kisco, New York
1977

Copyright © 1977
Futura Publishing Company, Inc.

Published by
Futura Publishing Company, Inc.
295 Main Street, P.O. Box 298
Mount Kisco, New York 10549

L.C.: 76-41062
ISBN: 0-87993-075-6

Printed by Noble Offset Printers, Inc., New York, N.Y. 10003

Dedication

To our wives, children,
families, and friends

Acknowledgments

In the preparation of this book the editor would like to express his appreciation to the excellent contributing authors. In addition, I am particularly grateful to my associate editors, friends and colleagues, Drs. Alan Forker and Gerald Wolf. They assisted in the conceptual, structural and editorial phases.

Simultaneously, I would recognize the support and inspiration of our publishers, Mr. Steven Korn and Mr. Jacques Strauss. Both worked very closely with the editors during the development of the text, providing added editorial assistance. Successful implementation of the text was a product of the administrative and secretarial dedication of Ms. Emily Salhany, Mrs. Vicki Aughe, Miss Darla Brown, Mrs. Laura Domboski, Mrs. Delores Reeve, and Mrs. Marge Virgilito.

I would also like to identify the assistance of Ms. Kristan Roskoski, whose editorial capabilities have been of great value in this and a previous text, (*The Practical Management of Hypertension*). If the book is lucid and reaches its mark, it is the product of all these capable individuals for which the author expresses his deepest appreciation.

Once again, our wives Phyllis, Susan and Lynn, ably and enthusiastically aided and abetted our efforts. They remain the unsung heroines of this endeavor.

Foreword

The physician in an affluent, industrialized society finds prevention of the majority of cardiac emergencies an unattainable goal. Of necessity, he frequently confronts cardiovascular disease in his patients on a virtual crisis basis. Until prevention becomes considerably less hypothetical, clinicians must seek information about cardiac emergencies that is directed to limiting the extent of each individual disaster.

This text was developed to provide current knowledge about the mechanisms, diagnosis, and management of cardiac emergencies. Our initial book on this topic resulted from a symposium on the same subject sponsored by the American College of Cardiology in 1972. The symposium has become an annual presentation of the College, reflecting both a rapid change in information and the desire of practitioners for continuing education in the management of these potential catastrophes.

We continue to believe that individual experts can best present selected topics with considerable experience of their own. Although single authored volumes possess many advantages, in our opinion the merits of uniform style weigh less heavily than emphasis on accurate content. Therefore, this book represents an edited collation of subjects of primary interest with each chapter written by experts in respective fields. Each author is a clinician as well as a productive investigator in his area of interest. All chapters have been prefaced by a brief editorial comment that is intended to summarize the content.

The book was born of the need for a comprehensive yet compact "state of the art" presentation addressing the pathophysiology, diagnosis, and management of cardiac emergencies. It is not an all-inclusive book. Priorities have been placed upon those subjects which physicians have indicated are their primary concern for further information and reference.

Topics selected for in-depth discussion include arrhythmias, pump failure, and cardiogenic shock by such leading authors as Gettes, Forrester, Swan and Mason. At times these presentations will not be light reading, yet they are invaluable resources for understanding clinical problems. In certain areas, understanding remains superficial and a panoramic overview most accurately presents the current state of knowledge. This is especially true for the management aspects of most cardiac emergencies.

The book is thus designed and developed for the practicing physician who must know the subject of cardiac emergencies at its contemporary level of understanding. It is not intended for paramedical personnel or even beginning medical students for whom less sophisticated texts are already available. We believe it represents an accurate, readable, and appropriately comprehensive depiction of this frequent clinical problem.

R.S.E.
G.L.W.
A.D.F.

Contributors

Amsterdam, Ezra A., M.D.
  Director, Coronary Care Unit, Section of Cardiovascular Medicine, University of
  California School of Medicine, Davis, California
Baltaxe, Harold A.,
  Professor and Chairman, Department of Radiology, University of Nebraska
  Medical Center, Omaha, Nebraska
Baroldi, Giorgio, M.D.
  Chief, Cardiovascular Section of Pathology, C.N.R. Institute Fisiologia Clinica,
  University of Pisa; Associate Professor, Institute of Morbid Anatomy, University
  of Milan; Visiting Associate Professor of Cardiology and Pathology, University of
  Nebraska Medical Center, Omaha, Nebraska
Berman, Daniel S., M.D.
  Associate Professor of Nuclear Medicine, Director of Nuclear Cardiology, Depart-
  ment of Nuclear Medicine, University of California School of Medicine, Davis,
  California
Buell, James, M.D.
  Assistant Professor of Medicine, University of Nebraska College of Medicine,
  Chief, Cardiology Section, Veterans Administration, Omaha, Nebraska
Carley, James E., M.D.
  Fellow in Cardiology, University of Kansas Medical Center, Kansas City, Kansas
Chambers, Ward, M.D.
  Fellow in Cardiology, University of Nebraska College of Medicine, Omaha,
  Nebraska
Chen, Chia-Maou, M.D.
  Resident Associate, Division of Cardiology, Department of Medicine, University
  of Kentucky College of Medicine, Lexington, Kentucky
Crawford, Michael H., M.D.
  Assistant Professor of Medicine in Residence, University of California Medical
  Center, San Diego, California
Criley, J. Michael, M.D.
  Chief, Division of Cardiology, Harbor General Hospital, Professor of Medicine
  and Radiology, University of California, Los Angeles, California
Dalske, H. Frederick, Ph.D.
  Assistant Professor of Pharmacology, University of Nebraska College of Medicine,
  Omaha, Nebraska

da Luz, Protasio L., M.D.
Senior Research Associate, Department of Cardiology, Cedars-Sinai Medical Center, Los Angeles, California

DeMaria, Anthony N., M.D.
Associate Professor of Medicine, Director of Echocardiography, Director of Cardiac Rehabilitation, Co-Director of Coronary Care Unit, University of California School of Medicine, Davis, California

Dobry, Charles A., M.D.
Associate Professor of Radiology, University of Nebraska College of Medicine, Omaha, Nebraska

Dunn, Marvin I., M.D.
Professor of Medicine, Director, Division of Cardiovascular Disease, University of Kansas Medical Center, Kansas City, Kansas

Dzindzio, Barry S., M.D.
Assistant Professor of Medicine, University of Nebraska College of Medicine, Omaha, Nebraska

Eliot, Robert S., M.D., F.A.C.C.
Professor of Medicine and Director, Cardiovascular Center and Division of Cardiovascular Medicine, University of Nebraska Medical Center, Omaha, Nebraska

Forker, Alan D., M.D., F.A.C.C.
Associate Professor of Medicine, Director of Heart Station, Director of Medical Education of the Cardiovascular Center, University of Nebraska College of Medicine, Omaha, Nebraska

Forrester, James S., M.D.
Assistant Professor, University of California School of Medicine, Assistant Director of Cardiology, Cedars of Lebanon Hospital Division, Cedars-Sinai Medical Center, Los Angeles, California

Gettes, Leonard S., M.D., F.A.C.C.
Professor of Medicine and Pharmacology, University of Kentucky College of Medicine, Lexington, Kentucky

Harrison, Donald C., M.D.
Chief, Cardiology Division, School of Medicine, Stanford University, Stanford, California

Hofschire, Philip J., M.D.
Associate Professor of Pediatrics, University of Nebraska College of Medicine, Omaha, Nebraska

Krueger, Steven, M.D.
Research Associate in Cardiology, University of Nebraska College of Medicine, Omaha, Nebraska

Lee, Garrett, M.D.
Assistant Professor of Medicine, Assistant Director, Coronary Care Unit, Section of Cardiovascular Medicine, University of California, School of Medicine, Davis, California

Lewis, A. James, M.D.
Director, Cardiac Care Unit, Harbor General Hospital, Assistant Professor of Medicine, University of California, Los Angeles, California

Mason, Dean T., M.D., F.A.C.C.
Professor of Medicine, Professor of Physiology, Chief, Section of Cardiovascular Medicine, University of California at Davis, School of Medicine, Davis, California

McAllister, Russell, M.D.
Assistant Professor of Medicine, Division of Cardiology, Department of Medicine, University of Kentucky College of Medicine, Resident Associate, Veterans Administration Hospital, Lexington, Kentucky

Miller, Richard R., M.D.
  Associate Professor of Medicine, Director of Cardiac Catheterization Laboratories, Director of Cardiology Clinic, Section of Cardiovascular Medicine, University of California School of Medicine, Davis, California
Morgan, James, M.D.
  Fellow in Cardiology, University of Nebraska College of Medicine, Omaha, Nebraska
O'Rourke, Robert A., M.D.
  Associate Professor of Medicine, Director of Clinical Cardiology, University of California Medical Center, San Diego, California
Phalen, James J., M.D.
  Chief, Department of Radiology, Veterans Administration Hospital, Omaha, Nebraska
Price, James, M.D.
  Associate Professor of Medicine in Residence, University of California School of Medicine, Davis, California
Salel, Antone F., M.D.
  Associate Professor of Medicine, Director of the Lippid Clinics, Director of Cardiovascular Bioengineering, Co-Director of Nuclear Cardiology, Section of Cardiovascular Medicine, University of California School of Medicine, Davis, California
Sass, Hope, M.D.
  Fellow in Cardiology, University of Nebraska College of Medicine, Omaha, Nebraska
Schnee, Mark, B.Sc., M.R.C.P.
  Fellow in Cardiology, University of Nebraska College of Medicine, Omaha, Nebraska
Starke, Helen, M.D.
  Assistant Professor of Internal Medicine, Division of Cardiology, University of Nebraska College of Medicine, Omaha, Nebraska
Stoner, John, III, M.D.
  Fellow in Cardiology Division, School of Medicine, Stanford University, Stanford, California
Stratbucker, Robert A., M.D., Ph.D., P.E.
  Assistant Professor, Internal Medicine, University of Nebraska College of Medicine, Omaha, Nebraska
Swan, H. J. C., M.D., Ph.D., F.A.C.C.
  Professor of Medicine, University of California School of Medicine, Director of Cardiology, Cedars-Sinai Medical Center, Los Angeles, California
Tonkon, Melvin J., M.D.
  Assistant Professor of Medicine, Assistant Director, Coronary Care Unit, Section of Cardiovascular Medicine, University of California, School of Medicine, Davis, California
Vismara, Louis A., M.D.
  Associate Professor of Medicine, Director of Ambulatory Electrocardiography, Co-Director of Cardiology Clinics, Co-Director of Cardiac Catheterization Laboratories, University of California College of Medicine, Davis, California
Waters, David D., M.D.
  Research Fellow, Department of Cardiology, Cedars-Sinai Medical Center, Los Angeles, California
Williams, David O., M.D.
  Associate Professor of Medicine, Director of Cardiology Services, Martinez Veterans Administration Hospital, Section of Cardiovascular Medicine, University of California School of Medicine, Davis, California

Wolf, Gerald L., M.D., Ph.D.
Associate Professor of Pharmacology and Radiology, University of Nebraska College of Medicine, Director, Cardiovascular Radiology Research, Cardiovascular Center for Nebraska, Omaha, Nebraska

Zucker, Robert P.
Head ECHO, Heart Station Supervisor, University of Nebraska College of Medicine, Omaha, Nebraska

Contents

CHAPTER 1
The Pathophysiology of Coronary Heart Disease

Giorgio Baroldi, M.D.; Robert S. Eliot, M.D.

This Chapter reviews current controversial views of the pathologic basis for the major causes of cardiac emergencies, namely coronary heart disease and sudden cardiac death. It encompasses the significance and contemporary views of degrees of coronary obstruction, the collateral circulation, coronary thrombosis, coronary spasm, small vessel diseases, the various forms of myocardial necrosis and the pathology of the most frequent complications of acute myocardial infarction.

In 1912 Herrick presented his classic paper on the clinical and pathologic features of myocardial infarction[1]. Although he emphasized the role of coronary thrombosis, he clearly indicated that myocardial infarction did not develop in some animals and some individuals with sudden or chronic arterial obstruction. In Herrick's time, however, the coronary circulation was believed to be an end-arterial system. This led to the conclusion that arterial blockage was the *sine qua non* of sudden coronary death and myocardial infarction. On that basis, a variety of pathogenetic mechanisms causing obstruction at any level of the coronary tree was proposed. The most popular mechanism was, and remains, acute thrombosis of the epicardial coronary vessels. Recently, however, several authors have suggested that coronary thrombosis may be a secondary event[2-7]. The secondary thrombus formation has itself been rechallenged[8,9].

It would, therefore, be appropriate at this time to review the role of coronary obstruction and myocardial damage in the natural history of "coronary heart disease".

CORONARY THROMBOSIS

In an attempt to determine the incidence of acute occlusive thrombosis in patients who died of myocardial infarction, pathologic material from 100 consecutive autopsies was reviewed. In each case death occurred in a coronary care unit within 25 days of the onset of typical symptoms of acute myocardial infarction[10]. Postmortem histologic study revealed typical coagulation necrosis of the myocardium. In 7% no acute occulsion was observed, and only minimal or no luminal narrowing was present[10,11]. In

1

93% severe stenosis or occlusion of one or more coronary arteries was demonstrated. Of the entire group, an acute occlusive thrombus was seen in only 38%. Thus, more than 60% of the infarctions were not associated with acute coronary thrombosis.

Certain phenomena correlated well with the frequency of coronary thrombus formation. First, all thrombi were found in vessels with lumen reduced by at least 70% from long-standing atherosclerotic disease (Table I). Second, the increased length of the old stenosis was a significant factor

TABLE I

FREQUENCY OF THE OCCLUSIVE THROMBUS VS. PERCENT LUMEN REDUCTION CAUSED BY CORONARY STENOSIS.

Acute infarct with	Percent lumen reduction					Total
	<50	60	70	80	>90	
Occlusive thrombus	–	–	11	14	13	38
No acute occlusion	10	5	18	13	16	62
Total	10	5	29	27	29	100

associated with thrombosis (Table II). Third, the larger the size of the myocardial infarction (Table III) the more likely a thrombus would be found in the epicardial coronary vessel. Fourth, the amount of atheromatous material in the damaged vessel was directly proportional to the likelihood of thrombosis[10].

In addition, there is a correlation between severe coronary stenosis and enlargement of normal existing collateral vessels[12-14]. A significant increase in the diameter and length of the normal collaterals in all cases of acute infarction associated with old severe obstructive coronary damage was observed. This increase was proportional to the degree and extent of the coronary stenosis. An equal increase was also shown in cases with the same cor-

TABLE II

FREQUENCY OF THE OCCLUSIVE THROMBUS VS. LENGTH OF CORONARY STENOSIS.

Acute infarct with	Length of stenosis (mm)				Total
	<10	20	30	>30	
Occlusive thrombus	5	5	10	18	38
No acute occlusion	26	13	11	12	62
Total	31	18	21	30	100

TABLE III

FREQUENCY OF THE OCCLUSIVE THROMBUS VS.
SIZE OF THE INFARCT.

Acute infarct with	Percent of left ventricle infarcted						Total
	<10	11-20	21-30	31-40	41-50	>51-60	
Occlusive thrombus	4	7	10	5	9	3	38
No acute occlusion	25	13	15	6	3	—	62
Total	29	20	25	11	12	3	100

onary damage without infarction. Since an occlusive thrombus is never found in a normal coronary artery, the previous findings indicate that an infarct associated with severe, old coronary obstruction occurs in the presence of already enlarged collateral vessels. The satisfactory function of the collaterals can be deduced by the lack of clinical evidence of ischemic disease despite the presence of morphologic coronary damage which pre-exists long before the onset of clinical "coronary" disease.

The relationship of the coronary thrombus with all aforementioned factors suggests that the latter may be a secondary event[5-10]. This hypothesis is based on the following sequence of events. The earliest functional change in the infarcted area is the loss of contractility with passive stretching of the noncontracting myocardium due to the intraventricular pressure, combined with the contractile preserved portions of the left ventricular wall. Subsequent interstitial edema and exudation as well as thrombosis of the intramural vessels occur from the external to the medial zone of the infarct[15]. These functional and morphologic events result in a hindrance of the intramural flow which is proportional to the size of the infarct. In turn, the increased resistance of blood flow into the infarct may predispose to a hindrance of flow in the subepicardial supplying vessel. This further results in stasis at the level of the epicardial coronary stenosis. When this stasis is combined with the reduced or absent fibrinolytic activity at the atheromatous wall, there may result more favorable conditions for the formation of a thrombus in a secondary fashion[16]. If we accept this hypothesis we can conclude that despite numerous theories[17] there is no proof that either myocardial infarction or sudden "coronary" death is due to primary acute occlusion at some point in the coronary tree.

CHRONIC CORONARY OBSTRUCTION

If acute occlusion is either absent or a hemodynamically insignificant secondary event, what is the role of the chronic stenosis? One school of thought feels stenosis may predispose to myocardial ischemia at times of increased myocardial demand. It has been previously mentioned that there is an increase in the size of the normal collaterals in the presence of severe coronary stenosis. The adequacy of collateral compensatory capability is documented by specific studies. In particular, in more than 50% of patients that die in the hospital from noncardiac causes, severe obstructive coronary damage was demonstrated in the absence of any previous clinical or post-mortem evidence of ischemic heart disease[12]. Furthermore, in "coronary" patients the pathologic appearance of the vascular lesions suggests that they antedate the onset of the clinical disease.

The presence of adequate collateral circulation helps to explain the long delay between the establishment of severe coronary stenosis and the onset of ischemic disease (angina, myocardial infarction, or sudden death). On the other hand, it must be stated that there is no proof that failure of collateral circulation is responsible for the onset of the disease. At any given time, functioning collateral vessels may be demonstrated by cineangiography *in vivo*. This information is independent of that identifying healthy people who died accidental deaths with no records of cardiac disease; such groups demonstrate a high frequency (37%) of severe coronary obstruction in one or more vessels (Baroldi, unpublished data).

From these findings, the role of thrombosis, as well as of coronary stenosis, becomes questionable since both health and disease can exist with essentially the same degree of coronary stenosis. The observations demonstrate that there is not a direct cause and effect relationship between severe morphologic coronary damage and ischemic heart disease. This observation is also confirmed by the lack of relationship between the post-mortem size of myocardial infarction and the number of severely obstructed vessels (Table IV). If coronary stenosis were the *single* predisposing factor, there should be a direct correlation and proportional relationship between the extent of coronary stenosis and the size of myocardial infarction[10].

TABLE IV

LACK OF CORRELATION BETWEEN INFARCT SIZE AND
THE NUMBER OF MAIN CORONARY ARTERIAL VESSELS
WITH SEVERE STENOSIS.

Infarct Size %	Vessels with stenosis > 70%			Patients with all vessels <70% stenosis to normal	Total %
	1 (%)	2 (%)	3 (%)		
<20	16 (32.6)	19 (38.7)	9 (18.3)	5 (10.0)	49 (100)
>20	23 (45.0)	17 (33.3)	5 (9.8)	6 (11.7)	51 (100)
Total	39	36	14	11	100

Small Vessel Disease

Another attempt to explain the absence of coronary obstruction in the presence of angina, infarction or sudden death, is the hypothesis of disturbances of the microcirculation, or small vessel disease. In recent years it has been proposed that platelet aggregates block the circulation at the small vessel or capillary level. It is further proposed that myocardial damage can follow these events. However, an experiment of nature, thrombotic thrombocytopenic purpura mitigates.against this hypothesis. In this condition both hypoxic and ischemic factors are present. There is profound hemolysis frequently reducing hemoglobin levels to 25% of normal. In addition, there is hemorrhage, platelet aggregation, and widespread obstructive disease of the myocardial small vessels. Despite this, microfocal coagulation necrosis could be found in only rare instances and no clinical angina or ischemic electrocardiographic changes were noted[18].

Finally, true small vessel disease is not found in those dying of coronary heart disease. When present, the changes are secondary, and within and around the infarcted area[19]. It must be kept in mind that structural changes such as hyperplasia of the media with longitudinal disposition of the smooth muscle, and progressive fibrosis of both media and intima, are frequent findings in the trabecula carnae and papillary muscles and, less frequently, in the interventricular septum. These can be found in many conditions as well as in apparently healthy individuals. Their significance remains uncertain. They are possibly a consequence of aging, but no proof exists that this limited vascular change is related to ischemic heart disease. In conclusion, from a morphologic standpoint, there is presently no proof that vascular damage (large or small) by itself accounts for coronary heart disease (Figure 1).

The Role of Spasm

Recently, the concept that spasm may play a role has been re-introduced. This has been accomplished as a result of the imaging of coronary spasm in cases of atypical or Prinzmetal's angina[20]. It has not yet been shown, however, that spasm precedes or follows typical anginal pain. In the meantime, it remains difficult to accept spasm as the main cause of sudden coronary death or myocardial infarction since the best physiologic vasodilator is hypoxia. In addition, sixty minutes of coronary occlusion is required to produce a finite infarction experimentally[21]. In the presence of associated hypoxia, a potent stimulus for vasodilatation, it would seem unlikely that spasm could persist for one hour in duration. Thus it remains to be proven whether spasm can induce ventricular fibrillation, infarction, or both.

Other Theories

Many other theories including steal syndrome, coronary hypotension, and cardiac hypertrophy require a more substantial background of supporting data. Even when present, no uniform significant correlation can be found between these conditions and angina or infarction[17].

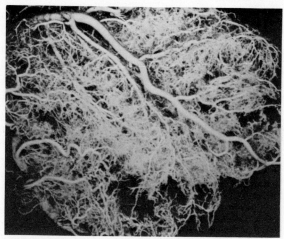

Figure 1 A plastic solution is injected into the coronary arteries and allowed to harden. The myocardial tissue is dissolved leaving a cast of the myocardial arterial circulation. It is interesting to note that there is a dense mass of interconnecting arterial branches. It is these branches that are responsible for the development of collateral blood flow. One can easily see how these extensive collateral channels could sustain an area of myocardium that is fed by gradually stenotic extramural coronary arterial lesion.

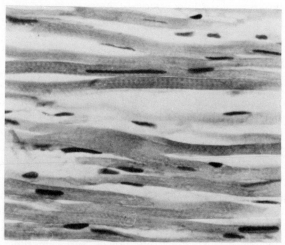

Figure 2 Coagulation Necrosis. Normal appearing myofibrils with thin muscle fibers and edema indicate a relative atonic state. The only visible necrosis is in the nuclei.

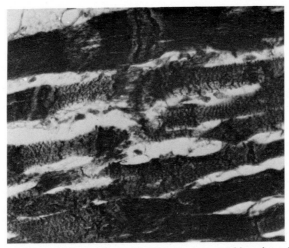

Figure 3   Coagulative Myocytolysis. The hypercontracted bands and broken myofibrils are prominent yet there is no associated nuclear change or exudative reaction.

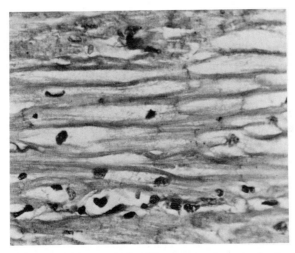

Figure 4   Colliquative Myocytolysis. The pattern here is dominated by intercellular edema without any inflammatory or destructive elements seen in the other forms.

Myocardial Necrosis

Previous statements reveal the complexity of coronary heart disease; perhaps it is more complicated than previously believed. Other nonvascular factors appear to play a role in its pathogenesis. This is particularly true when one considers the different types of myocardial necrosis found in coronary heart disease. The following three major forms of myocardial necrosis are observed in man with relation to distinct functional states[22,23]:

1. In one condition, the myocardial cell loses its contractility and seems to die in an atonic state. The earliest changes in this type of necrosis involve the nucleus, while the regular order of myofibrils is maintained even in the later stages of the repair process. The muscle fibers appear thinner as a result of passive overdistention. This type of necrosis, which is the fundamental lesion in a cardiac infarct, elicits an early exudation with the centripetal infiltration of polymorphonuclear leukocytes, subsequent wall damage, and secondary thrombosis of the vessels within the necrotic area. This type is the so-called *coagulation necrosis* (Figure 2).

2. In the second type, the myocardial cell dies in a hypercontracted state with early myofibrillar damage. The sarcomeres in the hypercontracted elements seem to clump together forming dense, anomalous, acidophilic crossbands, alternating with stretched and broken myofibrils in the contiguous segments. There is no early nuclear change, exudation, polymorphonuclear leukocytic infiltration, or vascular change. This type of myocardial damage characterizes many cardiomyopathies, particularly the form of myocardial necrosis seen with pheochromocytoma and the experimental catecholamine-induced necrosis. This type is called *coagulative myocytolysis*. It is related to irreversible hypercontraction and seems related to sympathetic overstimulation or a similar mechanism (Figure 3).

3. The third form is characterized by increasing intercellular edema with the dissolution of myofibrils but without nuclear or vascular change, inflammatory infiltration, or anomalous contraction bands. These findings appear to be the histologic landmark of the myocardial cell which dies in a progressively failing state. This is the type of pattern which is found in alcoholic cardiomyopathy or in the other low output states. It is called *colliquative myocytolysis* (Figure 4).

All three types of myocardial necrosis result in an "alveolar pattern" depicted by intact empty sarcolemmal tubes in which mononuclear cells and macrophages can be recognized. The healing process is accomplished by fibroplastic collagenation without granulation tissue formation[15].

In all cases of acute myocardial infarction, coagulation necrosis is the fundamental lesion. In all cases coagulative myocytolysis can be found in the external portion of the infarction and in the normal myocardium surrounding the infarct. In addition, 67% of cases of sudden coronary death displayed coagulative myocytolysis in the absence of demonstrable coagulation necrosis. Due to the histologic identity of this lesion in both sudden coronary death and myocardial infarction, as well as in catecholamine-induced myocardial necrosis, it can be inferred that the mechanisms are similar. Further, it is well-known that catecholamines may induce ventricular fibrillation. Therefore, the histologic finding of coagulative myocytolysis could indicate the likelihood of catecholamine-induced fatal ventricular fibrillation[22].

The third type of death (colliquative myocytolysis) has been found mainly in a few layers of the subendocardium and adjacent to surviving vessels in the infarcted area. It can be considered an expression of terminal failure of the cardiac pump in some instances since it was found in 43% of acute myocardial infarctions, generally with large areas of coagulation necrosis. It is also found in 10% of those dying of sudden coronary death. Usually it is associated with extensive myocardial fibrosis[22].

The clear histologic distinction between the three types of myocardial necrosis and their frequent association indicates that different pathogenetic mechanisms with different biochemical derangements occur in coronary heart disease[22].

The complexity of myocardial necrosis parallels that observed at the vascular level. Both the researcher and the clinician must be wary of the multifactorial nature of coronary heart disease. The findings suggest a clinical approach that favors attention to myocardial function balanced with coronary arterial morphology.

References

1. Herrick, J.B.: Clinical features of sudden obstruction of the coronary arteries. *JAMA*, **59**: 2015-2020, 1912.
2. Branwood, A.W. and Montgomery, G.L.: Observations on the morbid anatomy of coronary artery disease. *Scot. Med. J.*, **1**: 367-375, 1956.
3. Albertini, von A., Brunck, H.J., and Papernitzki, A.: Die Coronarsklerose in der schweizerischen bevolkerung. Eine statistische Erhebung an Hand der Sektionsfalle eines Jahres. *Bull. schweiz. Akad. med. Wissensch.*, **13**: 17-37, 1957.
4. Spain, D.M. and Bradess, V.A.: Frequency of coronary thrombi as related to duration of survival from onset of acute fatal episodes of myocardial ischemia. *Circulation*, **22**: 816, 1960.
5. Baroldi, G.: Acute coronary occlusion as a cause of myocardial infarct and sudden coronary heart death. *Am. J. Cardiol.*, **16**: 859-880, 1965.
6. Roberts, W.C.: Coronary arteries in fatal acute myocardial infarction. *Circulation*, **45**: 215-230, 1972.
7. Erhardt, L.R.: Clinical and pathological observations in different types of acute myocardial infarction. A study of 84 patients deceased after treatment in a coronary care unit. *Acta Med. Scandinav.*, Suppl. 560, 1974.
8. Chapman, I.: The cause-effect relationship between recent coronary artery occlusion and acute myocardial infarction. *Am. Heart J.*, **87**: 267-271, 1974.
9. Chandler, A.B., Chapman, I., Erhardt, L.R., Roberts, W.C., Schwartz, C.J., Sinapius, D., Sherry, S., Ness, P.M., and Simon, T.L.: Coronary thrombosis in

myocardial infarction. Report of a workshop on the role of coronary thrombosis in the pathogenesis of acute myocardial infarction. *Am. J. Cardiol.,* **34**: 823-833, 1974.

10. Baroldi, G., Radice, F., Schmid, G., and Leone, A.: Morphology of acute myocardial infarction in relation to coronary thrombosis. *Am. Heart J.,* **87**: 65-75, 1974.

11. Eliot, R.S., Baroldi, G., and Leone, A.: Necroscopy studies in myocardial infarction with minimal or no coronary luminal reduction due to atherosclerosis. *Circulation,* **49**: 1127-1131, 1974.

12. Baroldi, G. and Scomazzoni, G.: *Coronary Circulation in the Normal and Pathologic Heart.* U.S. Government Printing Office, 1967. American Registry of Pathology, Armed Forces Institute of Pathology, Washington, D.C. 20305.

13. Baroldi, G.: Functional morphology of the anastomotic circulation in human cardiac pathology. In E. Bajusz and G. Jasmin (Eds.): "Studies of functional morphology: selected examples". *Methods Achiev. Exp. Pathol.,* **5**: 438-473, Karger, Basel, 1971.

14. Myasnikov, A.L., Chazov, E.I., Koshevnikova, T.L., and Nikolaeva, L.F.: Some new data on the occurrence of coronary thrombosis in conjunction with atherosclerosis. *J. Atheroscl. Res.,* **1**: 401-402, 1961.

15. Baroldi, G. and Silver, M.D.: The healing of myocardial infarct in man. *Gior. It. Cardiol.,* **5**: 465-476, 1975.

16. Baroldi, G.: Coronary thrombosis: facts and beliefs. *A. Heart J.,* in press.

17. Baroldi, G.: Coronary heart disease: significance of the morphologic lesions. *Am. Heart J.,* **85**: 1-5, 1973.

18. Baroldi, G. and Manion, W.C.: Microcirculatory disturbances and human myocardial infarction. *Am. Heart J.,* **74**: 171-178, 1976.

19. Baroldi, G.: Histopathologic study of the intramural artery vessels in relation to the pathology of extramural coronary arteries and myocardial damage. *Cardiologia,* **41**: 364-380, 1962.

20. Oliva, P.B., Potts, D.E., and Pluss, R.G.: Coronary arterial spasm in Prizmetal's variant form of angia documentation of coronary arteriography. *N. Engl. J. Med.,* **288**: 745-751, 1973.

21. Jennings, R.B., Warthan, W.B., and Zudyk, A.F.: Production of an area of homogeneous myocardial infarction in the dog. *Arch. Path.,* **63**: 580-585, 1975.

22. Baroldi, G.: Different morphologic types of myocardial cell death in man. In A. Fleckenstein and G. Rona (Eds.): *Myocardial Cell Damage. Myocardiology,* University Park Press, Baltimore, 1976, in press.

23. Baroldi, G.: Different types of myocardial necrosis in coronary heart disease: a pathological review of their functional significance. *Am. Heart J.,* **89**: 742-752, 1975.

CHAPTER 2
Pathophysiology of Myocardial Infarction Shock*

Dean T. Mason, M.D.; Ezra A. Amsterdam, M.D.;
Richard R. Miller, M.D.; Anthony N. DeMaria, M.D.;
Louis A. Vismara, M.D.; James Price, M.D.;
Daniel S. Berman, M.D.; Antone F. Salel, M.D.;
David O. Williams, M.D.

This chapter depicts the major pathophysiologic subsets of shock resulting from myocardial infarction. It is an apt demonstration of the significant lessons derived when clinical observations are balanced with hemodynamic measurements. This comprehensive Chapter sets the stage for discussion of specific forms of therapy appropriate to those subsets described in Chapter 13.

Cardiogenic shock due to left ventricular pump failure is now the major cause of death in patients hospitalized with acute myocardial infarction. Myocardial infarction shock complicates about one in six in-hospital patients with acute transmural infarction and accounts for the loss of life in approximately 100,000 persons each year in the United States[1]. Since the implementation of the intensive coronary care unit monitoring concept in the past decade has provided effective management of potentially lethal ventricular tachyarrhythmias, thereby halving mortality in acute myocardial infarction from 30 to 15% in many medical centers[1], our efforts to overcome heart failure shock in myocardial infarction have been unsatisfactory and the remaining hospital deaths are largely the result of this grave complication which is fatal in more than four of five instances.

Although coronary arteriosclerosis is the leading killer of Americans, particularly in young adult men, and is responsible for one-third (675,000 deaths annually) of all national mortality and two-thirds of cardiovascular deaths[2], it has only been within the past decade that intensive investigation has been applied to coronary disorders. Further, the primary role of preventive cardiology is now recognized and population studies on the prevalence and control of coronary risk factors have recently been initiated. In addition,

*Supported in part by Research Program Project Grant HL 14780 from the National Heart and Lung Institute, NIH, Bethesda, Maryland and Research Grants from California Chapters of the American Heart Association.

the greatest (60% of total coronary deaths) and most perplexing of the coronary problems, sudden coronary death, is now under increased evaluation for identification of individuals at high risk, means of its prophylaxis, and the value of mobile coronary care units.

DEFINITION

Cardiogenic shock is a syndrome of extreme impairment of circulatory function resulting from severe, primary derangement of cardiac pump performance. Although, as in congestive heart failure, it is characterized by inadequate perfusion of vital organ systems, depression of cardiac and circulatory function is more severe in shock and, in contrast to congestive heart failure, untreated shock is generally incompatible with survival beyond several hours. Cardiogenic shock may be the clinical culmination of end-stage function of any disease of the heart, but it is most typically related to an abrupt, catastrophic complication of acute myocardial infarction.

The system of intensive coronary care has had little effect in improving survival in this syndrome. At present, mortality in acute myocardial infarction approximates 50 percent when associated with severe congestive failure[1,3] and rises to 80-100 percent when complicated by shock. These figures contrast with a mortality rate of less than 10 percent when myocardial infarction is uncomplicated[4], and commonly less than 20 percent when it is accompanied by signs of only mild left heart failure[5]. The diagnosis of cardiogenic shock[6] is made when clinical evidence of a severe low cardiac output state is present secondary to myocardial infarction (Table I).

TABLE I
DIAGNOSIS OF MYOCARDIAL INFARCTION SHOCK

1. Documentation of Acute Myocardial Infarction

2. Clinical Manifestations:

   Hypotension (systolic blood pressure < 80 mmHg)
   Oliguria (< 30 ml urine per hour)
   Diaphoresis, cyanosis
   Altered sensorium

3. Persistence of Shock Syndrome after

   Elimination of arrhythmias
   Abolition of pain
   Administration of oxygen
   Trial of volume expansion

LEFT VENTRICULAR DYSFUNCTION

The fundamental physiologic defect in myocardial infarction shock is depression of myocardial contractility due to loss of functioning cardiac muscle[7,8]. Marked impairment of cardiac pump function results with severely reduced perfusion of all organ systems. The inadequate functional performance of the heart is usually manifested by severe derangement of all parameters of cardiac pump function, such as systemic blood pressure, cardiac output, stroke output, cardiac work, stroke work, left ventricular ejection fraction, and elevation of left ventricular filling pressure[3,9-11]. Although these hemodynamic variables may be abnormal in the presence of uncomplicated myocardial infarction the degree of impairment is considerably greater when shock is present (Figure 1)[1,9-11]. Heart failure in acute myocardial infarction is usually characterized by clinical manifestations of pulmonary congestion. Derangement of underlying hemodynamic function may be marked in cardiac failure, but it is quantitatively less than in shock.

ACUTE MYOCARDIAL INFARCTION

	UNCOMPLICATED	CHF	SHOCK
BP:	N	N	↓
CO:	N	N/↓	↓/↓↓
LVEDP:	N/↑	↑/↑↑	↑↑/↑↑↑
PVR:	N	N/↑	↑
CVP:	N	N/↑	↑

Figure 1 Hemodynamics in acute myocardial infarction (MI): uncomplicated transmural MI, MI with congestive heart failure (CHF), and MI with cardiogenic shock. BP = systemic arterial blood pressure; CO = cardiac index; LVEDP = left ventricular end-diastolic pressure; PVR = peripheral vascular resistance; CVP = central venous pressure; N = normal value. (From Mason, D.T., Amsterdam, E.A., Miller, R.R. et al: Recent advances in pathophysiology and therapy of myocardial infarction shock. In H. Russek (Ed.): *Cardiovascular Disease: New Concepts in Diagnosis and Therapy*. University Park Press, Baltimore, 1974, pp. 143-157, with permission.)

A poor prognosis in myocardial infarction is portended by persistently low cardiac indices and marked elevation of left ventricular end-diastolic pressure, failure to augment stroke volume in response to plasma volume expansion, marked reduction of stroke work index, sustained systemic arterial desaturation, and low urine output[1,3,12,13]. Since right ventricular function is often normal in myocardial infarction, systemic venous pressure may be normal. However, right ventricular performance may be directly impaired in patients with right coronary occlusion and diaphragmatic infarction[14]. Pulmonary blood volume is usually increased, while total blood volume is normal, or even reduced, following treatment with sympathomimetic drugs. Systemic arterial hypoxemia is attributable to impaired alveolar-capillary diffusion and venous admixture caused by pulmonary edema[15]. Metabolic acidosis in cardiogenic shock is a consequence of marked reduction of cardiac output.

Depression of cardiac performance in acute myocardial infarction is, as a rule, directly related to the extent of myocardial damage. Thus, the anatomic basis for the extremely depressed cardiac function in the great majority of patients with myocardial infarction shock is the extensive loss of cardiac muscle. Whereas uncomplicated myocardial infarction is usually associated with relatively small quantitative damage, myocardial destruction in shock involves at least 40 percent, and usually more, of the ventricle as documented by postmortem studies[16-18]. Angiographic evaluation of the left ventricle, which we have performed in patients with acute myocardial infarction, has provided confirmation of these pathologic findings[9]. Thus, when shock accompanies acute myocardial infarction left ventriculography usually demonstrates severe dyssynergy of left ventricular myocardium, in contrast to the more modest involvement in uncomplicated infarction (Figure 2). The magnitude of the loss of left ventricular muscle in cardiogenic shock explains, to a large extent, the failure of conventional medical therapy in this syndrome.

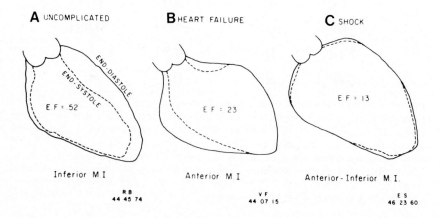

Figure 2 Diagrams of left ventricular angiograms of patients with acute myocardial infarction (M.I.). A: The inferior infarction is associated with inferior wall hypokinesis and is clinically uncomplicated. B: Congestive heart failure is associated with extensive anterior wall akinesis in the anterior infarction. C: The anterior-inferior infarction is complicated by shock resulting from the severe, diffuse impairment of contractile function. Ejection fraction (E.F.) is progressively decreased with increasing involvement of left ventricular myocardium. (From Amsterdam, E.A., Hughes, J.L., Iben, A., et al: Surgery for acute myocardial infarction. In R.M. Gunnar, H.S. Loeb, and S.H. Rahimtoola (Eds.): *Shock in Myocardial Infarction.* Grune & Stratton, Inc., New York, 1974, pp. 257-283, with permission.)

The extensive ventricular damage associated with cardiogenic shock represents cumulative myocardial loss sustained in past and present. Thus, total nonviable myocardial mass in this setting may be composed of old and new infarction as well as recent extension of infarction[17]. The essential factor resulting in shock is net loss of critical mass of left ventricular muscle, whether it evolves over an extended period and is related to multiple, separate infarctions or occurs acutely from a single, massive infarction. Experimental evidence suggests that the size of the infarction is related to myocardial oxygen requirements at the time of coronary occlusion[19]. Although ventricular compliance may be transiently increased in the first day following infarction[20], compliance is usually diminished throughout the initial five days of the acute episode[20-22]. This increased stiffness of the chamber actually tends to improve the lowered stroke volume from the dysfunctioning ventricle by raising left ventricular end-diastolic pressure and preload, and by diminishing ventricular distensibility during ejection[22].

Ventricular function is diminished in nearly all patients with acute transmural myocardial infarction[23-25]. Thus there is a range of depression of ventricular performance in transmural infarction: most extreme in cardiogenic shock, intermediate in congestive heart failure without hypotension, and least in uncomplicated infarction. In addition to the loss of contractile units, cardiac dysfunction results from a diminished inotropic state in ischemic areas and from regional ventricular dyssynergy. Viewed in terms of the Frank-Starling principle which relates cardiac performance to ventricular filling pressure (Figure 3), the ventricular function curve is most

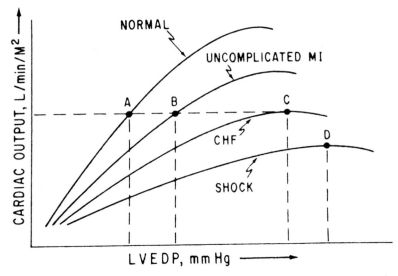

Figure 3 Ventricular function curves in normal subject, acute uncomplicated transmural myocardial infarction (MI), acute MI with congestive heart failure (CHF), and acute MI with cardiogenic shock. Points A, B, and C all represent the same cardiac output, but each is at a different level of left ventricular end-diastolic pressure (LVEDP) shown by the vertical broken lines. In shock, despite operation of the ventricle at the apex of its function curve (point D) with marked elevation of LVEDP, an adequate cardiac output cannot be delivered and hypotension results. (From Mason, D.T., Amsterdam, E.A., Miller, R.R. et al: Recent advances in pathophysiology and therapy of myocardial infarction shock. In H. Russek (Ed.): *Cardiovascular Disease: New Concepts in Diagnosis and Therapy.* University Park Press, Baltimore, 1974, pp. 143-157, with permission.)

depressed and flattened in cardiogenic shock. Thus, despite operation of the heart at the apex of this abnormal curve in cardiogenic shock, cardiac output is reduced to such a marked degree that organ perfusion is too low to maintain life[26].

Predisposing Factors

In addition to the high mortality rate (80-100%) and not infrequent occurrence (15%) of shock in myocardial infarction, certain other clinical findings are noteworthy. Although patients who develop shock in acute myocardial infarction may be slightly older than those without shock, no differences have been found in other predisposing factors such as prior myocardial infarction, cardiac failure, angina pectoris, or hypertension[3,18]. For shock and non-shock patients both drug therapy and the time between the onset of symptoms and hospital admission was similar[3]. However, while there was no difference in quantity of myocardium involved by previous myocardial infarction in the two groups, the magnitude of recent infarction was significantly greater in the shock patients[17]. Total mass of left ventricular tissue involved by infarction, therefore, was far greater in the shock patients (51% of left ventricle) than the non-shock group (23% of the left ventricle).

Time of Onset of Shock

Shock usually occurs early after infarction, though it may begin immediately or be delayed a week or more. Thus, several studies have demonstrated that the syndrome developed in half of shock patients within 24 hours and in two-thirds at 36 hours[3]; in one-third within 24 hours and half in less than three days[17]; and in three-fourths within 28 hours[18]. Further, the majority of patients in whom shock develops have clinically evident hemodynamic dysfunction on admission, ranging from mild cardiac failure to shock. It is also apparent from these data that late development of shock is not unusual in myocardial infarction. This has been attributed to continuing or new ischemic injury to the myocardium.

Duration of Shock

Cardiogenic shock is usually fatal within a short period. Of 73 patients in shock, Killip and colleagues noted 65% mortality in 24 hours and a median survival time of 10.2 hours[3]. In a second study of 21 patients with cardiogenic shock, all of whom died, the group was divided into 12 (57%) with rapid demise (duration of shock less than 24 hours, mean 12 hours), and nine (43%) with prolonged shock (duration of shock greater than 24 hours, mean 88 hours)[17].

Extension of Infarction

It has been proposed that progression of infarction is an important mechanism in the destruction of sufficient myocardial tissue to produce cardiogenic shock[17,18]. Killip et al observed that 18 of 22 shock patients had extension of infarct which was associated with the onset of shock[17]. However, infarct extension has also been considered the result rather than the cause of shock[16]. Progression of infarction contributes to the pathogenesis of cardiogenic shock, but this process may not be manifested clinically. In one study, symptoms and electrocardiographic evidence were usually absent, with diagnosis in most cases established by post-mortem dating of infarct zones[17]. Therapeutic interventions to interrupt extension of infarction must recognize this absence of clinical symptoms. Recognition may be enhanced by newer diagnostic techniques such as precordial ST-segment mapping[27] (Figure 4), serum myocardial enzyme creatine phosphokinase[28], and myocardial infarct scanning[29] (Figure 5) which may provide more sensitive analysis of alterations in the myocardium than conventional methods. Recent data are encouraging in this regard in demonstrating superiority of precordial ST-segment mapping over standard electrocardiography in detecting extension of infarction[30].

Infarct Location

While infarct size is uniformly acknowledged to be the major factor responsible for development of shock in acute myocardial infarction[16-18,31], opinions vary as to the significance of infarct location. Thus, there has been no relation noted between shock and location of infarction in some studies[3,16,31,32]. On the other hand, recent investigations have provided substantial evidence that derangement of cardiac pump function is greater and occurrence of shock more frequent in anterior infarction than in inferior[8,33,34,35]. This finding stems from anatomic and physiologic factors involving the relation of relative myocardial mass to coronary artery distribution.

In the human heart, the left coronary system supplies the predominant mass of myocardium, including the left ventricle. Further, in the majority of instances the left anterior descending artery supplies a greater quantity of left ventricular myocardium than either the right or left circumflex arteries[33,34]. Thus, the left anterior descending artery perfuses the left ventricular free wall, apex, and interventricular septum. The left circumflex artery supplies the lateral wall of the left ventricle and contributes variably to the supply of its inferior wall. In approximately ten percent of hearts it provides the major supply to this area. The left ventricular distribution of the right coronary artery varies reciprocally with that of the circumflex artery and involves the inferior wall and inferior aspect of the septum. It contributes the major portion of the blood supply to the inferior left ventricular wall in about 90 percent of human hearts. Anterior infarction, as localized electrocardiographically, is related to occlusive disease of the anterior descending artery and usually involves a relatively large quantity of left ventricular muscle[36]. By contrast, inferior infarction results from disease of the right coronary artery in the great majority (approximately 90%) of instances and is thereby usually associated with substantially less myocardial damage[36].

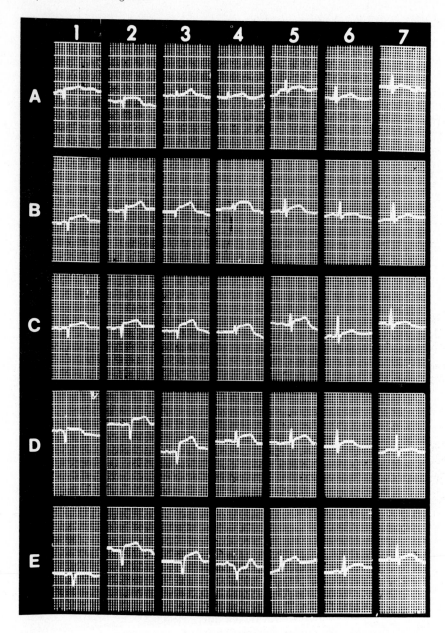

Figure 4 Precordial electrocardiographic ST-segment map in a patient with acute anterior myocardial infarction. Thirty-five precordial leads are utilized (5 horizontal rows of 7 adjacent leads) and the course of ischemic injury is followed by serial determination of the number of ST-segments which are elevated (NST), the sum of ST-segment elevation (Σ ST), and average ST-segment rise per lead demonstrating ST segment elevation (ST). For orientation with the standard precordial 6-lead ECG, D_{1-4} corresponds to V_{1-4} and E_5 and $_6$ corresponds to V_5 and $_6$.

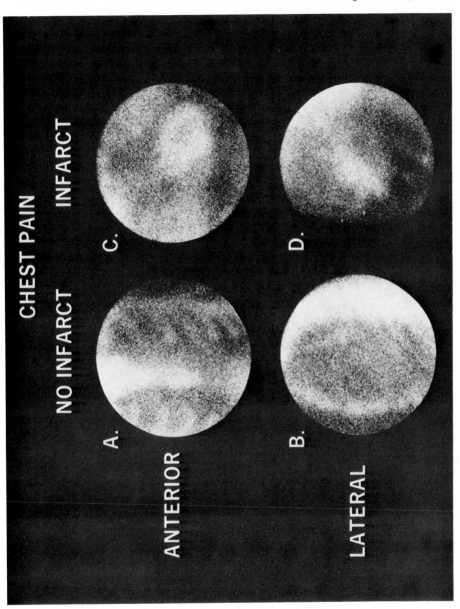

Figure 5 Precordial scintigraphic images obtained two hours after intravenous injection of Tc-99m pyrophosphate in two patients with chest pain. Anterior (A, C) and left lateral (B, D) views are shown. The patient in the left-hand column (A, B) had no clinical evidence of acute myocardial infarction (no infarct) corresponding to the scintigrams which demonstrated no abnormal concentration of radioactivity in the heart. In contrast, the patient in the right-hand column (C, D) had acute subendocardial myocardial infarction four days prior to the nuclear medicine study shown. The radionuclidic images revealed intense abnormal increased concentration of radioactivity throughout the anterior left ventricular wall (C and D).

Recent studies have supported the more serious implications on ventricular function of anterior compared to inferior infarction. Consistent findings have resulted from both clinical and hemodynamic investigation of this question in both stable coronary heart disease and acute myocardial infarction. Further, within broad limits the electrocardiogram identifies the presence and localizes left ventricular dyssynergy[36], affords estimation of the nature of dyssynergy[36] (Figure 6), provides a quantitative estimate of its extent[36] (Figure 7), and bears a consistent relation to left ventricular functional status[33,37-40]. Thus, the presence of pathologic Q waves correlates closely

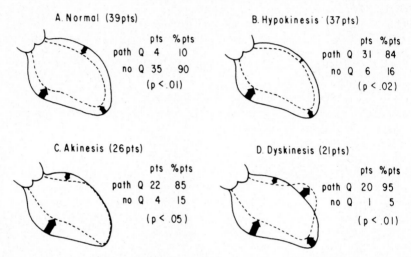

Figure 6 Nature of dyssynergy related to the presence (path Q) or absence (no Q) of ECG myocardial infarction. Normal contraction pattern (A) was associated with no Q (p < .01) while in hypokinesis (B) (p < .02), akinesis (C) (p < .05) and dyskinesis (D) (p .01) path Q was more common. (From Miller, R.R., Amsterdam, E.A., Bogren, H.G. et al: Electrocardiographic and cineangiographic correlations in assessment of the location, nature and extent of abnormal left ventricular segmental contraction in coronary artery disease. *Circulation,* **44**: 447, 1974, with permission.)

with left ventricular dyssynergy, whose site is localized by the electrocardiogram. Other electrocardiographic abnormalities, such as convex ST segment elevation and T wave inversion, in addition to Q waves, are associated not only with the presence of left ventricular aneurysm, as classically described, but with dyssynergy of considerably greater extent than is observed when these ST-T wave abnormalities are not present[36].

We have found a substantially greater incidence of shock in anterior myocardial infarction than in either inferior or non-transmural infarction[8,38] (Figure 8). Rackley and colleagues have demonstrated similar results[39]. In both series, differential frequency of shock relative to electrocardiographic infarct location paralleled the more severe hemodynamic dysfunction in the general infarct population associated with combined anterior-inferior and anterior infarction compared to inferior and non-transmural infarction

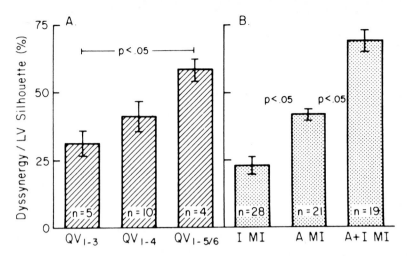

Figure 7 A. Relation of the percent of left ventricular perimeter demonstrating dyssynergy (dyssynergy/LV silhouette) to the extent of pathologic Q in 19 patients with isolated anterior infarction and QS deflections beginning in V_1 or V_2. With abnormal Q waves extending to V_5 or V_6, a greater quantity of left ventricle demonstrated abnormal motion than when pathologic Q reached only V_3 ($p < .05$). B. Relation of the area of dyssynergy to ECG location of infarction. The percent of left ventricular perimeter with dyssynergy was greater with anterior infarction (AMI) than inferior infarction: (IMI) ($p < .05$), and larger with combined anterior and inferior infarction (A + IMI) compared to AMI (p .05). (From Miller, R.R., Amsterdam, E.A., Bogren, H.G. et al: Electrocardiographic and cineangiographic correlations in assessment of the location, nature and extent of abnormal left ventricular segmental contraction in coronary artery disease. *Circulation*, **44**: 447, 1974, with permission.)

(Figure 9). Indeed, we have been impressed with the high proportion of patients with inferior and non-transmural infarction with normal hemodynamic function during the acute phase of infarction. Electrocardiographic evidence of combined anterior-inferior infarction is associated with the most severely impaired function and highest frequency of shock, a finding consistent with pathologic data previously noted relating the extent of involved myocardium to functional derangement[38]. Further, even in the presence of similar baseline hemodynamics in acute infarction, evaluation by volume loading and resultant ventricular function curves has demonstrated diminished performance in anterior compared to inferior infarction (Figure 10)[38], an observation also noted by Gunnar and colleagues[41]. On the basis of this experience, the occurrence of shock in inferior or non-transmural infarction suggests the not infrequent association of additional etiological factors such as a mechanical complication of infarction (rupture of papillary muscle, septum, or ventricular wall) (Figure 11) or intercurrent illness.

Electrocardiographic location of previous myocardial infarction in patients with chronic coronary heart disease yields similar results regarding

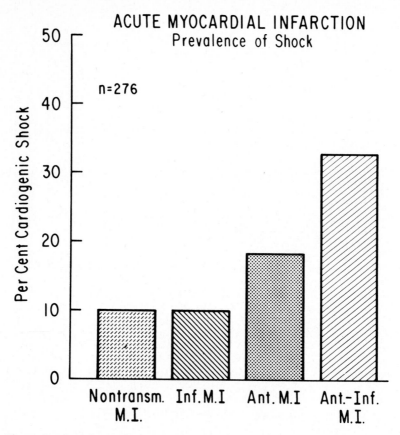

Figure 8 Prevalence of shock in acute myocardial infarction (MI) (shown as percent of patients with acute MI) in relation to electrocardiographic infarct location. Shock is most frequent in combined anterior-inferior (ant-inf) infarction. Prevalence in anterior (ant) infarction is approximately twice as great as that in inferior (inf) and nontransmural (nontransm) infarction. n = total number of acute MI patients.

ventricular function[36]. Thus, the extent and severity of left ventricular dyssynergy[36] and pump dysfunction are more severe in anterior than inferior infarction[35] and most impaired in combined anterior-inferior infarction[35]. These correlative angiographic studies have added a further dimension to the investigation of this question.

We have found that the infarct location itself is not the critical factor determining ventricular performance. When the extent of involvement by previous infarction is equivalent, as assessed by percent of left ventricular perimeter with abnormal contractile motion, function is similar regardless of infarct location[35]. The consistent difference in hemodynamic dysfunction associated with infarct location is related to the finding that anterior infarction is usually quantitatively greater than inferior[35,36], a result of involvement of the anterior descending coronary artery in the former and the right or circumflex coronary vessel in the latter.

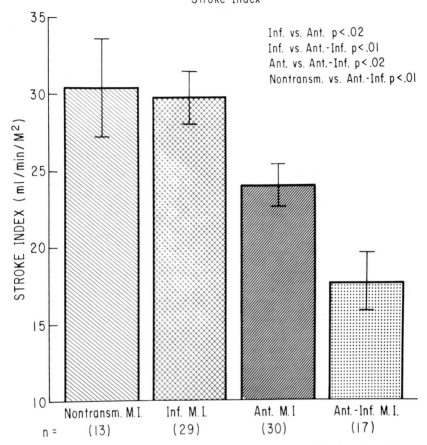

ACUTE MYOCARDIAL INFARCTION
Stroke Index

Inf. vs. Ant. p < .02
Inf. vs. Ant.-Inf. p < .01
Ant. vs. Ant.-Inf. p < .02
Nontransm. vs. Ant.-Inf. p < .01

STROKE INDEX (ml/min/M²)

	Nontransm. M.I.	Inf. M.I.	Ant. M.I	Ant.-Inf. M.I.
n =	(13)	(29)	(30)	(17)

Figure 9 Stroke work index related to electrocardiographic location of acute myocardial infarction. Stroke index is most impaired in combined anterior-inferior infarction and markedly reduced in anterior infarction compared to inferior and nontransmural infarction. n = number of patients with given location of acute MI.

MECHANICAL DISTURBANCES OF
LEFT VENTRICULAR FUNCTION

The mechanical complications of acute myocardial infarction may also exacerbate the depression of intrinsic cardiac function resulting from infarction. Thus mitral regurgitation, acute ventricular septal rupture, and a large paradoxically expansile or dyskinetic segment of myocardium may critically overload an injured ventricle and further impair pump performance.

Mitral Regurgitation

Rupture of papillary muscle is a relatively rare but catastrophic complica-

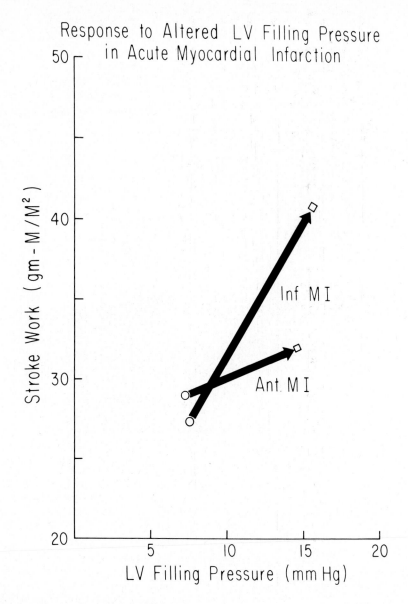

Figure 10 Effect of plasma volume expansion on left ventricular (LV) function (stroke work) in acute myocardial infarction. Although function prior to volume expansion is similar in the two groups, this intervention of increasing preload (elevation of LV filling pressure) with rapid dextran infusion resulted in substantial enhancement of left ventricular performance in inferior infarction (inf MI arrow) but little change in stroke work in anterior infarction (ant MI arrow), indicating more depression of left ventricular function in the latter compared to the former group of patients.

ACUTE DIAPHRAGMATIC
MYOCARDIAL INFARCTION
with RUPTURE

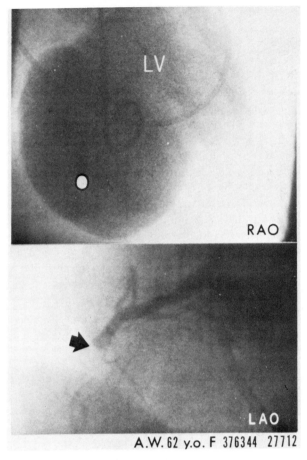

A.W. 62 y.o. F 376344 27712

O   **FALSE ANEURYSM**

➤   **TOTAL OCCLUSION RCA**

Figure 11   Left ventricular (LV) angiogram (top) (right anterior oblique position) and right coronary arteriogram (bottom) (left anterior oblique position) in a patient with intractable cardiac failure associated with acute inferior myocardial infarction related to total occlusion (arrow) of the right coronary artery (RCA). Angiography revealed rupture of the free inferior left ventricular wall indicated by opacification of a large area (the center of which is indicated by the open circle) beyond the inferior left ventricular border. Adhesion of pericardium to myocardium throughout the circumference of the rupture produced a false aneurysm. (From Mason, D.T., Amsterdam, E.A., Miller, R.R. et al: Recent advances in pathophysiology and therapy of myocardial infarction shock. In H. Russek (Ed.): *Cardiovascular Disease: New Concepts in Diagnosis and Therapy.* University Park Press, Baltimore, 1974, pp. 143-157, with permission.)

tion of acute myocardial infarction, occurring in approximately 1 percent of cases[42-44]. This lesion results in severe acute mitral regurgitation, from which mortality is 70 percent within 24 hours and 90 percent by 2 weeks[44]. Rupture of papillary muscle may involve severance of the body of the muscle, in which rapid onset of massive pulmonary edema and early death are common, or rupture of one or several heads of the muscle, in which the hemodynamic derangements, while severe, may be somewhat less so than with total separation. Rupture most commonly involves the posterior papillary muscle[44], consistent with its relatively less adequate blood supply than that of the anterior papillary muscle[45]. Electrocardiographic location of infarction is inferior with rupture of the posterior papillary muscle and anterolateral when the anterior muscle is affected. The unsupported, flail mitral leaflet is grossly incompetent, resulting in major mitral regurgitation, decreased cardiac output, and retrograde transmission of elevated pressure into the pulmonary circulation, with consequent pulmonary edema and low cardiac output. Quantitation of mitral insufficiency has indicated that in severe valvular incompetence the regurgitant blood volume comprises more than one-half of the total left ventricular stroke volume[46]. This hemodynamic burden, when superimposed on an already injured ventricle, has major significance even in a small infarct and can result in profound failure or shock in a larger infarct.

Papillary muscle dysfunction is more common than rupture[47] in acute myocardial infarction and can produce the entire clinical spectrum of mitral regurgitation from mild to severe[48]. This lesion is usually associated with ischemia (of varying degree) of the papillary muscle, and the clinical presentation differs accordingly from that of papillary muscle rupture[49]. Other factors contributing to mitral regurgitation in acute myocardial infarction, in addition to primary involvement of the valve apparatus, are ischemia and infarction of underlying myocardium, and ventricular dilatation[94].

Papillary muscle rupture or dysfunction usually occurs within the first 10 days after acute infarction. It is usually characterized by a loud holosystolic murmur at the cardiac apex, and may be accompanied by a thrill. However, severe mitral regurgitation may occur in myocardial infarction shock in the absence of a murmur[50]. A more common problem is the clinical differentiation of mitral regurgitation from ventricular septal rupture, and cardiac catheterization is required for definitive diagnosis. This can be accomplished by right heart catheterization, which can be performed at the bedside[51]. Identification of large V waves in the pulmonary capillary wedge pressure is consistent with mitral regurgitation (Figure 12). Negative findings on analysis of right ventricular blood oxygen content and indicator dilution curves exclude ventricular septal rupture.

Ventricular Septal Defect

Cardiac rupture accounts for approximately 7-9% of mortality in acute myocardial infarction[52,53]. This catastrophic event usually involves the left

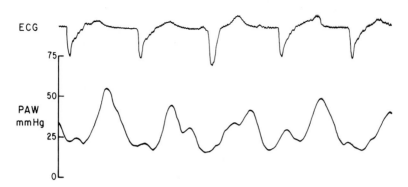

ECG

75

50
PAW
mmHg
25

0

Figure 12 Electrocardiogram (ECG) and pulmonary artery wedge pressure (PAW) in patient with acute myocardial infarction and severe mitral regurgitation. The prominent V waves in the pulmonary artery wedge pressure tracing indicate the presence of marked regurgitation.

ventricular free wall close to the interventricular septum[54]. However, in 12% of ruptures representing 1% of fatal infarctions, the perforation occurs through the interventricular septum[55,56]. Prognosis in this serious complication, which is usually associated with extensive infarction and results in rapid biventricular failure, is extremely grave. Mortality has been reported as 24 percent within 24 hours with the majority of patients dying within one week and only 13 percent surviving for 2 months[57]. The defect most frequently involves the lower portion of the muscular septum[58] but infarction in ventricular septal rupture is usually extensive and location almost always includes the anteroseptal area as well as the left ventricular free wall, and not uncommonly, the posterior region[59]. Size of the defect varies from minimal to more than 4.0 cm in its greatest dimension[58-60]. The rupture may consist of multiple perforations as found in 40 percent of patients in one series[60]. The magnitude of the left-to-right shunt is variable but in most cases is large, usually exceeding a pulmonary-to-systemic flow ratio of 2:1[15-61]. The resulting hemodynamic burden imposed on an infarcted, and thereby compromised, ventricle produces biventricular failure, pulmonary edema, and, commonly, shock. The extent of infarction in patients with rupture of the ventricular septum is indicated by the frequent association of large dyskinetic areas of the left ventricle, representing acute aneurysms of the infarcted segment of myocardium[59-63]. Thus, in one series of 57 patients with postinfarction septal rupture, aneurysms occurred in 35 percent[60]. In these cases the aneurysm may play a major role in the hemodynamic deterioration[59,64].

Acute rupture of the ventricular septum is characterized by abrupt clinical deterioration associated with the sudden appearance of a loud holosystolic murmur at the lower left sternal border often accompanied by a thrill. However, a thrill is commonly absent and the murmur may be most prominent at the cardiac apex, a phenomenon that may be related to inferoapical location of the septal defect[59]. Clinical differentiation of septal rupture from mitral regurgitation can thus be difficult or impossible. Definitive diagnosis, therefore, requires catheterization of the right side of the heart and analysis of right ventricular blood oxygen content and indicator dilution curves[61,64] (Figure 13).

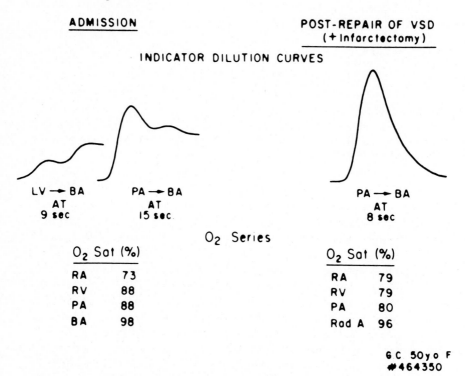

Figure 13 Indicator dilution curves and oxygen saturation (O_2Sat.) obtained by right heart catheterization in a patient with shock from acute myocardial infarction associated with ventricular septal rupture. The studies on admission indicate the presence of a left-to-right shunt at the ventricular level. After repair of the septal defect, there is no evidence of residual shunt. Infarctectomy was also performed. VSD = ventricular septal defect; LV = left ventricle; BA = brachial artery; PA = pulmonary artery; AT = appearance time; RA = right atrium; RV = right ventricle; Rad. A = radial artery. (From Amsterdam, E.A., Hughes, J.L., Iben, A., et al: Surgery for acute myocardial infarction. In R.M. Gunnar, H.S. Loeb, and S.H. Rahimtoola (Eds.): *Shock in Myocardial Infarction.* Grune & Stratton, Inc., New York, 1974, pp. 257-283, with permission.)

Factors which impose mechanical stress on the ventricular myocardium and impair its structural integrity are thought to relate to occurrence of cardiac rupture. Elevation of systolic blood pressure and an increase in end-diastolic volume augment intramyocardial wall stress and most patients with cardiac rupture have had hypertension[65]. Anticoagulants, although of uncertain significance in the pathogenesis of rupture, have been associated with a five-fold increase in cardiac perforation in some studies[66]. The softness of the infarcted area is another important factor,[54,67,68] and thus cardiac rupture usually occurs within the first few days of acute infarction[67]. The role of excessive early physical activity in the production of cardiac rupture remains controversial[69,70]. Finally, rupture is most commonly associated with the first transmural myocardial infarction in patients without previous coronary symptoms since such patients have neither diffuse ventricular fibrosis nor well-developed collateral vessels[54,67,68,71].

Abnormal Ventricular Segmental Contraction

Areas of acutely infarcted myocardium are manifested by localized disorders of left ventricular wall motion during systole. Dyssynergy is used in this review as a general term signifying any of the various patterns of abnormal regional ventricular movement[36] (Figure 6). Three specific patterns of dyssynergy are designated[72]; (1) hypokinesis: diminished regional systolic shortening in which there is less inward excursion of the disturbed segment (< 15-30% decrease of end-diastolic long and short diameters) than the remaining unaffected areas; (2) akinesis: absent systolic movement of a segment of the wall; and (3) dyskinesis: paradoxial outward systolic expansion (ventricular aneurysm) in which a portion of the end-systolic silhouette extends outside the end-diastolic perimeter.

Areas of dyssynergy contribute to disturbed ventricular function by more than the loss of the contribution of the infarcted zone to total ventricular contractile activity. Thus, the passive systolic expansion of acutely infarcted myocardium also may result in: (1) diversion of stroke volume and thereby reduced cardiac output; (2) increased end diastolic volume with elevation of myocardial oxygen requirements and augmentation of ischemia; (3) elevated left ventricular and diastolic pressure productive of pulmonary congestion; (4) impairment of papillary muscle function with consequent mitral valve incompetence; and (5) the provocation of serious arrhythmias from electrically unstable tissue. Cardiac pump dysfunction becomes manifest in the presence of coronary artery disease with ventricular dyssynergy when the involved area compromises more than 20 percent of the left ventricle[71-73].

ROLE OF CORONARY COLLATERAL CIRCULATION

The role of the coronary collateral circulation in ischemic heart disease is controversial. Although these vessels have been classically considered to have a protective effect on the myocardium[74] and experimental studies indicate enhancement of coronary blood flow by these auxiliary channels[75-77] recent investigations have produced variable findings both in chronic coronary heart disease and myocardial infarction[78-84]. Thus, postmortem studies demonstrating relation between collateral vessels and the presence and extent of myocardial infarction[85] are at variance with earlier conclusions indicating a protective effect of collaterals against infarction[74]. However, in myocardial infarction patients undergoing acute angiographic evaluation, we have recently correlated the presence of collateral vessels with reduced frequency of complications[86]. Thus, hemodynamic dysfunction (Figure 14), and incidence of shock and mortality (Figure 15) were greater in patients without collaterals than in those with collaterals. In the former group, shock developed in 71% (10/14 patients) and mortality was 57% (8/14), whereas in the latter group of six patients there was no shock and all patients survived.

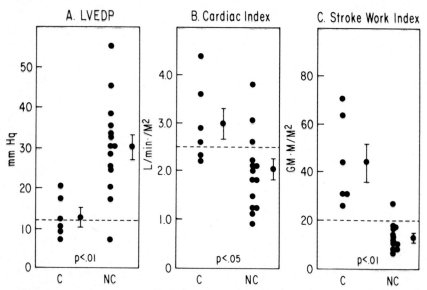

Figure 14 Left ventricular end-diastolic pressures (LVEDP) (panel A), cardiac indices (panel B) and stroke work indices (SWI) (panel C) in Group I acute myocardial infarction (AMI) patients with adequate collaterals (C) compared to Group II AMI patients with no or inadequate collaterals (NC). Mean values ± SEM are shown. Dashed horizontal line represents upper limit of normal LVEDP in panel A and lower limit of normal cardiac index in panel B. Dashed horizontal line in panel C represents the severely depressed level of SWI characteristic of AMI shock. (From Williams, D.O., Amsterdam, E.A., Miller, R.R., and Mason, D.T.: Functional significance of coronary collateral vessels in patients with acute myocardial infarction: relation to pump performance, cardiogenic shock and survival. *Am. J. Cardiol.*, **37**: 345-351, 1976, with permission.)

Many aspects of collateral vessel function remain uncertain, including the determinants of and capacity for blood flow in these channels. However, their documented ability, albeit limited, to augment regional myocardial perfusion[80] suggests a potential for maintenance of local cell viability in myocardial infarction and a critical reduction in the extent of damage which may be sufficient to avert shock in some patients.

ROLE OF THE PERIPHERAL CIRCULATION

Impairment of sympathetic reflex vasoconstriction in acute myocardial infarction has been demonstration experimentally[87-89] and clinically[90] (Figure 16). In experimental myocardial infarction this effect has been noted even in

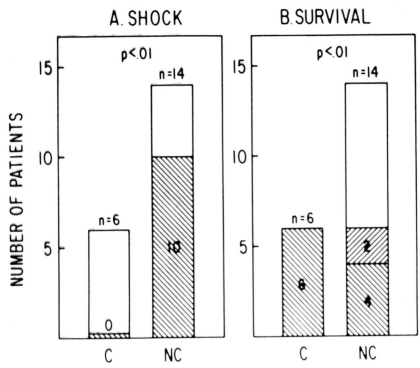

Figure 15 Number of patients who developed cardiogenic shock (panel A) and who survived acute myocardial infarction with subsequent hospital discharge (panel B) are indicated by the hatched portions of the vertical bars in Group I AMI patients with collaterals (C) compared to Group II AMI patients with no or inadequate collaterals (NC). The value of significance (p < .01) between the two patient groups refers to the incidence of shock (0/6 in I versus 6/14 in II). In the NC bar of panel B, downward-hatched portion represents surviving patients without surgery and upward-hatched portion indicates surviving patients who underwent surgical intervention. (From Williams, D.O., Amsterdam, E.A., Miller, R.R., and Mason, D.T.: Functional significance of coronary collateral vessels in patients with acute myocardial infarction: relation to pump performance, cardiogenic shock and survival. *Am. J. Cardiol.*, **37**: 345-356, 1976, with permission.)

the presence of systemic hypotension[87]-[89]. It has been attributed to inhibition of vasoconstriction[87,88,91] and competitive vasodilation[89] produced by inhibitory reflexes from receptors in the myocardium. It has been suggested that these receptors are activated by chemical[91] or mechanical[92] stimuli arising in injured cardiac muscle and mediated by vagal[93] or sympathetic[94] afferent pathways. This physiological defect has serious potential in acute myocardial infarction. The majority of patients with myocardial infarction have extensive coronary artery disease[95]. Coronary blood flow is thus dependent on the maintenance of perfusion pressure within a relatively narrow range since the normal autoregulatory function of the coronary circulation is impaired in the presence of obstructive coronary disease[96]. Inability to maintain blood pressure by compensating for reduced stroke volume with eleva-

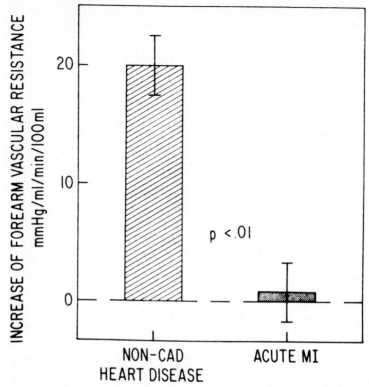

Figure 16 Reflex forearm vascular resistance responses to head-upright tilting in acute myocardial infarction (MI) compared to hospitalized cardiac patients without coronary artery disease (non-CAD). (From Mason, D.T., Amsterdam, E.A., Miller, R.R. et al: Recent advances in pathophysiology and therapy of myocardial infarction shock. In H. Russek (Ed.): *Cardiovascular Disease: New Concepts in Diagnosis and Therapy.* University Park Press, Baltimore, 1974, pp. 143-157, with permission.)

tion of peripheral vascular resistance may thus result in increased myocardial ischemia and necrosis with further deterioration of hemodynamic function.

HYPOVOLEMIA AND OTHER EXTRAMYOCARDIAL DEFECTS

Although cardiac pump dysfunction in acute myocardial infarction is principally related to the quantity of myocardium lost, other factors may also be operative in some patients. Thus, hypovolemia and impaired reflex sympathetic vasoconstriction in response to reduced systemic blood pressure may be important factors in circulatory failure accompanying myocardial infarction. The occurrence of these conditions in the presence of reduced myocardial contractility and loss of contractile units resulting from acute myocardial infarction, in themselves insufficient to cause shock, may further impair hemodynamic function and thereby play a role in the genesis of the shock syndrome.

Hypovolemia has been documented in myocardial infarction shock[97]. Hypovolemia of absolute or relative degree deprives the injured ventricle of the beneficial hemodynamic effect provided by utilization of the Starling mechanism. Thus, impairment of circulatory function due to depression of intrinsic cardiac capacity may be exacerbated by coexisting hypovolemia. The effect on cardiac performance is represented by a low point on an already depressed ventricular function curve. Hypovolemia in patients with acute myocardial infarction may be related to previous or current diuretic therapy, inadequate fluid intake or replacement, emesis, diarrhea, fever, or hyperventilation. In addition, alpha adrenergic stimulation by endogenous catecholamines, or exogenously administered sympathomimetic agents, may produce preferential, intense construction of post-capillary sphincters resulting in a loss of plasma volume by transudation of fluid to the extra-vascular space[98]. Severe hypoxia or acidosis may result in loss of structural or functional integrity in the micro-circulation with consequent escape of intra-vascular fluid.

Other extramyocardial factors may also be involved in the genesis of hypotension and circulatory failure when superimposed on only moderate intrinsic cardiac dysfunction in acute myocardial infarction. These include tachyarrhythmias or bradyarrhythmias, hypoxemia of noncardiac etiology, unmitigated pain and iatrogenic causes exemplified by drugs such as morphine, which depress cardiorespiratory function, and diuretic agents, the overzealous use of which can produce hypovolemia. Diagnostic evaluation should also include a search for concurrent or alternative etiologies for the shock syndrome such as cardiac tamponade, aortic dissection, pulmonary embolism, septicemia, hemorrhage, or abdominal catastrophe.

The extramyocardial alterations noted above may contribute to the depression of intrinsic myocardial function associated with myocardial infarction shock. Although shock in acute myocardial infarction can be directly related to the foregoing extramyocardial derangements in only a relatively small proportion of patients, these conditions, which may not be readily appreciated clinically, are emphasized since they are usually responsive to appropriate medical management in contrast to the characteristically refractory state of true cardiogenic shock.

CONCLUSION: SUBSETS OF CARDIOGENIC SHOCK

In at least one-half of patients with cardiogenic shock, shock occurs early within a few hours of the infarction[99]. These patients are usually relatively young, in their forties and fifties, with acute anterior myocardial infarction resulting from thrombotic occlusion of the left anterior descending coronary artery. Further, they often have accelerated coronary disease and athero-sclerosis risk factors. Cardiomegaly may be absent and usually is no more than moderate. Left ventriculography has demonstrated extensive dyskinesis of the anterior free wall and apex, usually greater than 50% of the ventricular silhouette, with increased extent and velocity of shortening of the posterior base of the chamber[9], as demonstrated in Figure 2B. Selective coronary arteriography has shown complete obstruction of the proximal left anterior descending coronary artery[9]. Pathologic examination has revealed that there is often distal patency of this vessel, although the patency may not be evident on angiography[9,99].

In approximately one-sixth of patients in cardiogenic shock, severe mechanical abnormalities are also present, such as mitral incompetence (Figure 12), ventricular septal defect (Figure 13), or cardiac tamponade[99]. In our experience it is unusual for a patient with diaphragmatic infarction to develop cardiogenic shock based solely on loss of left ventricular muscle; when shock occurs with this location of infarction it is usually caused by the added insult to cardiac function of a mechanical disturbance which should be identified (Figure 11).

In the remaining one-third of patients with myocardial infarction shock, this syndrome develops more slowly within several days of severe intractable congestive heart failure following acute infarction[99]. These patients usually have moderate to marked cardiomegaly (Figure 2C) and chronic symptomatology of ventricular pump dysfunction with previous episodes of myocardial ischemia and infarction. In addition, they usually are older, over 60 years, and have diffuse multivessel coronary disease. Pump dysfunction in these individuals can often be considered terminal, heart failure resulting from generalized left ventricular disease. On occasion, however, congestive heart failure and gradual development of shock occur with localized coronary stenosis in younger individuals in whom the extent of anterior infarction is less than that which produces acute onset of cardiogenic shock.

Acknowledgments

The authors gratefully acknowledge the technical assistance of Martie Wood, Robbie Brocchini, Robert Kleckner, Arthur Lewis and Leslie Silvernail.

References

1. Swan, H.J.C., Forrester, J.S., Danzig, R., and Allen, H.N.: Power failure in acute myocardial infarction. *Prog. Cardiov. Dis.,* **12**: 568, 1970.
2. Mason, D.T.: Face of the enemy. In D.T. Mason (Ed.): *Essays in Medicine: Cardiovascular Management.* Medcom Publishers, New York, 1974, pp. 8-11.
3. Scheidt, S., Ascheim, R., and Killip, T.: Shock after acute myocardial infarction. *Am. J. Cardiol.,* **26**: 556, 1970.
4. Wolk, M.J., Scheidt, S., and Killip, T.: Heart failure complicating acute myocardial infarction. *Circulation,* **45**: 1125, 1972.
5. Killip, T. and Kimball, J.T.: Treatment of myocardial infarction in a coronary care unit. *Am. J. Cardiol.,* **20**: 457, 1967.
6. Amsterdam, E.A., Zelis, R., Massumi, R.A., and Mason, D.T.: Evaluation and management of cardiogenic shock. Part I: Approach to the patient. *Heart and Lung 1,* **3**: 402, 1972.
7. Swan, H.J.C., Forrester, J.S., Diamond, G., et al: Hemodynamic spectrum of myocardial infarction and cardiogenic shock. A conceptual model. *Circulation,* **45**: 1097, 1972.

8. Amsterdam, E.A.: Function of the hypoxic myocardium. Experimental and clinical aspects. *Am. J. Cardiol.,* **32**: 461, 1973.
9. Amsterdam, E.A., Choquet, Y., Bonnanno, J.A., et al: Correlative hemodynamic and angiographic studies in acute coronary syndromes. *Clin. Res.,* **21**: 232, 1973.
10. Karliner, J.S. and Ross, J.: Left ventricular performance after acute myocardial infarction. *Progr. Cardiovasc. Dis.,* **13**: 374, 1971.
11. Gunnar, R.M., Loeb, H.S., Pietras, R.J., and Tobin, J.R., Jr.: Hemodynamic measurements in a coronary care unit. *Progr. Cardiovasc. Dis.,* **11**: 29, 1968.
12. Russell, R.O., Jr., Rackley, C.E., Pombo, J., et al: Effects of increasing left ventricular filling pressure in patients with acute myocardial infarction. *J. Clin. Invest.,* **49**: 1539, 1970.
13. Ramo, B.W., Myers, N., Wallace, A.G., et al: Hemodynamic findings in 123 patients with acute myocardial infarction on admission. *Circulation,* **42**: 567, 1970.
14. Vismara, L., Mason, D.T., Amsterdam, E.A., and Zelis, R.: Right ventricular muscle mechanics in myocardial infarction: implications concerning indices of left ventricular filling. *Circulation,* **46 (Suppl. 2**:: 232, 1972.
15. Loeb, H.S., Chuquima, R., Sinno, M.Z., et al: Effects of low flow oxygen on hemodynamics and left ventricular function in patients with uncomplicated acute myocardial infarction. *Chest,* **60**: 352, 1971.
16. Page, D.L., Caulfield, J.B., Kastor, J.A., et al: Myocardial changes associated with cardiogenic shock. *N. Engl. J. Med.,* **285**: 133, 1971.
17. Alonso, D.R., Scheidt, S., Post, M., and Killip, T.: Pathophysiology of cardiogenic shock. Quantification of myocardial necrosis; clinical, pathologic and electrocardiographic correlations. *Circulation,* **48**: 588, 1973.
18. Weber, K.T., Ratshin, R.A., Janicki, J.S., et al: Left ventricular dysfunction following acute myocardial infarction. A clinopathologic and hemodynamic profile of shock and failure. *Am. J. Med.,* **54**: 697, 1973.
19. Maroko, P.R., Kjekshus, J.K., Sobel, B.E., et al: Factors influencing infarct size following experimental coronary artery occlusions. *Circulation,* **43**: 67, 1971.
20. Forrester, J.S., Diamond, G., Parmley, W.W., and Suran, J.J.C.: Early increase in left ventricular compliance following acute myocardial infarction. *J. Clin. Invest.,* **51**: 598, 1972.
21. Hood, W.B., Jr., Bianco, J.A., Kumar, R., and Whiting, R.B.: Experimental myocardial infarction: IV. Reduction of left ventricular compliance in the healing phase. *J. Clin. Invest.,* **49**: 1316, 1970.
22. Swan, H.J.C., Forrester, J.S., Diamond, G., et al: Hemodynamic spectrum of myocardial infarction and cardiogenic shock: a conceptual model. *Circulation,* **45**: 1097, 1972.
23. Shillingford, J. and Thomas, M.: Hemodynamic effects of acute myocardial infarction in man. *Prog. Cardiov. Dis.,* **9**: 571, 1967.
24. Ratshin, R.A., Rackley, C.A., and Russell, R.O., Jr.: Hemodynamic evaluation of left ventricular failure in cardiogenic shock complicating acute myocardial infarction. *Am. J. Cardiol.,* **26**: 655, 1970.
25. Hamosh, P. and Cohn, J.N.: Left ventricular function in acute myocardial infarction. *J. Clin. Invest.,* **50**: 523, 1971.
26. Mason, D.T., Amsterdam, E.A., Miller, R.R., et al: Recent advances in pathophysiology and therapy of myocardial infarction shock. In H. Russek (Ed.): *Cardiovascular Disease: New Concepts in Diagnosis and Therapy.* University Park Press, Baltimore, 1974, pp. 143-157.
27. Awan, N., Amsterdam, E.A., Vera, Z., et al: Reduction of ischemic injury in patient with acute myocardial infarction by sublingual nitroglycerin. Submitted.

28. Norris, R.M., Whitlock, R.M.L., Barratt-Boyes, C., and Small, C.W.: Clinical measurement of myocardial infarct size: modification of a method for the estimation of total creatine phosphokinase release after myocardial infarction. *Circulation*, **51**: 614, 1975.

29. Berman, D.S., Amsterdam, E.A., Salel, A.F., et al: Diagnostic accuracy of Tc-99m-pyrophosphate scintigraphy in the detection of acute myocardial infarction. *(abstr) Circulation*, **52**: (Suppl II): 53, 1975.

30. Reid, P.R., Taylor, D.R., Kelly, D.T., et al: Myocardial-infarct extension detected by precordial ST-segment mapping. *N. Engl. J. Med.*, **290**: 123, 1974.

31. Buja, L.M. and Roberts, W.C.: The coronary arteries and myocardium in acute myocardial infarction shock. In R. Gunnar, H.S. Loeb and S.H. Rahimtoola (Eds.): *Shock in Myocardial Infarction.* Grune & Stratton, New York, 1974, pp. 1-21.

32. Watson, A., Hackel, D.B., and Estes, E.H.: Acute coronary occlusion and the "power failure" syndrome. *Am. Heart J.*, **79**: 613, 1970.

33. Ratshin, R.A., Massing, G.K., and James, T.N.: The clinical significance of the location of acute myocardial infarction. In E. Corday and H.J.C. Swan (Eds.): *Myocardial Infarction.* Williams & Wilkins Co., Baltimore, 1973, pp. 77-85.

34. Amsterdam, E.A., Miller, R.R., Foley, D.H., and Mason, D.T.: Pathophysiology and treatment of coronary artery disease. In R. Zelis (Ed.): *The Peripheral Circulation.* Grune & Stratton, New York, 1975, pp. 363-394.

35. Miller, R.R., Olson, H.G., Vismara, L.A., et al: Determinants of pump dysfunction following myocardial infarction: importance of location, extent and pattern of abnormal left ventricular segmental contraction. *Am. J. Cardiol.*, in press, 1976.

36. Miller, R.R., Amsterdam, E.A., Bogren, H.G., et al: Electrocardiographic and cineangiographic correlations in assessment of the location, nature and extent of abnormal left ventricular segmental contraction in coronary artery disease. *Circulation*, **49**: 447, 1974.

37. Russell, R.O., Hunt, D., and Rackley, C.E.: Left ventricular hemodynamics in anterior and inferior myocardial infarction. *Am. J. Cardiol.*, **26**: 658, 1970.

38. Hughes, J.C., Salel, A.F., Massumi, R.A., et al: The electrocardiogram as a predictor of ventricular function and cardiogenic shock in acute myocardial infarction. *Circulation*, **44**: II-179, 1971.

39. Ratshin, R.A., Rackley, C.E., and Russell, R.O.: Hemodynamic evaluation of left ventricular function in cardiogenic shock complicating myocardial infarction. *Circulation*, **45**: 127, 1972.

40. Hamby, R.I., Hoffman, I., Hilsenrath, J., et al: Clinical, hemodynamic and angiographic aspects of inferior and anterior myocardial infarctions in patients with angina pectoris. *Am. J. Cardiol.*, **34**: 513, 1974.

41. Loeb, H.S., Rahimtoola, S.H., Rosen, K.M., et al: Assessment of ventricular function after acute myocardial infarction by plasma volume expansion. *Circulation*, **47**: 720, 1973.

42. Cederquidt, L. and Soderstrom, J.: Papillary muscle rupture in myocardial infarction. *Acta Med. Scand.*, **176**: 287, 1964.

43. Robinson, J.S., Stannard, M.M., and Long, M.: Ruptured papillary muscle after acute myocardial infarction. *Am. Heart J.*, **70**: 233, 1965.

44. Sanders, R.J., Neuberger, K.T., and Ravin, A.: Rupture of papillary muscles: occurrence of rupture of posterior muscle in posterior myocardial infarction. *Dis. Chest*, **31**: 316, 1957.

45. Estes, E.H., Jr., Dalton, F.M., Entman, M.L., et al: Anatomy of blood supply of papillary muscles of left ventricle. *Am. Heart J.*, **71**: 356, 1966.

46. Miller, G.A.H., Kirklin, J.W., and Swan, H.J.C.: Myocardial function and left ventricular volumes in acquired valvular insufficiency. *Circulation*, **31**: 374, 1965.

47. Heinkkila, J.: Mitral incompetence complicating acute myocardial infarction. *Brit. Heart J.,* **29**: 162, 1967.
48. Burch, G.E., DePasquale, N.P., and Phillips, J.H.: The syndrome of papillary muscle dysfunction. *Am. Heart J.,* **75**: 399, 1968.
49. Burch, G.E., DePasquale, N.P., and Phillips, J.H.: Clinical manifestations of papillary muscle dysfunction. *Arch. Intern Med.,* **112**: 112, 1963.
50. Forrester, J.S., Diamond, G., Freedman, S., et al: Silent mitral insufficiency in acute myocardial infarction. *Circulation,* **44**: 877, 1971.
51. Swan, H.J.C., Ganz, W., Forrester, J., et al: Catheterization of the heart in man with use of a flow directed balloon-tipped catheter. *N. Engl. J. Med.,* **283**: 447, 1970.
52. Oblath, R.W., Lievinson, D.C., and Griffith, G.C.: Factors influencing rupture of the heart after myocardial infarction. *JAMA,* **149**: 1276, 1952.
53. Griffith, G.C., Hedge, B., and Oblath, R.W.: Factors in myocardial rupture. *Am. J. Cardiol.,* **8**: 792, 1961.
54. London, R.E. and London, S.B.: Rupture of the heart. *Circulation,* **31**: 202-208, 1965.
55. Bernard, P.M. and Kennedy, J.H.: Post-infarction ventricular septal defect. *Circulation,* **32**: 76, 1965.
56. Van Tassel, R.A. and Edwards, J.E.: Rupture of the heart complicating myocardial infarction. *Chest,* **61**: 104, 1972.
57. Sanders, R.J., Kern, W.H., and Blount, S.G., Jr.: Perforation of the interventricular septum complicating myocardial infarction. *Am. Heart J.,* **51**: 736, 1956.
58. Swithinbank, J.M.: Perforation of the interventricular septum in myocardial infarction. *Brit. Heart J.,* **21**: 562, 1959.
59. Selzer, A., Gerbode, F., and Kerth, W.J.: Clinical hemodynamic and surgical considerations of rupture of the ventricular septum after myocardial infarction. *Am. Heart J.,* **78**: 598, 1969.
60. Kitamura, S., Mendez, A., and Kay, J.H.: Ventricular septal defect following myocardial infarction. Experience with surgical repair through a left ventriculotomy and a review of the literature. *J. Thorac. Cardiovasc. Surg.,* **61**: 186, 1971.
61. Iben, A.B., Miller, R.R., Amsterdam, E.A., et al: Successful immediate repair of acquired ventricular septal defect and survival in patients with acute myocardial infarction shock using a new double patch technique. *Chest,* **66**: 665, 1974.
62. Buckley, M.J., Mundth, E.D., Daggett, W.M., et al: Surgical therapy for early complications of myocardial infarction. *Surgery,* **70**: 814, 1971.
63. Mundth, E.D., Buckley, M.J., Daggett, W.M., et al: Surgery for complications of acute myocardial infarction. *Circulation,* **45**: 1279, 1972.
64. Amsterdam, E.A., Hughes, J.L., Iben, A., et al: Surgery for acute myocardial infarction. In R.M. Gunnar, H.S. Loeb, and S.H. Rahimtoola (Eds.): *Shock in Myocardial Infarction.* Grune & Stratton, Inc., New York, 1974, pp. 257-283.
65. Roberts, W.C., Ronan, J.A., and Harvey, W.P.: Rupture of the left ventricular free wall or ventricular septum secondary to acute myocardial infarction: an occurrence virtually limited to the first transmural myocardial infarction in a hypertensive individual. *Am. J. Cardiol.,* **35**: 166, 1975.
66. Lee, K.T. and O'Neal, R.M.: Anticoagulant therapy of acute myocardial infarction. *Am. J. Med.,* **21**: 555, 1956.
67. Lautsch, E.V. and Lanks, K.W.: Pathogenesis of cardiac rupture. *Arch. Path.,* **84**: 264, 1967.
68. Naeim, F., DeLaMaza, L.M., and Robbins, S.L.: Cardiac rupture during myocardial infarction. *Circulation,* **45**: 1231-1239, 1972.
69. Jeller, W.W. and White, P.D.: Rupture of the heart in patients in mental institutions. *Ann. Intern. Med.,* **21**: 783, 1944.

70. Kavelman, D.A.: Myocardial rupture: a study in psychotic and nonpsychotic patients. *Canad. Med. Assoc. J.,* **82**: 1105, 1960.
71. Awan, N.A., Ikeda, R., Olson, H., et al: Intraventricular free wall dissection causing acute interventricular communication with intact septum in myocardial infarction. *Chest,* in press, 1976.
72. Mason, D.T., Zelis, R., Amsterdam, E.A., and Massumi, R.: Clinical determinations of left ventricular contractility by hemodynamics and myocardial mechanics. In P. Yu and J. Goodwin (Eds.): *Progress in Cardiology.* Lea & Febiger, Philadelphia, 1972, pp. 121-153.
73. Klein, M.D., Herman, M.V., and Gorlin, R.: A hemodynamic study of left ventricular aneurysm. *Circulation,* **35**: 614, 1967.
74. Zoll, P.M., Wessler, S., and Schlesinger, M.J.: Interarterial coronary anastomoses in the human heart, with particular reference to anemia and relative cardiac anoxia. *Circulation,* **4**: 797, 1951.
75. Chimoskey, J.E., Szentivanyi, M., Zakheim, R., et al: Temporary coronary occlusion in conscious dogs: Collateral flow and electrocardiogram. *Am. J. Physiol.,* **212**: 1025, 1967.
76. Haft, J.I. and Damato, A.N.: Measurement of collateral blood flow after myocardial infarction in the closed-chest dog. *Am. Heart J.,* **77**: 641, 1969.
77. Elliot, E.C., Bloor, C.M., Jones, E.L., et al: Effect of controlled coronary occlusion on collateral circulation in conscious dogs. *Am. J. Physiol.,* **220**: 857, 1971.
78. Amsterdam, E.A., Most, A.S., Wolfson, S., et al: Relation of degree of angiographically documented coronary artery disease to mortality. *Ann. Intern. Med.,* **72**: 780, 1970.
79. Helfant, R.H., Vokonas, P.S., and Gorlin, R.: Functional importance of the human coronary collateral circulation. *N. Engl. J. Med.,* **284**: 1277, 1971.
80. Smith, S.C., Gorlin, R., Herman, M.V., et al: Myocardial blood flow in man: effects of coronary collateral circulation and coronary artery bypass surgery. *J. Clin. Invest.,* **10**: 2556, 1972.
81. Miller, R.R., Amsterdam, E.A., Zelis, R., et al: Determinants and functional significance of the coronary collateral circulation in ischemic heart disease. In H. Russek (Ed.): *Cardiovascular Disease.* University Park Press, Baltimore, 1974, pp. 75-83.
82. Carroll, R.J., Verani, M.S., and Falsetti, H.L.: The effect of collateral circulation on segmental left ventricular contraction. *Circulation,* **50**: 7-9, 1974.
83. Banka, V.S., Bodenheimer, M.M., and Helfant, R.H.: Determinants of reversible asynergy. *Circulation,* **50**: 714, 1974.
84. Levin, D.C.: Pathways and functional significance of the coronary collateral circulation. *Circulation,* **50**: 831, 1974.
85. Snow, P.J.D., Jones, A.M., and Daber, K.S.: Coronary disease: a pathological study. *Brit. Heart J.,* **17**: 503, 1955.
86. Williams, D.O., Amsterdam, E.A., Miller, R.R., and Mason, D.T.: Functional significance of coronary collateral vessels in patients with acute myocardial infarction: relation to pump performance, cardiogenic shock and survival. *Am. J. Cardiol.,* **37**: 345-357, 1976.
87. Agress, C.M., Rosenberg, M.J., Jacobs, H.I., et al: Protracted shock in the closed chest dog following coronary embolization with graded microspheres. *Am. J. Physiol.,* **170**: 536, 1952.
88. Toubes, D.B. and Brody, M.J.: Inhibition of reflex vasoconstriction after experimental coronary embolization in the dog. *Circ. Res.,* **26**: 211, 1970.
89. Hanley, H.G., Costin, J.C., and Skinner, N.S.: Differential reflex adjustments in cutaneous and muscle vascular beds during experimental coronary artery occlusion. *Am. J. Cardiol.,* **27**: 513, 1971.
90. Hughes, J.L., Amsterdam, E.A., Mason, D.T., et al: Abnormal peripheral

vascular dynamics in patients with acute myocardial infarction: diminished reflex arteriolar constriction. *Clin. Res.*, **19**: 321, 1971.

91. Constantin, L.: Extracardiac factors contributing to hypotension during coronary occlusion. *Am. J. Cardiol.*, **11**: 205, 1963.

92. Sleight, P. and Widdicombe, J.G.: Action potentials in fibers from receptors in the epicardium and myocardium of the dog's left ventricle. *J. Physiol.*, **181**: 235, 1966.

93. Kezdi, P., Misra, S.N., Kordenat, R.K., et al: The role of vagal afferents in acute myocardial infarction. *Am. J. Cardiol.*, **26**: 642, 1970.

94. Brown, A.M.: Excitation of afferent cardiac sympathetic nerve fibers during myocardial ischemia. *J. Physiol.* (London), **190**: 35, 1967.

95. Blumgart, H.L., Schlesinger, M.J., and Davis, D.: Studies in the relationship of the clinical manifestations of angina pectoris, coronary thrombosis and myocardial infarction to pathologic findings. *Am. Heart J.*, **19**: 1, 1940.

96. Berne, R.M.: Regulation of coronary blood flow. *Physiol. Rev.*, **44**: 1, 1964.

97. Loeb, H.S., Pietras, R.J., Tobin, J.R., Jr., and Gunnar, R.M.: Hypovolemia in shock due to acute myocardial infarction. *Circulation*, **40**: 653, 1969.

98. Finnerty, F.A., Jr., Bucholz, J.H., and Guilkauden, R.L.: The blood volumes and plasma protein during levarterenol-induced hypertension. *J. Clin. Invest.*, **37**: 425, 1958.

99. Swan, H.J.C.: Cardiogenic Shock, Abstracts of Papers: *Fifth Asian-Pacific Congress of Cardiology*, Oct. 8-13, 1972, Singapore, p. 21, 1972.

CHAPTER 3
The Pathophysiology of Congestive Heart Failure

James S. Forrester, M.D.; Protasio L. daLuz, M.D.; David D. Water, M.D.; H.J.C. Swan, M.D.

To properly treat congestive heart failure the clinician must recognize and grasp the pathophysiologic categories that present unique clinical features and display different hemodynamic measurements. Rational therapy thus requires the indepth understanding of the multifaceted basis for this common clinical entity well defined by Forrester et al. It forms the basis for therapeutic management presented by these authors in Chapter 12.

Heart failure is an imprecise term. Conceptually, heart failure is a reduction of cardiac performance below the normal level, and therefore any discussion of the pathophysiology of disordered cardiac function must begin with a clear understanding of those factors which regulate normal cardiac function.

REGULATORY FACTORS FOR NORMAL CARDIAC FUNCTION

The factors controlling function of the intact heart are most precisely defined by a study of the mechanisms which regulate the function of a segment of cardiac muscle. When an isolated mammalian heart muscle is stimulated to contract, how much it shortens is determined by three factors: its length at the onset of contraction ("preload"), the vigor of its contraction ("contractility"), and the tension that it is required to develop during contraction ("afterload"). As the resting length of a cardiac muscle is increased, the force it develops during contraction increases[1]. This effect of increased preload on force of contraction is most commonly termed the "Starling relationship." The relationship is not linear: as the unstretched muscle initially lengthens, it shortens proportionately more; but with further increase in length, a plateau is reached beyond which no further increase in force of contraction occurs. Thus, the amount of muscle shortening is markedly affected by its length prior to contraction.

Once contraction begins, shortening is also determined by the load against which the muscle must contract[2], and by the intrinsic contractility of the muscle.

As shown in Figure 1a, a progressive increase in afterload results in progressive reduction in shortening at any given preload. When afterload in-

41

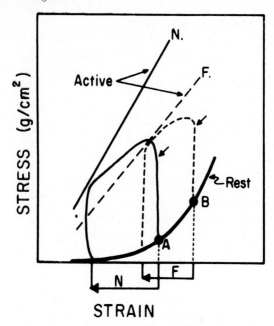

Figure 1a The relationship between stress and strain for a hypothetical sarcomere within a normal (N) and failing (F) left ventricular wall. The lower curve (heavy line) represents resting end-diastolic length. The upper solid and dash lines represent the tension which would be developed during the contraction at each end-diastolic length.

From a normal diastolic length (point A), the sarcomere develops force until the force developed equals the afterload. At this point the aortic valve opens (indicated by the arrow), and the sarcomere begins to shorten as developed force exceeds afterload. Relaxation begins when continued shortening leads to an intersection with the predicted active tension-length relationship. Point B represents an increased end-diastolic sarcomere length associated with a hypothetical failing left ventricle. As with Point A, force begins to develop with activation, and rises steeply until the developed force is equal to the afterload, at which point the aortic valve opens (arrow). Because the left ventricle is larger, a greater force development is required than in the normal heart. Concomitant with this need for greater force development, there is a decrease in the extent of shortening during ejection. Thus, heart failure associated with cardiac dilatation leads to an increase in required force development and a decrease in the magnitude of shortening during systole.

creases to the point where it is equal to or greater than the force the muscle can develop at a given preload, no shortening occurs, although the muscle still develops tension. This phenomenon of force development without shortening, termed isometric contraction, has allowed further studies of "contractile state" in which preload and afterload are held constant and shortening does not occur. In these studies, the addition of inotropic agents, such as digitalis or catecholamines, uniformly results in a substantial increase in the force developed during isometric contraction.

Analogous forces operate in the intact heart, although for practical reasons truly direct measurements of preload, afterload, and contractility are seldom made (Table I). In the intact heart, preload is proportional to the

TABLE I

ASSESSMENT OF FUNDAMENTAL DETERMINANTS
OF CARDIAC FUNCTION BY HEMODYNAMICS

Physiologic Parameter	Hemodynamic Analog
Preload	LVEDV, LVEDP, PCP
Afterload	LVs, APs
Contractility	LV dp/dt

LVEDV = left ventricular end-diastolic volume
LVEDP = left ventricular end-diastolic pressure
PCP = pulmonary capillary pressure
LVs = left ventricular systolic pressure
APs = systolic arterial pressure

volume of the left ventricle at end-diastole, and is most commonly estimated clinically by the correlative distension pressure, left ventricular end-diastolic pressure. Afterload is represented by the force the left ventricle develops during contraction and is estimated clinically by arterial or left ventricular systolic pressure. Contractility cannot be readily measured in the intact heart, since it represents an undefined biochemical state rather than a physical force. All hemodynamic parameters of contractility, therefore, are influenced to various degrees by preload and afterload. Clinically, however, the most widely used and readily obtained index of contractility is "max LV dP/dt," the maximum rate of pressure development during cardiac contraction. Muscle shortening (i.e., change in length) is best represented in the intact heart by a cubic function of length, for instance, cubic centimeters, which is expressed as stroke volume. The inverse relationship between increasing afterload and decreased shortening during contraction of an isolated muscle is expressed in the intact heart as "stroke work," the product of stroke volume (for shortening) and arterial systolic pressure (for afterload). In the intact heart, as in the isolated muscle, a "family" of Starling function curves results from these interrelationships, and the effect of a change in one of the factors controlling cardiac function is shown in Figure 1b.

The interaction of these factors in normal man is highly complex. Reduction in cardiac performance secondary to an alteration in one determinant of cardiac function generally leads to a series of regulatory responses in the other determinants which tend to return cardiac performance toward normal levels. For example, an increase in afterload by vasoconstriction will activate the Starling mechanism. Thus, increased resistance to ejection causes

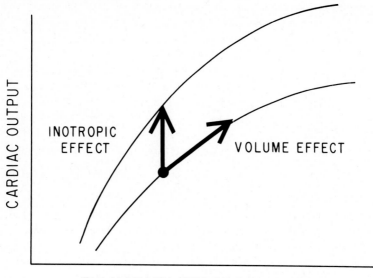

Figure 1b Effects of altered preload ("volume loading") and altered contractility ("inotropic agents") upon cardiac performance. Increased preload increases cardiac output by means of the Frank-Starling mechanism. Inotropic agents often increase cardiac output at the same preload, moving the heart to a new Starling function curve.

a decrease in stroke volume and a subsequent increase in end-diastolic volume (preload). Conversely, a decrease in preload activates the autonomic nervous system; decreased end-diastolic volume causes a decrease in stroke volume, activating the carotid baro-receptors and causing a subsequent increase in peripheral vascular resistance and heart rate.

The sequence of events that results in a change in cardiac function in normal man is, therefore, to a large extent, dictated by the initiating stimulus. For instance, during exercise the need for an immediate and substantial increase in cardiac output is met predominantly by an increase in autonomic tone, with an increase in heart rate, selective regional vasoconstriction and dilatation, and an increase in contractility. The Starling mechanism is not utilized in the exercise response in normal man, and end-diastolic volume generally diminishes. In contrast, the response to a change of position from the supine to upright position initiates an immediate need for control of blood flow distribution. The resulting selective peripheral vasomotor response, particularly in the lower extremities, causes increased total systemic vascular resistance. This increased resistance causes a decrease in stroke volume, which is immediately counterbalanced by the resulting increase in end-diastolic volume, returning stroke volume toward normal. By the continuous interplay of these regulatory factors, cardiac output is readily maintained at a level appropriate to the requirements of metabolizing tissues, so that a fairly large change in any one of the regulatory mechanisms can be well tolerated in normal man.

Heart failure occurs when a change in one or more of the determinants of cardiac performance exceeds the ability of the other mechanisms to compensate. Because there are several determinants of cardiac function and a plethora of manifestations of heart failure, it is impossible to develop an explicit definition satisfactory to all investigators and to all circumstances. In practical clinical terms, however, heart failure may be considered to be that state in which an abnormality of myocardial performance is responsible for the inability of the heart to pump blood at a rate commensurate with the requirements of metabolizing tissues.

The transition from normal cardiac function to heart failure is therefore a subtle continuum, in which each of the mechanisms responsible for maintaining cardiac output is used with increasing intensity to maintain effective cardiac performance at near normal levels. Initially, the "excessive" use of compensatory responses may be detected only during a substantial stress upon the heart. As heart failure increases, signs become apparent at rest. At this point, other compensatory responses, not normally used in the regulation of cardiac performance, are also recruited. As a generalization, therefore, the acute compensatory responses are those which control normal cardiac function, whereas chronic compensatory responses are encountered only in nonphysiologic conditions.

Although no rigid or quantitative description for the progression from normal function to heart failure is possible, there is a usual sequence of clinical events. In general, the autonomic nervous system and the Starling response are the first to be employed in response to acute heart failure. Increased autonomic tone increases peripheral vascular resistance, heart rate, and myocardial contractility. As a result of both primary reduction in function and the compensatory increased vascular resistance, the Starling mechanism is activated through the mechanism of decreased stroke volume leading to an increased end-diastolic volume. When these mechanisms fail to return cardiac output to normal levels, additional responses, such as renal retention of sodium and water, occur. As heart failure persists beyond several days, the acute compensatory responses tend to diminish in intensity and effectiveness, and are replaced by cardiac dilatation and hypertrophy.

ACUTE HEART FAILURE

The Autonomic Nervous System

Reduced myocardial contractility plays a major role in the genesis of heart failure. Thus, the papillary muscles of cats with either left ventricular failure or cardiac hypertrophy exhibit depression in LV max dp/dt (an index of myocardial contracility) and, as a consequence, a reduction in their ability to develop force during contraction[3]. Left ventricular papillary muscles removed from heart failure patients at surgery show similar reduction in the maximum tension that can be developed during contraction. This depression in intrinsic contractility may be homogeneous, as in the cardiomyopathies, or localized, as in coronary heart disease.

In response to depressed intrinsic cardiac performance, increased sympathetic activity is used to restore cardiac function toward normal. Three separate mechanisms are employed: increased contractility, increased heart rate, and altered peripheral vascular tone. The inotropic effect of the sympathetic neurotransmitter, norepinephrine, augments the force of cardiac contraction at any level of end-diastolic volume. Normally, the heart's supply of norepinephrine comes from two sources: 90% of it is synthesized in the heart itself, from the precursor amino acid tyrosine[4], plus the heart can readily extract norepinephrine from the circulating blood. Profound alterations in both cardiac and circulating norepinephrine occur in heart failure. Biopsies of atrial[5] and papillary muscle tissues[6] of patients undergoing open-heart surgery reveal substantial reduction in norepinephrine concentration as compared to patients who do not have failure. This depression in cardiac norepinephrine concentration is related to a significant decrease in the enzyme tyrosine hydroxylase, which catalyzes the first reaction in the transformation of tyrosine to norepinephrine[7].

Although the myocardial stores of norepinephrine are depleted, the clinical findings of pallor, tachycardia, and peripheral vasoconstriction suggest increased activity of the sympathetic nervous system. Indeed, when the concentration of arterial norepinephrine is measured in patients with heart failure, both at rest and during exercise, substantially increased values are found[8,9], and the 24 hour urinary excretion of norepinephrine also increases in heart failure.

These data suggest that the sympathetic nervous system exerts a substantial supportive role when cardiac function is depressed, but that the magnitude and duration of the cardiac compensatory response may be limited by intrinsic myocardial norepinephrine depletion. Additional support for this hypothesis comes from the demonstration that suppression of sympathetic activity by small doses of either propranolol or guanethidine causes little change in cardiac performance in normal man, but causes substantial accentuation of the symptoms and signs of heart failure when cardiac function is chronically depressed[10,11].

The second mechanism, increased heart rate, increases cardiac output so long as the concomitant shortening of the time available for diastolic filling does not result in a substantial diminution of end-diastolic volume. Increased heart rate is most frequently a result of decreased carotid baroreceptor stretch secondary to the reduced stroke volume of heart failure. Although this increase in heart rate has been classically attributed to activation of the sympathetic nervous system, recent evidence suggests that a concomitant withdrawal of parasympathetic activity also plays an important role[4].

A third compensatory response in which the autonomic nervous system plays a crucial role is redistribution of blood flow. Under acute stress, either

physiologic or pathologic, the increased demand for oxygen is met by alterations in vascular tone throughout the body induced by both local and sympathetic nervous system stimuli. Thus skin, gut, and inactive muscle receive
proportionately less cardiac output than more essential organs, as brain,
kidney, and heart. As part of this phenomenon, when blood flow to an organ
decreases, the organ itself can compensate by increasing its extraction of
nutrients from the blood. Different tissues have strikingly different oxygen
extraction ratios at rest, and thus marked differences in reserve capacity. For
instance, the kidney normally extracts only 10% of the oxygen from the
blood passing through it, whereas the normal heart extracts approximately
70% of arterial oxygen even at rest. Since the kidney can substantially increase its oxygen extraction, it is relatively invulnerable to decrease in flow,
but the heart has little capacity to withstand a primary decrease in perfusion
by increasing oxygen extraction.

Activation of the sympathetic nervous system, as with every compensatory
mechanism, carries physiologic costs. An increase in heart rate, contractility, and total peripheral resistance each serve to augment myocardial oxygen demand: in the presence of acute myocardial ischemia, compensatory
responses to improve myocardial coronary performance may aggravate the
imbalance between myocardial oxygen supply and demand[12].

The Starling Response

Early in the course of left ventricular failure, changes in end-diastolic
volume can compensate for depressed contractility, maintaining stroke
volume within the normal range[13-15]. At this stage, although heart failure
may not be immediately apparent, analysis of the ratio of stroke volume to
the end-diastolic volume, i.e., the ejection fraction, will reveal reduced cardiac performance. The normal ejection fraction is approximately 70%,
When the ejection fraction drops to less than 50%, heart failure is present[16].

The effectiveness of the Starling mechanism as a method for maintaining
stroke volume diminishes progressively as end-diastolic volume is increased,
in a manner directly analogous to the response of the isolated cardiac muscle
to increasing length. This response has a well defined ultrastructural basis[1].
The fundamental contractile unit of the muscle fiber is the sarcomere. The
normal resting sarcomere measures approximately 1.9 micra and the length
at which maximal contractile response occur is 2.2 micra. When ventricular
volume is increased to the point that sarcomere length exceeds 2.2 micra, a
further increase in diastolic volume does not lead to increased shortening.
Clinically, although the Starling mechanism causes a substantial increase in
stroke volume when the heart is operating on the steep portion of the
ventricular curve, this mechanism has a limit of effectiveness set by the maximum effective sarcomere length. Thus, the Starling mechanism, like increased autonomic tone and increased contractility, constitutes an important, rapidly activated compensatory response of the failure myocardium,
but it is ultimately of limited capacity.

As with all compensatory mechanisms, the Starling response carries substantial costs. The most important disadvantage associated with ventricular dilatation is the increase in ventricular diastolic pressure which accompanies it. This increased pressure backs up through the left atrium and pulmonary veins to the pulmonary capillaries where it may cause symptoms of pulmonary congestion. In addition, an increase in ventricular preload increases ventricular wall tension. This increase in wall tension substantially increases myocardial oxygen consumption, and may therefore aggravate myocardial ischemia in acute coronary heart disease[17].

Chronic Mechanism

All of the aforementioned mechanisms may be enlisted within seconds to prevent the appearance of overt cardiac failure. In chronic heart failure these adjustments may still remain active, but structural changes within the heart provide additional reserves. The dilated failing heart hypertrophies in response to the increased tension placed on muscle fibers by increased left ventricular volume. Although the contractile performance of each muscle unit is depressed, total cardiac output can be maintained by the increased number of units. The effectiveness of cardiac hypertrophy as a compensatory mechanism is limited by the ability of the coronary vasculature to provide oxygen to the increased muscle mass, and by the increase in ventricular diastolic pressure that accompanies both cardiac dilatation and hypertrophy.

THE RELATIONSHIP OF ALTERED CARDIAC FUNCTION
TO THE CLINICAL STATE

The clinical presentation of a patient with acute heart failure is a complex constellation of decreased cardiac performance, plus the acute and chronic cardiac and extra-cardiac compensatory responses to this primary decrease in function. Regardless of either the etiology of the heart failure, or the magnitude of compensatory responses, three fundamental alterations in cardiac hemodynamics determine the type of presentation, prognosis, and therapy: an increase in right atrial pressure, an increase in pulmonary capillary pressure, and a decrease in cardiac output. Each of these parameters may change independently, and each is responsible for a different set of symptoms (Table II).

Increased Right Atrial Pressure: The Cause of Venous Congestion

Right atrial pressure reflects both right ventricular diastolic pressure (when the tricuspid valve is open, the right atrium and right ventricle are common chambers) and the central venous pressure. When right ventricular diastolic volume increases with right heart failure, right ventricular diastolic pressure, right atrial and central venous pressure all increase. The increased right atrial pressure presents clinically as jugular venous distention, hepatic enlargement, and peripheral edema.

TABLE II
NORMAL AND ABNORMAL CARDIAC HEMODYNAMICS

Measurement	Normal Range	Increased in:	Signs & Symptoms
RA	0-8 mmHg	RV Failure: PE, COPD Tricuspid valve abn. Pericardial tamponade	Engorged neck veins Enlarged liver Peripheral edema
PA	15-30 mmHg 5-12*	Systolic: ↑ Resistance: PE, COPD ↑ Flow: VSD Diastolic: ↑Resistance: PE, COPD All causes of ↑ PCP	RV heave Palpable PA impulse Increased P_2
PCP	5-12* mmHg	LV Failure Mitral valve disease Tamponade ↓ LV compliance: hypertrophy, infarct	Rales Dyspnea
		Decreased in:	
CI	2.7-4.3 L/min/M²**	Shock	Oliguria Obtundation Cold skin Hypotension Tachycardia

RV = right ventricle, PE = pulmonary embolus, TI = tricuspid insufficiency, MI = mitral insufficiency, COPD = chronic obstructive pulmonary disease, VSD = ventricular septal defect, LV = left ventricle, P_2 = pulmonary component of the second heart sound.

* Although clinical signs of pulmonary congestion begin at approximately 18 mmHg, the generally accepted upper limit of normal is 12 mmHg.
** Although clinical signs of peripheral hypoperfusion begin at approximately 2.2 L/min/M², the generally accepted lower limit of normal is 2.7 L/min/M².

Increased Pulmonary Capillary Pressure: The Cause of Pulmonary Congestion

When left ventricular diastolic volume increases with acute heart failure, so does left ventricular diastolic pressure. This increased pressure backs up through the pulmonary venous system and results in increased pulmonary capillary pressure. This increase in pulmonary capillary pressure is the direct hemodynamic cause of pulmonary congestion, since it is the hydrostatic pressure that forces fluid out of the intravascular space into the pulmonary interstitium and alveoli. This process results in the symptoms of shortness of breath and dyspnea, the signs of rales, and the radiologic manifestations of pulmonary congestion. The severity of acute pulmonary congestion is closely related to the magnitude of elevation in pulmonary capillary pressure, as follows:

> 18-20 mm Hg — onset of pulmonary congestion
> 21-25 mm Hg — moderate congestion
> 26-30 mm Hg — severe congestion
> 30 mm Hg — onset of acute pulmonary edema

The radiologic manifestations of acute pulmonary congestion occur in a specific sequence that relates directly to the amount of elevation in pulmonary capillary pressure[18]. The first radiologic change that follows an increase in pulmonary capillary pressure is *redistribution of flow* to the upper lobes of the lung. As pulmonary capillary pressure is further increased, fluid passes out of the capillaries into perivascular and interstitial tissue, resulting in *diminished clarity of the borders of medium-sized pulmonary veins* and the development of *perihilar haze.* As pressure increases still further, fluid moves to the perialveolar space, resulting in the appearance of radiolucent grapelike clusters surrounded by radiodense fluid, called *"peri-acinar rosettes".* Finally, with very high pulmonary capillary pressure, the rosettes coalesce and other signs are accentuated, resulting in the radiologic appearance of *alveolar pulmonary edema.*

Although this sequence remains unchanged in chronic pulmonary congestion, the amount of pulmonary capillary pressure elevation required to produce such signs may increase significantly. The walls of small pulmonary vessels thicken markedly in response to chronic pressure elevation and serve to resist the passage of fluid into the interstitial space. Thus, it is possible to encounter an asymptomatic patient with pulmonary capillary pressure levels of as high as 30 mm Hg when pulmonary capillary pressure is chronically elevated in disease states such as mitral stenosis.

Decreased Cardiac Output: The Cause of Peripheral Hypoperfusion

Reduction in cardiac output manifests clinically as decreased perfusion of all organs, most dramatically the skin, kidney, and brain, resulting in cold clammy skin, oliguria, anxiety, lethargy, or coma. The severity of peripheral hypoperfusion relates to the depression in cardiac output (expressed as cardiac index in order to normalize for differences due to body size)*. Cardiac index (CI) relates to acute hypoperfusion as follows:

> 2.7-4.3 L/min/M^2 — "normal" range
> 2.0-2.2 L/min/M^2 — onset of peripheral hypoperfusion
> 1.8-2.0 L/min/M^2 — onset of cardiogenic shock

As with pulmonary congestion, the ability of the body to withstand chronic depression of cardiac output can be remarkable. Occasionally, a patient with moderately severe chronic heart failure presents with a level of cardiac index that would be lethal in acute heart failure.

*Cardiac index equals cardiac output divided by body surface area.

Since increased pulmonary capillary pressure causes pulmonary congestion and decreased cardiac index leads to peripheral hypoperfusion, it is possible to predict the range of both pulmonary capillary pressure and cardiac
index by clinical evaluation[19]. Figure 2 illustrates the level of pulmonary
capillary pressure and cardiac index in 200 patients with acute myocardial
infarction. Fifty-two percent of the patients with clinical evidence of
pulmonary congestion had a pulmonary capillary pressure more than 18
mm Hg, and 45% of those with peripheral hypoperfusion had a cardiac index less than 2.2 L/min/m². As a consequence of this high correlation between clinical and hemodynamic state, it is possible to accurately predict the
level of both pulmonary capillary pressure and cardiac index by clinical
evaluation in approximately 70% of patients with acute myocardial infarction.

In summary, there are many pathophysiologic responses to deteriorating
cardiac function. Nevertheless, this highly complex biological phenomenon
manifests itself through a limited number of important hemodynamic
changes, which in turn produce three clearly recognizable groups of clinical

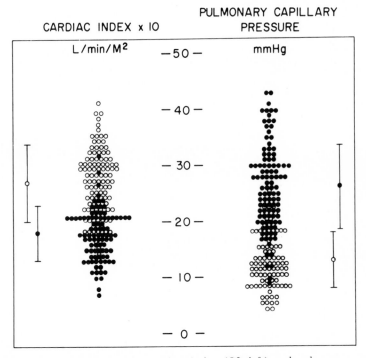

Figure 2 The distribution of cardiac index (CI, left) and pulmonary capillary
pressure (PCP, right) in 200 patients with acute myocardial infarction. In the left
panel, closed circles represent those patients with clinical evidence of peripheral
hypoperfusion, and in the right panel closed circles represent those patients with
clinical pulmonary congestion. Mean values + SD are located to the outside of the
data. When a CI of 2.2 L/min/M² and a PCP of 18 mm Hg are used to separate
these two groups, a correct "prediction" of the presence or absence of peripheral
hypoperfusion and pulmonary congestion can be obtained in over 80% of patients.

signs. It is this correlation between the clinical and hemodynamic manifestations of heart failure that forms the basis for evaluation of prognosis and selection of therapy.

References

1. Braunwald, E., Ross, J., Jr., and Sonnenblick, E.H.: *Mechanism of Contraction of the Normal and Failing Heart,* 2nd edition. Little, Brown and Company, Boston, 1975.
2. Sonnenblick, E.H., Ross, J., Jr., Spotnitz, H.M., et al: The ultrastructure of the heart in systole and diastole: changes in sarcomere length. *Circ. Res.,* **21**: 423-431, 1967.
3. Spann, J.F., Jr., Buccino, R.A., Sonnenblick, E.H., et al: Contractile state of cardiac muscle obtained from cats with experimentally produced ventricular hypertrophy and heart failure. *Circ. Res.,* **21**: 341-354, 1967.
4. Braunwald, E.: The autonomic nervous system in heart failure. In *The Myocardium: Failure and Infarction.* HP Publishing Co., Inc., New York, 1974, p. 3.
5. Chidsey, C.A., Braunwald, E., Morrow, A.G., et al: Myocardial norepinephrine concentration in man: effects of reserpine and of congestive heart failure. *N. Engl. J. Med.,* **269**: 653-658, 1963.
6. Chidsey, C.A., Sonnenblick, E.H., Morrow, A.G., et al: Norepinephrine stores and contractile force of papillary muscle from failing human heart. *Circulation,* **33**: 43-51, 1966.
7. Pool, P.E., Covell, J.W., Levitt, M., et al: Reduction of cardiac tyrosine hydroxylase activity in experimental congestive heart failure: its role in depletion of cardiac norepinephrine stores. *Circ. Res.,* **20**: 349-353, 1967.
8. Chidsey, C.A., Harrison, D.C., and Braunwald, E.: Augmentation of plasma norepinephrine response to exercise in patients with congestive heart failure. *N. Engl. J. Med.,* **267**: 650-654, 1962.
9. Chidsey, C.A., Braunwald, E., and Morrow, A.G.: Catecholamine excretion and cardiac stores of norepinephrine in congestive heart failure. *Am. J. Med.,* **39**: 442-451, 1965.
10. Gaffney, T.E. and Braunwald, E.: Importance of adrenergic nervous system in support of circulatory function in patients with congestive heart failure. *Am. J. Med.,* **34**: 320-324, 1963.
11. Epstein, S.E. and Braunwald, E.: Effect of beta adrenergic blockade on patterns of urinary sodium excretion: studies in normal subjects and in patients with heart disease. *Ann. Intern. Med.,* **65**: 20-27, 1966.
12. Ross, J., Jr., Covell, J.W., and Sonnenblick, E.H.: Mechanics of left ventricular contraction in acute experimental cardiac failure. *J. Clin. Investigation,* **46**: 299-312, 1967.
13. Starling, E.H.: The Linacre Lecture on the Law of the Heart, Given at Cambridge, 1915. Longmans, London, 1918, p. 27.
14. Patterson, S.W. and Starling, E.H.: On mechanical factors which determine output of ventricles. *J. Physiol.,* **48**: 357-379, 1914.
15. Sarnoff, S.J. and Mitchell, J.H.: Control of function of heart. In *Handbook of Physiology.* Section 2, Circulation, Vol I. Edited by W.F. Hamilton and P. Dow. Chapt. 15, American Physiological Society, Washington, D.C., 1962, pp. 489-532.
16. Dodge, H.T. and Baxley, W.A.: Hemodynamic aspects of heart failure. *Am. J. Cardiol,* **22**: 24, 1968.
17. Braunwald, E.: Control of myocardial oxygen consumption; physiologic and clinical consideration. *Am. J. Cardiol.,* **27**: 416, 1974.

18. McHugh, T.J., Forrester, J.S., Adler, L., et al: Pulmonary vascular congestion in acute myocardial infarction: hemodynamic and radiologic correlations. *Ann. Intern. Med.*, **76**: 29-33, 1972.

19. Forrester, J.S., Diamond, G.A., and Swan, H.J.C.: A correlative classification for clinical and hemodynamic abnormalities associated with acute myocardial infarction. Submitted for publication, *Circulation*.

CHAPTER 4

Electrophysiology of Cardiac Arrhythmias*

Leonard S. Gettes, M.D.

The inquiring clinical mind seeks and utilizes knowledge of the basis for the clinical problems faced. This Chapter provides a comprehensive resource which reviews the current state of understanding in impulse formation, arrhythmias, and conduction disturbances. Some will elect to read and review this vital field in its entirety; all will have occasion to refer to specific portions of this Chapter pertinent to a current clinical problem.

INTRODUCTION

In the last ten years, a veritable explosion of new information has expanded our appreciation of the electrophysiologic abnormalities participating in the genesis of cardiac arrhythmias. We now understand more completely the causes of the alterations in impulse formation, conduction and refractoriness which permit ectopic spontaneous foci to arise and which lead to the development of "heart block" and reentry. This is not to imply that all problems have been solved or that all arrhythmias can be catalogued according to their mechanisms. Indeed, much of the new information has yet to be fully incorporated into our understanding of clinically encountered arrhythmias. Nonetheless, we are coming closer to achieving the goal. An arbitrary listing of some of the new information would include: (1) an appreciation of the slow calcium sensitive inward (depolarizing) current and a more complete appreciation of the kinetics of the rapid sodium inward current, (2) an elucidation of the voltage and time dependent characteristics of the outward (repolarizing) currents, and (3) an understanding of the functional characteristics of the AV junction and the His-Purkinje system. In this chapter I shall briefly review some of the electrophysiologic concepts considered important in the genesis of cardiac arrhythmias, illustrate the use of these concepts in an analysis of some of the more commonly occurring arrhythmias, consider the electrophysiology of arrhythmias occurring in specific clinical settings, and discuss some problems in clinical diagnosis. A

*Studies reported in this review were supported by a grant from NIHL 5R01-HL13321-06.

more complete treatment of these various topics may be found in several recent reviews[1-6].

ELECTROPHYSIOLOGIC CONCEPTS

Impulse Formation

There are now reasons to believe that spontaneous impulse formation may result from several different mechanisms. These have in common the ability of the cells to spontaneously depolarize to that level of membrane potential from which a propagated action potential occurs, i.e., the threshold potential for the rapid or slow inward current system. Spontaneous depolarization during diastole is the mechanism underlying the repetitive activity of pacemaker cells in the sinus node, AV junction, and His-Purkinje system. However, it has been shown that pacemaker activity can occur in virtually all cardiac fibers in the appropriate situation. Table I lists the various methods which have been used to induce or enhance this activity in the various fiber types.

TABLE I
AGENTS CAPABLE OF CAUSING SPONTANEOUS
IMPULSE FORMATION IN VARIOUS CARDIAC FIBERS

I.   Atrial Fibers

         a.   Low K and Low Ca[7]
         b.   Ba[8]

II.   Ventricular Fibers

         a.   Low K and Low Ca[7]
         b.   Stretch[9]
         c.   Depolarizing Currents[3,10,11]
         d.   Ba[12]

III.   Purkinje Fibers

         a.   Low K[13]
         b.   Digitalis[14,15,16,17]
         c.   Catecholamines[18]
         d.   Ba[8,19]
         e.   Sr[20]
         f.   Depolarizing Current[3,21,22,23]
         g.   Stretch[19]

Spontaneous diastolic depolarization indicates that there is a net inward (depolarizing) current during diastole. This could result from either an absolute increase in inward current with no change in outward (repolarizing) current or an absolute decrease in outward current with no change in inward current. Pacemaker activity in Purkinje fibers has been attributed[24] to a time dependent decrease in outward current carried by potassium. It is most likely that the enhancement of pacemaker activity caused by a decrease in extracellular potassium is due to a further decrease in this current (Figure 1). It is also possible that in some instances spontaneous depolariza-

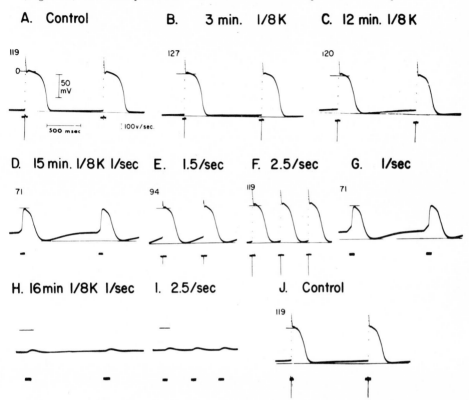

Figure 1   Effect of a decrease of extracellular K+ on action potentials recorded from the right bundle in the pig moderator band. The action potentials are recorded during the continuous impalement of the same cell. The downward spikes below each action potential are the differentiated upstrokes. Note the progressive increase in spontaneous depolarization during diastole following a change of extracellular K+ from 4.8 mEq/1 (control) to 0.6 mEq/1 (1/8 K). In E and F the rate of stimulation is increased. In H and I, the fiber becomes depolarized to a level from which it is unexcitable. In J, following perfusion with the control solution, the fiber is again excitable and the action potential is almost normal. (From Gettes, L.S. and Surawicz, B.: *Effects of low and high concentrations of potassium on the simultaneously recorded Purkinje and ventricular action potentials of the perfused pig moderator band. Circ. Res.,* **23**: 717, 1968, with permission.)

tion results from an absolute increase in inward current. The pacemaker activity induced by barium[8,19] and strontium[20] may be due to this mechanism. It is thought that catecholamines[18], digitalis[14], and depolarizing currents[3,10,21,22,23] (Figure 2) may also exert their effect on pacemaker activity at least partially by increasing the inward current.

The current system responsible for the rapid upstroke of the action poten-

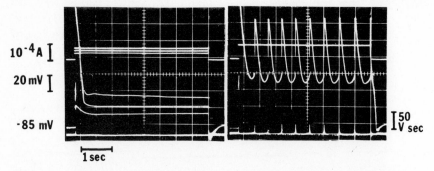

Figure 2 Effect of 4 sec depolarizing current pulses on guinea pig papillary muscle. Depolarizations below -40 mV do not induce spontaneous activity. However, when the fiber is depolarized to approximately -20 mV, repetitive spontaneous activity occurs. (From Imanishi, S. and Surawicz, B.: Automatic activity in depolarized guinea pig ventricular myocardium: characteristics and mechanism. In preparation, with permission.)

tial in pacemaker fibers depends upon the membrane potential range in which the spontaneous depolarization occurs. At membrane potentials more negative than -60 mV the rapid sodium inward current is probably the responsible mechanism. However, at less negative potentials the sodium system is inactivated and depolarization is due to the slow calcium sensitive inward current system whose threshold is between -40 and -50 mV[3]. An appreciation of the differences in these two types of spontaneously occurring action potentials has broadened our understanding of both normal and abnormal rhythms. The rapid upstroke of both the SA nodal and AV junctional cells are believed due to slow channel activity[25,26]. These depolarizations are blocked by specific inhibitors of the slow inward current system such as verapamil and mangenese but not by tetrodotoxin, a specific inhibitor of the rapid sodium inward current. Slow channel depolarization is also held responsible for the action potentials generated by depolarizing currents in the level of -50 mV or less, both in the absence and presence of sodium in the bathing medium[3,11,27] (Figure 2).

A second mechanism responsible for spontaneous activity has been recently labelled transient or after-depolarizations[3]. These depolarizations may occur singly or repetitively as a series of oscillations. If these oscillations reach the threshold potential or are brought to threshold by summation with a second subthreshold depolarization, a propagated action potential will occur[28]. If the anatomical arrangement permits the summating impulses to exit through a branch of excitable tissue, the impulse may then promote the development of reentry. In the absence of this anatomical arrangement, two colliding subthreshold impulses may result in inhibition and contribute to the development of conduction block. These after-depolarizations have been attributed both to a time dependent decrease in the potassium outward current[29] and to an increase in the slow channel inward current[3], and have been demonstrated after a variety of interventions in both Purkinje and ventricular fibers.

The current responsible for the propagated depolarization depends, as in the case of pacemaker fibers, on the level of membrane potential at which the oscillations occur. Since these after-depolarizations depend upon the preceding action potential, they may contribute to the development of premature responses which are coupled to a preceding response.

Slowed Conduction

Slowed conduction, coupled with unidirectional block and a refractory period of appropriate duration, has long been recognized as one of the requisites for reentry. Of the various factors contributing to conduction velocity, the rate of depolarization of the individual cell is most important. In atrial, ventricular, and Purkinje fibers the depolarization is accomplished by the rapid inward movement of sodium ions. The resting membrane potential determines the magnitude of available steady-state current[30] and the time course of recovery of this steady-state current[31]. The steady-state relationship between the membrane potential and the rapid inward current is characterized by the S-shaped curve shown in Figure 3. The curve illustrates that the magnitude of the inward sodium current decreases as the resting potential is reduced from -90 mV to approximately -50 mV. This will result in a decrease in the maximum rate of rise of the action potential and a slowing of conduction, and will be observed at all rates and in premature as well as in non-premature responses.

The membrane potential also determines the recovery characteristics of the maximum rate of rise of the action potential upstroke. The recovery characteristics may be defined as the time required for the maximum upstroke velocity to regain its steady-state value after the fiber has undergone a depolarization-repolarization sequence and the membrane potential has returned to its resting value. When the resting potential is normal, that is, when it is more negative than -80 mV, the recovery time of the upstroke velocity is very short and the upstroke of the action potentials arising within a few milliseconds of the end of the preceding action potential will be close to the steady-state value. When the fiber is depressed and the resting potential falls towards -60 mV, the recovery time becomes progressively longer and 100 to 200 milliseconds may be required following the completion of repolarization before the upstroke velocity in the subsequent response regains its steady-state value[32] (Figures 4 and 5). This time-dependent factor will be an important determinant of conduction velocity in premature responses and at rapid heart rates[32]. When a premature response arises from an incompletely repolarized fiber, the upstroke velocity will reflect the time-dependent factor and will be slower than predicted by the steady-state effect of the lowered membrane potential (Figure 6).

In the intact heart, slowing of conduction is seen when the serum potassium is raised[5,33,84]. Experiments now in progress in our laboratory show that

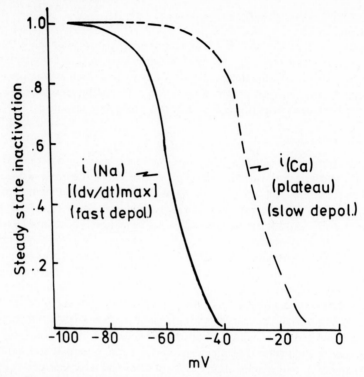

Figure 3 Schematic reconstruction of steady-state inactivation curves of rapid sodium inward current, i (Na) (solid line), and slow calcium sensitive inward current, i (Ca) (broken line). (dV/dt) max refers to the maximum rate of rise of the action potential. The vertical axis is normalized for each current. The horizontal axis represents the membrane potential at the onset of the action potential. (See Text.)

an increase in serum potassium not only causes a slowing of intra-ventricular conduction causing widening of the QRS complex in the non-premature beats (as demonstrated in Figure 10), but also causes even more marked slowing of conduction in premature responses arising after the end of the T wave[33]. This indicates the importance of the time dependent factor.

When the membrane potential is depolarized to less than -60 mV the sodium current becomes totally inactivated. Action potential arising from such levels of membrane potential are then dependent on the slow, calcium sensitive inward current system. The steady-state and kinetic characteristics of the slow inward current system are also voltage dependent but are quantitatively different than those of the rapid inward current (Figures 3 and 5). These characteristics will contribute to the upstroke velocity of "slow channel" action potentials[3] and to the plateau duration particularly in ventricular fibers[31] (See below). The rate of rise of these potentials is approximately 10 V/sec[3,11] when the resting potential is approximately -40 mV as compared to 100-300 V/sec for ventricular muscle and 500-1000 V/sec for Purkinje fibers when the resting potential is approximately -85 mV. Conduction velocity associated with slow responses is less than 0.1 m/sec[3] compared to conduction velocities associated with rapid responses of more than 0.5 m/sec in ventricular muscle and 3-4 m/sec for Purkinje fibers. Because of the extremely slow conduction velocity, the length of reentry pathway may be very short in fibers whose membrane potential is in the -40 mV range, the actual distance being determined by the product of the conduction velocity in the depressed area and the refractory period (approximately 250 msec) in the nondepressed area[1,2,3].

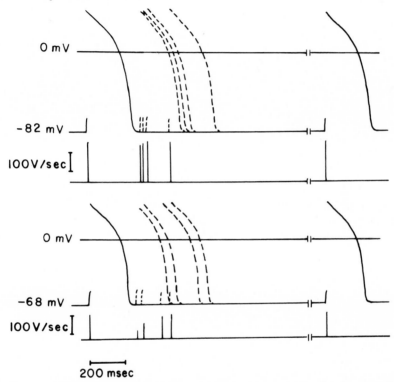

Figure 4 Effect of a change in resting membrane potential on the recovery of the action potential upstroke in guinea pig papillary muscle. The action potentials traced in solid lines are obtained at the basic rate of 0.2/sec. Those traced in broken lines are premature action potentials. The vertical spikes below the action potentials are the electronically differentiated upstrokes. The magnitude of these spikes represents the maximum upstroke velocity [(dV/dt) max]. In the upper traces, the extracellular K+ is 4.8 mM, the resting potential is -82 mV, and (dV/dt) max is 250 V/sec. In the lower traces the K+ is 10 mM, the resting potential is -68 mV, and (dV/dt) max is 130 V/sec. This represents the steady-state decrease in (dV/dt) max associated with the K+ induced decrease in resting potential (Figure 3). When the resting potential is -82 mV, (dV/dt) max in the premature responses regains the steady-state value within 30 msec of the end of the non-premature action potential. When the resting potential is -68 mV, recovery of the steady-state value requires more than 100 msec after the end of the non-premature action potential, illustrating the dependence of the resting membrane potential on recovery kinetics. (From Gettes, L.S. and Reuter, H.: *J. Physiol.*, **240**: 703, 1974, with permission.)

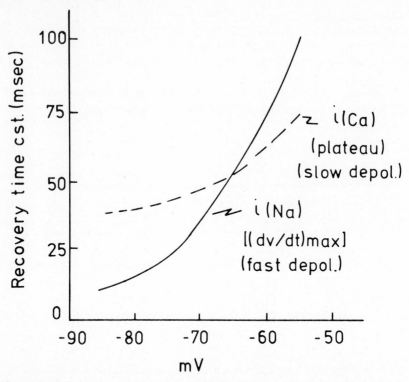

Figure 5 Schematic reconstruction of relationships between the membrane potential at the onset of the action potential (horizontal axis) and the time constant of recovery of the rapid (solid line) and slow (broken line) inward current systems. (See Text.) (From data in Gettes, L.S. and Reuter, H.: *J. Physiol.*, **240**: 703, 1974.)

As mentioned above, slow channel dependent action potentials are now believed to be present normally in fibers of the SA node and AV junction and can be induced in Purkinje fibers and muscle fibers by combinations of high potassium (which depolarizes the fiber to a level at which the sodium inward current is inactivated) and by catecholamines or other agents which increase the magnitude of the slow inward current[3,10,11]. Slow channel depolarization, like pacemake activity, can be induced in all fiber types by appropriate treatment.

Refractory Period

The refractory period defines the time required for a cell to regain its excitability after it is once depolarized. As noted above, the steady-state and kinetic determinants of both depolarizing current systems are voltage dependent and neither current will be active at membrane potentials more positive than the plateau of the action potential. For the sodium current to be reactivated, the membrane potential must be returned to at least -50 to -60 mV and for the calcium current, to approximately -20 mV. Although the time re-

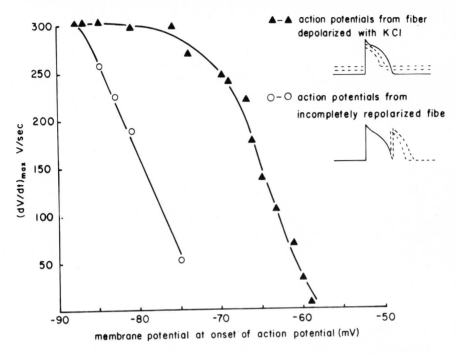

Figure 6 Relationship between membrane potential at the onset of depolarization (horizontal axis) and maximum rate of rise of the action potential upstroke — (dV/dt) max (vertical axis) in the guinea pig papillary muscle. The solid line represents the steady-state curve obtained by K+ induced depolarization of the fiber driven at 0.2/sec (insert — upper trace). The broken line shows the values obtained when premature responses arise from the same fiber before it is completely repolarized, i.e. the membrane responsiveness curve (insert — lower trace). Note that at any given membrane potential, (dV/dt) max is slower in the premature response. This is attributed to the added effect of the recovery characteristics of the action potential upstroke. (From Gettes, L.S. and Reuter, H.: *J. Physiol.*, **240**: 703, 1974, with permission.)

quired for the membrane potential to return to these values is determined primarily by the duration of the action potential plateau, the refractory period will also depend upon the recovery kinetics of the appropriate depolarizing current system and may be longer than the duration of the action potential. Such time dependent refractoriness has been demonstrated in the AV junction[34], in the fibers surrounding the SA node[35] and in ventricular and Purkinje fibers following coronary ligation[36] and/or exposure to lidocaine[37]. In general, factors which shorten the action potential plateau will shorten refractory period (rapid rate, hypoxia, heat, etc.) and vice versa (slow rate, cold, low calcium, etc.).

The effects of prematurity on action potential duration and refractoriness are complex since they depend more on the interval from the repolarization phase of the preceding non-premature response to the onset of the premature response, the diastolic interval, and on the duration of the preceding non-premature action potential than on the coupling interval itself, that is, the interval between depolarization of the preceding non-premature response and depolarization of the premature response[38,39]. Thus, the effects of prematurity are not the same as those of increasing rate. Moreover, there are differences in the effect of prematurity on Purkinje and ventricular fibers. These differences are explained by the dependence of the plateau of the Purkinje fiber on the slowly activated potassium outward current[39,40] and of the ventricular fiber on inactivation of the slow inward current[41,42,43]. In both types of fibers, however, the action potential duration in an early premature response becomes markedly shorter than the duration of the action potential in the preceding non-premature response, particularly when the premature response arises from an incompletely repolarized fiber[38]. The difference between the durations of the non-premature and premature responses becomes exaggerated when the duration of the preceding action potential is prolonged. This effect may be one reason why bradycardia, which prolongs the action potential duration, may be associated with an increased incidence of tachyarrhythmias. Action potential duration is also influenced by electrotonic interaction with adjacent cells and is markedly altered if such interaction is absent[44].

The difference between the duration of action potentials in the various portions of the ventricular myocardium[45] results in a inhomogeneity in the recovery of excitability. This inhomogeneity is increased in early premature beats and by other factors such as ischemia and unilateral sympathetic stimulation[46].

ELECTROPHYSIOLOGIC MECHANISMS UNDERLYING CERTAIN ARRHYTHMIAS

Atrial and Ventricular Fibrillation

These arrhythmias are considered by most observers to be due to reentry. They can be initiated by properly timed single premature response and require a minimum muscle mass in order to be maintained[6]. The malignancy of extrasystoles arising from the apex to the end of the T wave (the vulnerable period) is probably due to the changes in conduction and refractoriness which occur when the premature response arises from an incompletely repolarized fiber (Figure 7). Because the fibers are incompletely repolarized the membrane potential at the onset of depolarization will be decreased. Thus, the upstroke of the action potential will be slowed reflecting both the voltage and time dependent characteristics referred to above. The slowing will not be uniform throughout the ventricle, however, because the normal differences in ventricular action potential durations will result in the onset of the premature action potential from slightly different levels of membrane potential in the various fibers. If some of the fibers are inexcitable, unidirectional block may occur. Shortening of the refractory

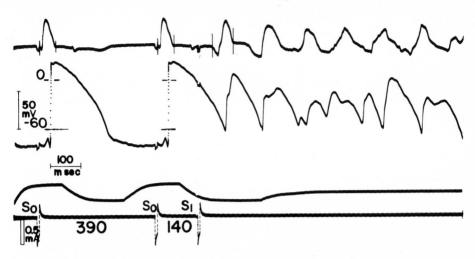

Figure 7 Bipolar ECG (top line), epicardial right ventricular action potential (2nd line), ventricular contractility recorded with a strain guage (3rd line), and stimulus artifact (bottom line) recorded from perfused isolated rabbit heart. S_0 is the basic driving stimulus. S_1 is the premature stimulus applied 140 msec after S_0. Note that the premature response originates from an incompletely repolarized fiber and that its action potential has a slowed upstroke and shortened duration. The corresponding QRS complex is widened indicating diffusely slowed intraventricular conduction and ventricular fibrillation follows. See Text. (From Surawicz, B., Gettes, L.S., and Ponce-Zumino, A.: *Relation of vulnerability to ECG and action potential characteristics of premature beats. Amer. J. Physiol.*, **212**: 1519-1528, 1967, with permission.)

period in the premature response will occur because of the shortened interval between the onset of the premature response and the repolarization phase of the preceding non-premature response, but will be inhomogeneous, again reflecting differences in the duration of the non-premature action potential. Thus, the dispersion of recovery of excitability in the premature response will be increased. In acute ischemia, ventricular fibrillation can also be induced by a premature beat occurring beyond the vulnerable period[47]. This probably reflects the slowed conduction and time dependent prolongation of refractoriness induced by ischemia itself (See below). Although ventricular fibrillation can be induced in the isolated heart by a single premature stimulus[48], its spontaneous occurrence in man in the absence of factors such as ischemia or complete AV block, i.e., factors which exaggerate the normally occurring inhomogeneity in both conduction and refractoriness, is undoubtedly extremely rare.

Paroxysmal Supraventricular Tachycardia

This common arrhythmia which occurs in adults and children, in the presence or absence of underlying heart disease, and in the presence and absence of WPW, is also generally accepted to result from reentry[49]. In patients with WPW, one of the conduction pathways comprising the reentry circuit is outside of the AV junction. Such an anomalous AV connection may be present but unrecognized clinically and serve as a pathway for retrograde activation only[50,51]. Anomalous atrial ventricular pathways such as the James and Maheim fibers may also involve portions of the AV junction and facilitate the development of a reentry circuit[52]. It is important to realize that the normal functional dissociation of AV junctional tissue[53] also permits this arrhythmia to occur in normal hearts[54,55]. The multiplicity of potential reentry pathways may result in several forms of reentry in the same patients. In patients with sinus rhythm it may be initiated by a sinus beat or by a single atrial premature beat[55]. The PR interval of the initiating beat is usually prolonged (Figure 8) but may be normal. In the latter situation, a critical acceleration of the heart rate is usually required[49]. In the laboratory the arrhythmia can be initiated and/or terminated by a single atrial or ventricular

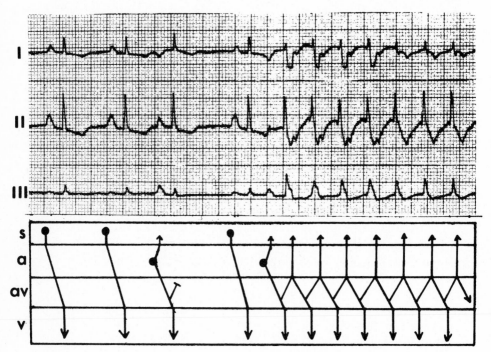

Figure 8 ECG recorded from 24 year old female with repetitive paroxysmal supraventricular tachycardia. The first two beats are sinus with PR of 0.18 sec. The third is a premature atrial beat with PR of 0.20 sec and initiates the tachycardia. Note that the premature P wave which initiates the tachycardia has a different vector (negative in I, positive in II and III) than the P wave recorded during the tachycardia (negative in I and II and isoelectric in III). Note also the aberrant QRS complexes which initiate the tachycardia. The ladder diagram below illustrates the AV junctional reentry postulated as the mechanism. (From Gettes, L.S. and Yoshonis, K.F.: *Rapidly recurring supraventricular tachycardia: a manifestigation of reciprocating tachycardia and indication for propranolol therapy. Circulation*, **41**: 689-700, 1970, with permission.)

premature beat which establishes or interrupts the reentry circuit[56]. Clinically the arrhythmia may end when either pathway is blocked. Thus, on the electrocardiogram the arrhythmia may terminate following a P wave or QRS complex[55]. The arrhythmia should be suspected in all cases of paroxysmal or sustained supraventricular tachycardia exhibiting 1:1 AV conduction. The diagnosis should also be entertained in all cases of supraventricular arrhythmia which respond readily to vagal maneuvers and/or treatment with propranolol and digitalis.

Extrasystoles

In spite of or perhaps because of the frequency with which extrasystoles occur, their many possible electrophysiologic explanations, and the ease with which they can be induced, no single causative mechanism has been uniformly accepted. The two situations on which most observers agree are parasystole[57] and extrasystoles with fixed coupling. The former is attributed to spontaneous impulse formation and the latter to reentry. However, the appearance of both types of extrasystoles in the same patient[58,59] clearly suggest that the same mechanism (presumably spontaneous impulse formation) may cause both types of extrasystoles. Laboratory studies showing that spontaneous impulse formation can be induced by a single premature response[60] also suggest that both mechanisms may contribute to a single arrhythmia.

Ventricular Tachycardia

As with premature beats, both reentry and spontaneous impulse formation can be postulated to explain the occurrence of this arrhythmia. The ability to induce and terminate such an arrhythmia by a single premature stimulus would suggest a reentry circuit[61]. In those situations in which the ectopic rhythm is similar in rate to the sinus and in which the coupling interval of the first ectopic beat is the same as the rate of the tachycardia, as often occurs in the accelerated idioventricular arrhythmias associated with myocardial infarction[62], it is reasonable to suspect spontaneous impulse formation as the etiology.

AV Block

Slowed conduction between atria and ventricle may occur in the AV junction, the common His bundle, or the bundle branches. It may be incomplete or complete. Incomplete block resulting in prolongation of the AH or HV intervals or in hemiblock may occur when conduction is slowed. It is possible to postulate several mechanisms for this phenomenon:

1. A sudden acceleration of the rate such that the interstimulus interval is shorter than the refractory period. This may be considered as physiological AV block.

2. A decrease in resting membrane potential causing a steady-state or voltage dependent change.

3. The presence of spontaneously depolarizing fibers or of fibers with after-depolarizations such that the membrane potential of the onset of the action potential is decreased causing another example of voltage dependent slowing.

4. Prolongation of the refractory period beyond the end of the action potential without a change in action potential duration thereby causing an increase in time dependent slowing.

5. Prolongation of the refractory period due to prolongation of the action potential duration resulting in the depolarization of incompletely repolarized fibers and thus, both voltage and time dependent slowing.

6. Concealed retrograde reflection of the impulse into a functionally discrete retrograde pathway[63]. Such reflection would result in slowed conduction of the subsequent impulse.

7. Combinations of the above.

These mechanisms would explain the AV block induced by vagal stimulation and tachycardia, Wenckebach periodicity in the AV junction and the intraventricular conducting system, as well as tachycardia and bradycardia induced infranodal AV blocks. When complete atrio-ventricular block is located in or below the common His bundle, the rate of escape pacemaker may be slowed by atrial tachycardia perhaps due to the incomplete penetration of the impulse into the area of the escape pacemaker[64].

ARRHYTHMIAS OCCURRING IN SPECIFIC CLINICAL SETTINGS

Myocardial Ischemia

Acute interruption of flow through a coronary artery causes a complex series of incompletely defined but interrelated biochemical, mechanical, and electrophysiological changes which are expressed clinically as both brady and tachyarrhythmias. The decrease in myocardial flow causes myocardial hypoxia which induces anaerobic metabolism, lactic acid production, and acidosis. The combination of hypoxia and acidosis results in a decrease in intracellular and an increase in extracellular K^+ concentrations as well as changes in other electrolyte concentrations, fatty acids, and ATP. The rapid development of hypoxia, acidosis, and hyperpotassemia in the ischemic zone stimulates sympathetic and parasympathetic nerve endings and depresses contractility. This latter factor leads to a further decrease in myocardial perfusion and a worsening of myocardial ischemia.

The following points concerning ischemia related arrhythmias are now generally accepted.

1. AV block following inferior infarctions may be reflexly mediated and is almost invariably transient.

2. Parasystole is generally a benign arrhythmia[65].

3. Ventricular arrhythmias occurring early in the course of acute infarction are probably reentrant while those occurring later may represent enhanced automaticity[66,67].

4. Ventricular fibrillation may occur without infarction[68], may follow either an early or late ventricular premature beat and may occur without any preceding warning arrhythmia[47,69,70].

In the sections which follow some of the electrophysiologic mechanisms underlying the ischemia related arrhythmias will be reviewed.

Changes in Spontaneous Impulse Formation

Depression. Parasympathetic stimulation will lead to the accumulation of acetylcholine in the parasympathetic nerve endings which are concentrated about the SA node, atrium, and AV junction. This will decrease the rate of spontaneous depolarization of the cells in the sinus node and AV junction[71,72] and cause bradycardia. This effect has been attributed to the acetylcholine induced increase in K^+ conductance[71,73] and possibly a decrease in inward current[72].

Enhancement. Sympathetic stimulation will lead to accumulation of norepinephrine in the ischemic myocardium and an increase in circulating catecholamines which will increase the rate of induced spontaneous depolarization in cells of the specialized conducting system. This effect may be particularly important in the surviving Purkinje fibers located in the subendocardial region of the ischemic zone[36,74,75,75]. The depolarization of fibers which occurs as a result of the changes in extracellular and intracellular K^+ concentration may enhance or induce spontaneous activity by (1) creating a battery between cells depolarized to different degrees and producing a flow of DC current which may enhance diastolic depolarization of cells within a specialized conducting system[21], and (2) by lowering the membrane potential to the threshold of the slow inward depolarizing current (approximately -40 mV) which, in combination with the effect of the catecholamines liberated from the ischemic myocardium, may result in repetitive spontaneous "slow channel" depolarizations[3,10,11]. These several mechanisms may be responsible for some of the ectopic beats and tachyarrhythmias associated with myocardial ischemia.

Slowed Conduction The acetylcholine liberated as a result of parasympathetic stimulation will lead to slowing of the action potential upstroke in cells of the AV junction. This mechanism combined with a K^+ induced depolarization probably contributes to the delay in AV conduction which not infrequently occurs in association with inferior myocardial infarctions.

The decrease in resting membrane potential which occurs as a result of the K^+ changes will result in a decreased rate of depolarization in the action potential and a slowing of conduction due to the voltage dependent characteristics of the rapid Na^+ inward current system. The decreased resting potential will also slow the recovery of the inward current. In cells depolarized to levels of -40 millivolts, the Na^+ system will be totally inactivated. In this situation a propagated depolarization may result from the slow inward Ca^{++} sensitive current system, particularly when this current is increased by the sympathetic catecholamines liberated from the ischemic area. The slow conduction velocity in such responses[3] probably contributes to the marked slowing of conduction which occurs within the ischemic zone[77-80] and which has been shown to be rate dependent[81].

Changes in Refractoriness

Hypoxia and an increase in extracellular K^+ shorten the action potential duration and would be expected to shorten the refractory period. The catecholamines may also alter action potential duration[82]. The action potential duration of early premature action potentials will be shortened particularly when the premature action potentials arise from partially depolarized fibers. These changes may contribute to the increase in inhomogeneity of the recovery of excitability which accompanies myocardial ischemia[46] and which, in combination with the changes in conduction referred to above, may be responsible for the development of reentrant arrhythmias, particularly ventricular fibrillation.

Arrhythmias Associated with Digitalis

In considering the effects of digitalis, it is necessary to remember that the indirect, vagally mediated effects and the direct effects of the drug occur simultaneously, and that the direct effects of the drug may result in spontaneous impulse formation, shortened refractory period, and a decrease in membrane potential leading to slowed conduction (Table II). These actions

TABLE II
SIMULTANEOUSLY OCCURRING EFFECTS OF DIGITALIS

	Vagally Mediated	Direct
Spontaneous Impulse Formation	Depress	Stimulate
Refractory Period (Excluding AV node)	Shorten	Shorten
a. AV Node	Lengthen	No Change
Conduction in AV Node	Slow	No Change

may sometimes produce opposite effects and help to explain the occurrence of atrial tachycardia with block, complete atrio-ventricular block and junctional tachycardia, and the ability of digitalis to cause virtually all arrhythmias. Propranolol, an agent which increases vagal tone by blocking sympathetic effects, acts additively with digitalis in slowing AV transmission (Figure 9) or causing SA block. Hypopotassemia which by itself has electrophysiologic effects similar to many of the direct digitalis effects, potentiates the arrhythmogenic effects of digitalis in ventricular and atrial fibers.

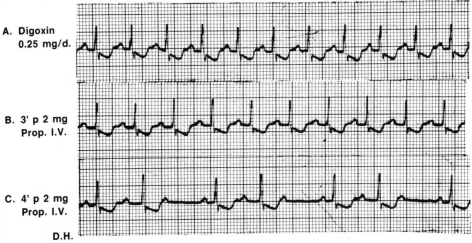

A. Digoxin 0.25 mg/d.

B. 3' p 2 mg Prop. I.V.

C. 4' p 2 mg Prop. I.V.

D.H.

Figure 9 Lead II ECG recorded in 46 year old female following mitral valve replacement. In A, the rate is 140/min and the PR is 0.16 sec. In B, 3 minutes after propranolol, the rate is 130/min and the PR is 0.19 sec. In C, taken 1 minute after B, the atrial rate is still 130/min but there is a 3:2 AV block of the Wenckebach type, which, in the absence of propranolol therapy would have been compatible with a diagnosis of digitalis toxicity. (See Text.)

The diseased myocardium may be very sensitive both to the vagally mediated and direct electrophysiologic effects of digitalis because of pre-existing areas of depressed conduction or ectopic spontaneous impulse formation. In this situation, manifestations of digitalis toxicity may appear in association with digitalis blood levels well within the range considered therapeutic.

Arrhythmias Associated with Electrolyte Disturbance

Hyperpotassemia

An increase in extracellular K^+ decreases the resting potential, shortens the action potential plateau, speeds rapid repolarization, and depresses spontaneous diastolic depolarization in fibers of the His-Purkinje system. Although the changes in repolarization cause the earliest electrocardiographic manifestations of hyperpotassemia, (peaking of the T wave and shortening of the QT interval), and occur at a K^+ concentration of approximately 6 mEq/l, it is the changes resulting from the decrease in resting potential and the decrease in spontaneous diastolic depolarization which are more important in the arrhythmogenic effects of hyperpotassemia.

When the K^+ concentration is above 6 mEq/l, the decrease in resting potential causes a decrease in the rate of depolarization and both a voltage and time dependent slowing of intra-atrial, atrio-ventricular, and intra-ventricular conduction. These changes are manifested on the ECG by a widening and decrease in amplitude of the P wave and by prolongation of the PR, AH, and HV intervals and QRS duration[33,83,84,85]. Intra-atrial conduction may be abolished at K^+ concentrations which still permit atrioventricular and intra-ventricular conduction. When this occurs, impulses arising in the SA nodal fibers, the least sensitive of the various fiber types to an increase in extracellular K^+, may travel to the ventricles through specialized atrial conducting fibers. This may result in sino-ventricular conduction in the presence of sino-atrial block[86,87] (Figure 10).

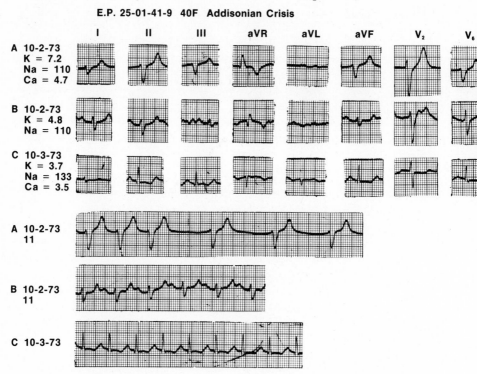

E.P. 25-01-41-9 40F Addisonian Crisis

Figure 10 ECG's recorded from 40 year old female with Addisonian Crisis. The Lead II rhythm strips associated with each tracing are below. In A, when K is 7.2 and Na 110 mEq/1, no P waves can be seen. The QRS complex is compatible with the right bundle branch block with left axis deviation (left anterior hemiblock). The rhythm strips below suggests sino-ventricular conduction with intermittent 2:1 AV block. In B, when K is 4.8 and Na 110 mEq/1, P waves are easily identified. The rate is almost the same as in A and the PR interval is 0.24 sec. The QRS complex shows RBBB with less left axis than in A. In C, when K is 3.7 and Na is 133, the rate is faster and the PR shorter (0.20 sec). The IV conduction disturbance is no longer present.

Hyperpotassemia may cause ventricular standstill or ventricular fibrillation from two mechanisms. When K^+ elevation occurs slowly, intra-ventricular conduction becomes progressively depressed. This results in a generalized widening of the QRS complex although shifts in electrical axis have also been reported[88,89] (Figure 9). Ultimately the ventricular myocardium loses its excitability. When K^+ is elevated rapidly, suppression of pacemaker cells may occur before conduction abnormalities become apparent[90] and cardiac standstill may occur. Ventricular fibrillation may occur when ventricular conduction becomes so slow that some fibers recover their excitability before depolarization through the entire ventricle is completed thereby permitting reentry to occur[91].

Hypopotassemia

A decrease in extracellular K^+ to within clinically applicable concentrations results in a more negative resting potential, shortens the action potential plateau, slows the slope of rapid repolarization, and increases the slope of spontaneous diastolic depolarization. The effects on repolarization and diastolic depolarization are similar to those of digitalis. It is not surprising therefore, that hypopotassemia should potentiate the tachyarrhythmias induced by digitalis. However, even in the absence of digitalis, hypopotassemia promotes supraventricular and ventricular arrhythmias and AV conduction disturbances[92] (Figure 11). In the isolated heart, a decrease in extracellular K^+ to less than 1 mEq/1 invariably induces AV conduction disturbances, atrial and ventricular premature beats, and ventricular fibrillation[93].

Calcium

An increase in extracellular Ca^{++} shortens the action potential plateau, which is associated with shortening of the QT interval on the electrocardiogram. It also increases slightly the rate of diastolic depolarization of pacemaker fibers and increases the excitability threshold[94]. In the experimental animal, hypercalcemia increases QRS duration and produces ectopic beats and ventricular fibrillation. Clinically, severe hypercalcemia may be associated with prolongation of the QRS complex and of the PR interval. Occasionally, higher degrees of AV block may occur. Although it is postulated that patients with hypercalcemia may develop ventricular fibrillation, direct evidence confirming this relationship is not available.

A decrease in extracellular Ca^{++} lengthens the action potential and prolongs the QT interval on the electrocardiogram[94], but is not associated with arrhythmias. On the contrary, hypocalcemia induced by the infusion of Na2 EDTA has been found effective in suppressing ventricular ectopic beats in about 50% of both digitalized and non-digitalized patients[95].

The effect of changes in Ca^{++} concentration depends on the serum concentration of K^+ and vice versa. Increasing serum Ca^{++} restores the resting membrane potential[71] and abolishes the intraventricular conduction disturbances induced by hyperpotassemia. In experimental animals, the AV conduction disturbances and ventricular arrhythmias, including ventricular fibrillation, induced by perfusion with low K^+ solution can be abolished and prevented by simultaneously lowering Ca^{++} concentration of the perfusate[93]. However, the ionic concentrations of both potassium and calcium required to demonstrate this interaction are not compatible with life.

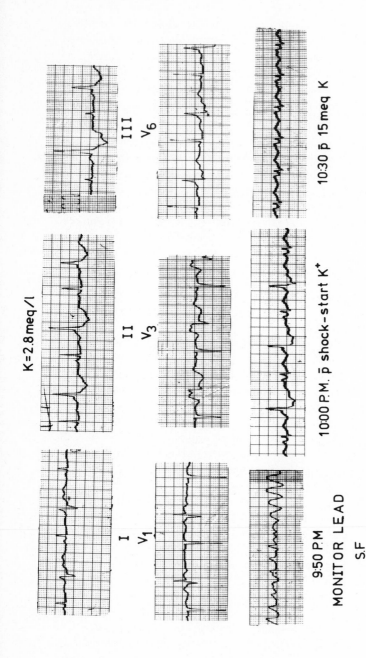

Figure 11 Leads I, II, III, V1, V3, V6 (upper 2 rows) and monitored lead (lower row) recorded from 32 year old female who was a chronic laxative user. K⁺ on admission was 2.8 mEq/1 and the ECG showed frequent ventricular ectopic beats in bigeminal pattern, as well as ST, T and U waves changes compatible with hypopotassemia. Three hours after admission, (9:50 pm) an episode of ventricular fibrillation occurred. After countershock (10 pm) VEB's were again noted. Thirty minutes later (10:30 pm) following the intravenous administration of 15 mEq KCl(0.5 mEq/min) the ectopic beats were suppressed and the patient proceeded to have an uneventful recovery. There was no heart disease documented by history, physical examination or ECG, chest x-ray or echocardiogram, and no other cause of hypopotassemia.

Sodium and Chloride

While alterations of NA^+ and Cl- concentrations are capable of altering electrophysiologic properties of single fibers, clinically observed changes in the plasma concentrations of the ions are not associated with arrhythmias. However, it is possible that hyponatremia if present, may contribute to the QRS widening and intraventricular conduction disturbances associated with hyperpotassemia[88] (Figure 10).

Magnesium

Although hypermagnesemia (3-5 mm/l) may cause atrio-ventricular conduction disturbances[94] there is no conclusive evidence implicating alterations in Mg^{++} concentration *per se* in the genesis of cardiac arrhythmias. However, there is evidence to suggest that hypomagnesemia decreases the dose of digitalis required to induce ectopic tachyarrhythmias in both experimental animals and in man[96,97].

DIAGNOSIS OF ARRHYTHMIAS

In my estimation, the failure to diagnose arrhythmias correctly can usually be attributed to one of several pitfalls. Two of these are technical and include: (1) failure to record long enough strips of electrocardiogram and (2) failure to record the onset and termination of the arrhythmia. Long strips will permit the determination of intraectopic intervals and in this way permit the diagnosis of parasystole, for example. By recording long strips, it is also possible to determine whether extrasystoles are uniform or multiform and will assist in aiding in the analysis of the causes of changes in conduction. Recording the onset and/or termination of an arrhythmia will give information needed to diagnose the reciprocating tachycardias (Figure 8) and may show changes in the QRS configuraiton necessary to determine if an arrhythmia is of ventricular or supraventricular origin. Recording the onset of arrhythmias may also provide information concerning the conditions predisposing to an arrhythmia such as a long pause, sino-atrial or AV block, or extrasystoles and thereby allow more rational therapy.

Other frequent causes of misdiagnosis include failure to look for or to recognize P waves, failure to employ maneuvers which increase vagal tone, failure to recognize WPW, and failure to recognize aberrant ventricular conduction. Failure to recognize P waves is of particular importance in the diagnosis of atrial flutter with 2:1 AV block and reciprocating tachycardias when the P waves may be located in the T wave (Figure 8). Carotid sinus massage and other maneuvers to increase vagal tone will help in both situations. In addition, the use of an intracardiac atrial lead will help to establish the correct diagnosis. Failure to recognize WPW and aberrant ventricular conduction will lead to an incorrect diagnosis of ventricular arrhythmia (Figure 12). In these situations a high index of suspicion is most important. Intracardiac recordings may also help. In both WPW and aberrant conduction each QRS

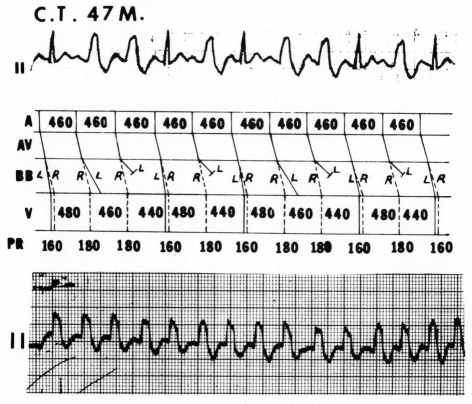

Figure 12 Lead II ECG from 47 year old male with recurrent tachycardia. The upper strip, retouched for clarity, and the corresponding ladder diagram below shows intermittent left bundle branch block appearing with no changes in sinus rate. Note that when two LBBB complexes appear consecutively, the second is slightly wider than the first suggesting a Wenckebach type of conduction delay within the left bundle. After complete LBBB, the subsequent QRS is normal. The lower strip recorded during an episode of paroxysmal atrial fibrillation with LBBB could easily have been mistaken for ventricular tachycardia if the nature of the aberrant conduction was not appreciated.

will be associated with an atrial spike whereas in ventricular tachycardia the atrial spikes and the QRS complexes will be independent of one another. His bundle recordings will also aid in the diagnosis of aberrancy since each QRS will be preceded by a His spike. This will not occur in WPW however, since the His spike will usually be lost in the QRS complex. The response to various drugs such as digitalis and lidocaine may also assist in the differential of supraventricular and ventricular arrhythmias, since digitalis and other agents which increase vagal "tone" will be more effective when the arrhythmia is supraventricular and lidocaine more useful when the arrhythmia is ventricular.

CONCLUSION

The purpose of this chapter has been to give a rather broad overview of some of the current thinking regarding the genesis of cardiac arrhythmias. Various combinations of the electrophysiologic changes alluded to could be utilized to explain most of the clinically encountered cardiac arrhythmias. However, the correctness of these explanations is still unknown. It is encouraging that many of the hypotheses formulated by electrophysiologists and electrocardiographers in the premicroelectrode era have been confirmed. It is reasonable to anticipate that many of the hypotheses currently proposed will be confirmed in the future.

References

1. Wit, A.L., Rosen, M.R., and Hoffman, B.F.: Electrophysiology and pharmacology of cardiac arrhythmias. II. Relationship of normal and abnormal electrical activity of cardiac fibers to the genesis of arrhythmias. B. Reentry. Section I and II. *Am. Heart J.*, **88**: 664, 1974.
2. Hoffman, B.F., Rosen, M.R., and Wit, A.L.: Electrophysiology and pharmacology of cardiac arrhythmias. III. The causes and treatment of cardiac arrhythmias. Part A. *Am. Heart J.*, **89**: 115, 1975.
3. Cranefield, P.F.: *The Conduction of the Cardiac Impulse.* Futura, New York, 1975.
4. Gettes, L.S.: Electrophysiologic basis for arrhythmias in acute myocardial ischemia. In M.F. Oliver (Ed.): *Modern Concepts in Cardiology.* Butterworths, London, 1975, Chapter 8.
5. Gettes, L.S.: Role of ionic changes in the appearance of arrhythmias. In *International Encyclopedia of Pharmacology and Therapeutics.* In press.
6. Surawicz, B. and Steffens, T.: Cardiac vulnerability. In A.N. Brest (Ed.): *Cardiovascular Clinics,* **5**: 159, 1973.
7. Mueller, P.: Ca- and K-free solution and pacemaker activity in mammalian myocardium. *Helv. Physiol. Acta,* **23**: 38, 1965.
8. Masher, D.: Electrical and mechanical responses in ventricular muscle fibres during barium perfusion. *Pfleugers Archiv.,* **342**: 325, 1973.
9. Kaufmann, R. and Theophile, U.: Automatic-fordernde dehnungseffekte an Purkinje-faden, papillarmuskeln and vorhoftrabekelm von rhesus-affen. *Pfleugers Archiv.,* **297**: 174, 1967.
10. Imanishi, S. and Surawicz, B.: Automatic activity in depolarized guinea pig ventricular myocardium: characteristics and mechanism. In preparation.
11. Katzung, B.: Effects of extracellular calcium and sodium in depolarization-induced automaticity in guinea pig papillary muscle. *Circ. Res.,* **37**: 118, 1975.
12. Reid, J.A. and Hecht, H.H.: Barium-induced automaticity in right ventricular muscle in the dog. *Circ. Res.,* **21**: 849, 1967.
13. Gettes, L.S. and Surawicz, B.: Effects of low and high concentrations of potassium on the simultaneously recorded Purkinje and ventricular action potentials of the perfused pig moderator band. *Circ. Res.,* **23**: 717, 1968.
14. Vassalle, M., Karis, J., and Hoffman, B.F.: Toxic effects of ouabain on Purkinje fibers and ventricular muscle fibers. *Am. J. Physiol.,* **203**: 433, 1962.
15. Kassebaum, D.G.: Electrophysiological effects of strophanthin in the heart. *J. Pharmacol.,* **140**: 329, 1963.
16. Ferrier, G.R., Saunders, J.H., and Mendez, C.: A cellular mechanism for the generation of ventricular arrhythmias by acetylstrophanthidin. *Circ. Res.,* **32**: 600, 1973.
17. Rosen, M.R., Gelband, H., Merker, C., and Hoffman, B.F.: Mechanisms of

digital toxicity. Effects of ouabain on phase four of canine Purkinje fiber transmembrane potentials. *Circulation,* **47**: 681, 1973.

18. Kassebaum, D.G. and Van Dyke, A.R.: Electrophysiological effects of isoproterenol on Purkinje fibers of the heart. *Circ. Res.,* **19**: 940, 1966.

19. Antoni, H. and Oberdisse, E.: Elektrophysiologische untersuchungen uber die Barium-induzierte Schrittmacher-Aktivitat im isolierten Saugetier-myokard. *Pfleugers Archiv.,* **284**: 259, 1965.

20. Vereecke, J. and Carmeleit, E.: Sr action potentials in cardiac Purkinje fibres. *Pfleugers Archiv.,* **322**: 60, 1971.

21. Trautwein, W. and Kassebaum, D.G.: On the mechanism of spontaneous impulse generation in the pacemaker of the heart. *J. Gen. Physiol.,* **45**: 317, 1961.

22. Reuter, H. and Scholz, H.: Ueber den einfluss des extracellularen Cakonzentration auf membranpotential und rena kontraktion isolierter herzpraparte bei graduierter depolarisation. *Pfleugers Archiv.,* **300**: 87, 1968.

23. Imanishi, S.: Calcium-sensitive discharges in canine Purkinje fibers. *Jap. J. Physiol.,* **21**: 443, 1971.

24. Vassalle, M.: Analysis of cardiac pacemaker potential using a "voltage clamp" technique. *Am. J. Physiol.,* **210**: 1335, 1966.

25. Zipes, D.P. and Mendez, C.: Action of manganese ions and tetrodotoxin on atrioventricular nodal transmembrane potentials in isolated rabbit hearts. *Circ. Res.,* **32**: 447, 1973.

26. Zipes, D.P. and Fischer, J.C.: Effects of agents which inhibit the slow channel on sinus node automoticity and atrioventricular conduction in the dog. *Circ. Res.,* **34**: 184, 1974.

27. Surawicz, B.: Calcium responses ("Calcium Spikes"). *Am. J. Cardiol.,* **33**: 689, 1974.

28. Cranefield, P.F. and Hoffman, B.F.: Conduction of the cardiac impulse. II. Summation and inhibition. *Circ. Res.,* **28**: 220, 1971.

29. Hauswirth, O., Noble, D., and Tsien, R.W.: The mechanism of oscillatory activity at low membrane potentials in cardiac Purkinje fibres. *J. Physiol.,* **200**: 255, 1969.

30. Weidmann, S.: The effect of the cardiac membrane potential on the rapid availability of the sodium-carrying system. *J. Physiol.,* **127**: 213, 1955.

31. Gettes, L.S. and Reuter, H.: Slow recovery from inactivation of inward currents in mammalian myocardial fibres. *J. Physiol.,* **240**: 703, 1974.

32. Chen, C.M. and Gettes, L.S.: Combined effects of rate, membrane potential and drugs on (dV/dt) max. *Circ. Res.,* in press.

33. Buchanan, J., Chen, C.M., Saito, S., and Gettes, L.S.: Time dependent effects of hyperpotassemia on conduction in intact dog hearts. *Circulation (Suppl. II),* **52**: 18, 1975.

34. Merideth, J., Mendez, C., Mueller, W.J., and Moe, G.K.: Electrical excitability of atrioventricular nodal cells. *Circ. Res.,* **23**: 69, 1968.

35. Strauss, H.C. and Bigger, J.T.: Electrophysiological properties of the rabbit sino-atrial perinodal fibers. *Circ. Res.,* **31**: 490, 1972.

36. Lazzara, R., El-Sherif, N., and Scherlag, B.J.: Disorders of cellular electrophysiology produced by ischemia of the canine His bundle. *Circ. Res.,* **36**: 444, 1975.

37. Chen, C.M., Gettes, L.S., and Katzung, B.: Effect of lidocaine and quinidine on steady-state characteristics and recovery kinetics of (dV/dt) max in ventricular action potentials. *Circ. Res.,* **37**: 20, 1975.

38. Gettes, L.S., Morehouse, N., and Surawicz, B.: Effect of premature depolarization on the duration of action potentials in Purkinje and ventricular fibers of the moderator band of the pig heart. Role of proximity and the duration of the preceding action potential. *Circ. Res.,* **30**: 55, 1972.

39. Hauswirth, O., Noble, D., and Tsien, R.W.: The dependence of plateau cur-

rents in cardiac Purkinje fibres on the interval between action potentials. *J. Physiol.*, **222**: 27, 1972.

40. Noble, D. and Tsien, R.W.: Outward membrane currents activated in the plateau range of potentials in cardiac Purkinje fibres. *J. Physiol.*, **200**: 205, 1969.

41. Beeler, G.W. and Reuter, H.: Voltage clamp experiments on ventricular myocardiol fibres. *J. Physiol.*, **207**: 165, 1970.

42. Giebisch, G. and Weidmann, S.: Membrane currents in mammalian ventricular heart muscle fibres using a voltage-clamp technique. *J. Gen. Physiol.*, **57**: 290, 1971.

43. New, W., and Trautwein, W.: Inward membrane currents in mammalian myocardium. *Pflugers Arch. Ges. Physiol.*, **334**: 1, 1972.

44. Sasyniuk, B.I. and Mendez, C.: A mechanism for reentry in canine ventricular tissue. *Circ. Res.*, **28**: 3, 1971.

45. Moore, E.N., Preston, J.B., and Moe, G.K.: Duration of transmembrane action potentials and functional refractory periods of canine false tendon and ventricular myocardium. *Circ. Res.*, **17**: 259, 1965.

46. Han, J.: Mechanisms of ventricular arrhythmias associated with myocardial infarction. *Am. J. Cardiol.*, **24**: 800, 1969.

47. Williams, D.O., Scherlag, B.J., Hope, R.R., El-Sherif, N., and Lazzara, R.: The pathophysiology of malignant ventricular arrhythmias during acute myocardial ischemia. *Circulation*, **50**: 1163, 1974.

48. Surawicz, B., Gettes, L.S., and Ponce-Zumino, A.: Relation of vulnerability to ECG and action potential characteristics of premature beats. *Am. J. Physiol.*, **212**: 1519, 1967.

49. Coumel, P.: Junctional reciprocating tachycardias. The permanent and paroxysmal forms of AV nodal reciprocating tachycardias. *J. Electrocardiology*, **8**: 79, 1975.

50. Slama, P.R., Coumel, P., and Bouvrain, Y.: Les syndromes de Wolff-Parkinson-White de Type A inapparentus au latents en rythme sinusal. *Arch. Mal. Coeur*, **66**: 639, 1973.

51. Spurrell, R.J., Krikler, D.M., and Sowton, E.: Concealed bypasses of the atrio-ventricular node in patients with paroxysmal supraventricular tachycardia revealed by intracardiac stimulation and Verapamil. *Am. J. Cardiol.*, **33**: 590, 1974.

52. Durrer, D., Schuilenburg, R.M., and Wellens Hein, J.J.: Pre-excitation revisited. *Am. J. Cardiol.*, **25**: 690, 1970.

53. Moe, G.K. and Mendez, C.: The physiologic basis of reciprocal rhythm. *Prog. Cardiovasc. Dis.*, **8**: 461, 1966.

54. Denes, P., Wu, D., Dhingra, R.C., Chuquimia, R., and Rosen, K.M.: Demonstration of dual AV nodal pathways in patients with paroxysmal supraventricular tachycardia. *Circulation*, **48**: 549, 1973.

55. Gettes, L.S. and Yoshonis, K.F.: Rapidly recurring refractory supraventricular tachycardia. A manifestation of reciprocating tachycardia and an indication for propranolol therapy. *Circulation*, **41**: 468, 1970.

56. Bigger, J.T. and Goldreyer, B.N.: The mechanism of supraventricular tachycardia. *Circulation*, **42**: 673, 1970.

57. Steffens, T. and Gettes, L.S.: Parasystole. *Cardiovasc. Clinics*, **6**: 100, 1974.

58. Langendorf, R. and Pick, A.: Parasystole with fixed coupling. *Circulation*, **35**: 304, 1967.

59. Cohen, H., Langendorf, R., and Pick, A.: Intermittent parasystole-mechanism of protection. *Circulation*, **48**: 761, 1973.

60. Wit, A.L., Fenoglio, J.J., Wagner, B.M., and Bassett, A.L.: Electrophysiological properties of cardiac muscle in anterior mitral valve leaflet and the adjacent atrium in the dog. *Circ. Res.*, **32**: 731, 1973.

61. Wellens, Hein J.J., Lie, K.I., and Durrer, D.: Further observations on

ventricular tachycardia as studied by electrical stimulation of the heart. *Circulation,* **49**: 647, 1974.

62. Rothfeld, E.L., Zucker, I.R., Parsonnet, V., and Alinsonorin, C.A.: Idioventricular rhythm in acute myocardial infarction. *Circulation,* **37**: 203, 1968.
63. Damato, A.N., Varghese, P.J., Lau, S.H., Gallagher, J.J., and Bobb, G.A.: Manifest and concealed reentry. *Circ. Res.,* **30**: 283, 1972.
64. Aravindakshan, V., Surawicz, B., and Daoud, F.S.: Depression of escape pacemakers associated with rapid supraventricular rate in patients with atrioventricular block. *Circulation,* **50**: 255, 1974.
65. Kotler, M.N., Tabatznik, B., Mower, M.M., and Tominaga, S.: Prognostic significance of ventricular ectopic beats with respect to sudden death in the late postinfarction period. *Circulation,* **47**: 959, 1973.
66. Waldo, A.L. and Kaiser, G.A.: A study of ventricular arrhythmias associated with acute myocardial infarction in the canine heart. *Circulation,* **47**: 1222, 1973.
67. Scherlag, B.J., El-Sherif, N., Hope, R., and Lazzara, R.: Characterization and localization of ventricular arrhythmias resulting from myocardial ischemia and infarction. *Circ. Res.,* **35**: 372, 1974.
68. Baum, R.S., Alvarez, H., and Cobb, L.A.: Survival after resuscitation from out-of-hospital ventricular fibrillation. *Circulation,* **50**: 1231, 1974.
69. Dhurandhar, R.W., MacMillan, R.L., and Brown, K.W.G.: Primary ventricular fibrillation complicating acute myocardial infarction. *Am. J. Cardiol.,* **27**: 347, 1971.
70. Lie, K.I., Wellens, Hein J.J., Downer, E., and Durrer, D.: Observations on patients with primary ventricular fibrillation complicating acute myocardial infarction. *Circulation,* **52**: 755, 1975.
71. Hoffman, B.F. and Cranefield, P.F.: Electrophysiology of the Heart. *McGraw Hill, New York,* 1960.
72. Paes de Carvalho, A., Hoffman, B.F., and de Paula Carvalho, M.: Two components of the cardiac action potential. I. Voltage-time course and the effect of acetylcholine on atrial and nodal cells of the rabbit heart. *J. Gen. Physiol,* **54**: 607, 1969.
73. Ware, F. and Graham, G.D.: Effects of acetylcholine on transmembrane potentials in frog ventricle. *Am. J. Physiol.,* **212**: 451, 1967.
74. Friedman, P.L., Stewart, J.R., Fenoglio, J.J., and Wit, A.L.: Survival of subendocardial Purkinje fibers after extensive myocardial infarction in dogs. In vitro and in vivo correlations. *Circ. Res.,* **33**: 597, 1973.
75. Friedman, P.L., Stewart, J.R.,and Wit,A.L.: Spontaneous and induced cardiac arrhythmias in subendocardial Purkinje fibers surviving extensive myocardial infarction in dogs. *Circ. Res.,* **33**: 612, 1973.
76. Lazzara, R., El-Sherif, N., and Scherlag, B.J.: Early and late effects of coronary artery occlusion on canine Purkinje fibers. *Circ. Res.,* **35**: 391, 1974.
77. Bagdonas, A.A., Stuckey, J.H., Piera, J., Amer, N.S., and Hoffman, B.F.: Effects of ischemia and hypoxia on the specialized conducting system of the canine heart. *Am. Heart J.,* **61**: 206, 1961.
78. Scherlag, B.J., Helfant, R.H., Haft, J.I., and Damato, A.N.: Electrophysiology underlying ventricular arrhythmias due to coronary ligation. *Am. J. Physiol.,* **219**: 1665, 1970.
79. Boineau, J.P. and Cox, J.L.: Slow ventricular activation in acute myocardial infarction. *Circulation,* **48**: 702, 1973.
80. Cox, J.L., Daniel, T.M., and Boineau, J.P.: The electrophysiologic time-course of acute myocardial ischemia and the effects of early coronary artery reperfusion. *Circulation,* **48**: 971, 1973.
81. Hope, R.R., Williams, D.O., El-Sherif, N., Lazzara, R., and Scherlag, B.J.: The efficacy of antiarrhythmic agents during acute myocardial ischemia and the role of heart rate. *Circulation,* **50**: 507, 1974.

82. Giotti, A., Ledda, F., and Mannaioni, G.: Effects of noradrenaline and iso-prenaline in combination with α and B-receptor blocking substances on the action potential of cardiac Purkinje fibres. *J. Physiol.*, **229**: 99, 1973.

83. Surawicz, B.: Relationship between electrocardiogram and electrolytes. *Am. Heart J.*, **73**: 814, 1967.

84. Ettinger, P.O., Regan, T.F., Oldewirtel, H.A., and Khan, M.I.: Ventricular conduction delay and asystole during systemic hyperkalemia. *Am. J. Cardiol.*, **33**: 876, 1974.

85. Cohen, H.C., Gozo, E.G., and Pick, A.: The nature and type of arrhythmias in acute experimental hyperkalemia in the intact dog. *Am. Heart J.*, **86**: 777, 1971.

86. Vassalle, M. and Hoffman, B.F.: The spread of sinus activation during potassium administration. *Circ. Res.*, **17**: 285, 1965.

87. Bellet, S. and Jedlicka, J.: Sinoventricular conduction and its relation to sinoatrial conduction. *Am. J. Cardiol.*, **24**: 831, 1969.

88. Ewy, J.A., Karliner, J., and Bedynek, J.L.: Electrocardiographic QRS axis shift as a manifestation of hyperkalemia. *JAMA*, **215**: 429, 1971.

89. Bashour, T., Hsu, I., Gorfinkel, H.J., Wickramesekaran, R., and Rios, J.C.: Atrioventricular and intraventricular conduction in hyperkalemia. *Am. J. Cardiol.*, **35**: 199, 1975.

90. Surawicz, B. and Gettes, L.S.: Two mechanisms of cardiac arrest produced by potassium. *Circ. Res.*, **12**: 415, 1963.

91. Surawicz, B.: Arrhythmias and electrolyte disturbances. *Bull. N.Y. Acad. Sci.*, **43**: 1160, 1967.

92. Davidson, S. and Surawicz, B.: Ectopic beats and atrioventricular conduction disturbances in patients with hypopotassemia. *Arch. Intern. Med.*, **120**: 280, 1967.

93. Gettes, L.S., Surawicz, B., and Kim, K.H.: Role of myocardial K and Ca in initiation and inhibition of ventricular fibrillation. *Am. J. Physiol.*, **211**: 699, 1966.

94. Surawicz, B. and Gettes, L.S.: Effect of electrolyte abnormalities on the heart and circulation. In H.L. Conn and O. Horowitz (Eds.): *Cardiac and Vascular Diseases*. Lea and Febiger, Philadelphia, 1971.

95. Surawicz, B., MacDonald, M.G., Kaljot, V., and Bettinger, J.D.: Treatment of cardiac arrhythmias with salts of ethylenediamine tetraacetic acid (EDTA). *Am. Heart J.*, **58**: 493, 1959.

96. Seller, R.H., Cangrario, J., Kim, K.E., Mendelssohn, D., Rust, A.N., and Schwartz, C.: Digitalis toxicity and hypomagnesemia. *Am. Heart J.*, **79**: 57, 1970.

97. Beller, J.A., Hood, W.D., Smith, T.W., Abelmann, W.H., and Wacker, W.E.L.: Correlation of serum magnesium levels and cardiac digitalis intoxication. *Am. J. Cardiol.*, **33**: 225, 1974.

CHAPTER 5

The Bedside Diagnosis of the Complications of Myocardial Infarction

Michael H. Crawford, M.D.; Robert A. O'Rourke, M.D.

Recognition of impending catastrophe remains in many instances the province of astute clinical observation. Despite technical advances in both non-invasive and invasive monitoring, these techniques can only be initiated, adjusted, and interpreted in light of clinical acumen. This Chapter reviews the clinical arts required in the initial and continuing evaluation of myocardial infarction patients who may require urgent intervention.

The most common complication of acute myocardial infarction is arrhythmia. However, due to the widespread utilization of coronary care units, the use of intravenous antiarrhythmic agents, and the feasibility of rapid pacemaker insertion, these arrhythmias are an uncommon primary cause of death in hospitalized patients with myocardial infarction. Currently, most hospital deaths are due to complications directly related to cardiac structural damage. Left ventricular failure, cardiac rupture, mitral regurgitation, emboli, and pericarditis are early complications of myocardial infarction that occur as a result of structural heart damage. These conditions are seen frequently in the coronary care unit and are occasionally the presenting features of a recent myocardial infarction. With the advent of newer inotropic agents, mechanical circulatory assist, and improved surgical techniques, some of these complications are less likely to be lethal. Therefore, the prompt bedside recognition of the early complications of myocardial infarction is important for optimal patient management (Table I).

TABLE I
COMPLICATIONS OF MYOCARDIAL INFARCTION

1. ARRHYTHMIAS
2. POWER FAILURE
3. CARDIAC RUPTURE
4. MITRAL REGURGITATION
5. PERICARDITIS
6. EMBOLI

POWER FAILURE

Left ventricular power failure is second only to arrhythmias as a cause of death in patients with acute myocardial infarction. The most severe manifestations of left ventricular failure are pulmonary edema and cardiogenic shock. These conditions are not difficult to diagnose and are the subject of other sections of this book. Mild left ventricular failure often precedes the development of pulmonary edema and shock; and the early recognition of mild left ventricular dysfunction may be important for instituting therapy which will prevent the development of more severe cardiac decompensation.

The physical signs of early left ventricular failure can be divided into two groups; those due to myocardial dysfunction itself and those produced by the activation of compensatory reserve mechanisms. An early sign of myocardial dysfunction is *pulsus alternans*, which is an alternation in the amplitude of the peripheral arterial pulse despite a regular rhythm. Pulsus alternans may be initially noted in the first few beats following a premature ventricular contraction, but as left ventricular failure worsens it becomes a persistent finding during sinus rhythm or sinus tachycardia. Pulsus alternans is best appreciated in a distal artery (e.g. radial) which has a slightly wider pulse pressure than the more central arteries (e.g. carotid). The patient should be instructed to hold his breath in mid-expiration to eliminate the small changes in arterial pressure caused by normal respiration. Often patients with mild left ventricular failure have a low blood pressure with a small pulse pressure, which makes pulsus alternans difficult to appreciate. In this situation pulsus alternans can be documented by a sphygmomanometer; the difference in millimeters of mercury between the alternating pressure levels allows one to quantitate the degree of alternans. The mechanism of this physical finding is controversial. Some believe that it is related to a variation in left ventricular end diastolic volume, which causes an alternation in the force of contraction[1]. Others feel that there is a failure of electromechanical coupling on alternate beats in certain damaged regions of the heart which results in an alternation in the amount of muscle cells participating in contraction[2]. Of course, both mechanisms may be at work in patients with myocardial infarction.

Decreased myocardial performance leads to a rise in left atrial pressure which is transmitted to the pulmonary capillaries and eventually results in the transudation of fluid into the alveoli. Alveolar fluid produces audible pulmonary rales. *Rales* are not specific for left ventricular failure and can be due to primary lung disease which often presents a diagnostic problem in the post-infarction patient. However, rales due to lung disease can usually be differentiated from those due to left ventricular dysfunction by their failure to migrate to the most dependent part of the lungs with changes in body position. The effect of gravity on the rales of heart failure is best demonstrated by positioning the patient on one side for thirty minutes or more and then auscultating the lung fields again. Rales will be most prominent over the posterior lung field on the side upon which the patient has been lying.

Elevation of the *jugular venous pressure* (JVP) may parallel an increase in left atrial pressure because of the resultant pulmonary hypertension, since the most common cause of right heart failure is left heart failure. However, an elevation in the JVP may also be a sign of right ventricular dysfunction secondary to infarction of the right ventricle. Right ventricular infarction is not uncommon and may lead to serious consequences if significant left ventricular failure also develops. In this situation the right ventricle is unable to provide the volume needed for adequate left ventricular output and excessive amounts of fluid may need to be administered to the patient, despite right ventricular failure[3]. In patients suspected of having right ventricular failure in whom the JVP is normal, firm pressure over the right upper quadrant of the abdomen for 30 to 60 seconds will enhance venous return to the right heart and cause a rise in the JVP if the right ventricle cannot accommodate this increased volume. This maneuver has been called *"hepato-jugular reflux"* and is an early sign of right ventricular decompensation. It should be pointed out that a normal JVP does not exclude left ventricular failure or increased left atrial pressure[4].

One of the earliest signs of left ventricular failure is the ventricular *diastolic gallop*, or third heart sound, which is coincident with rapid filling of the ventricle. *The third sound* is best heard with the patient in the left lateral decubitus position with the bell of the stethoscope placed lightly over the apex of the left ventricle. This low frequency sound can also be heard over the right ventricle in patients with right ventricular failure.

The third heart sound is not specific for ventricular failure and can be heard in normal young individuals, in high output states and in patients who have atrioventricular valvular regurgitation and are not in heart failure. A presystolic gallop, or *fourth heart sound*, is almost always heard in patients with myocardial infarction who are in sinus rhythm[5]. The fourth sound is associated with decreased diastolic compliance of the ventricle and is not in itself a sign of ventricular decompensation. When tachycardia is present the third and fourth sounds may merge during diastole producing a loud *summation gallop*.

Myocardial infarction is often associated with a diminished audibility of the first heart sound which may alternate in intensity if pulsus alternans is present. When left ventricular performance is severely depressed, left ventricular ejection can be delayed long enough relative to right ventricular ejection that the pulmonic component of the second sound may precede the aortic component, causing audible splitting of the two components of the second sound during expiration. With inspiration the pulmonic sound is delayed and the second sound will close, resulting in reversed splitting of the second sound. This auscultatory phenomenon may be difficult to elicit in patients with a large chest and hyperinflation of the lungs. However, the most common cause of a *paradoxically split second sound* in patients with myocardial infarction is left bundle branch block and not left ventricular failure.

One of the earliest compensatory mechanisms activated after acute myocardial infarction is an increase in sympathetic tone which results in tachycardia and arterial constriction. Thus, during the acute phase of myocardial infarction patients often exhibit increased systemic blood pressure, decreased skin temperature, and even cyanosis of the extremities. Increased sympathetic tone also produces venoconstriction which may contribute to an increase in the jugular venous pressure. Persistent tachycardia and signs of decreased peripheral perfusion after the first few hours suggest impaired left ventricular function. However, some patients with persistent tachycardia never demonstrate other signs of left ventricular decompensation.

If the increase in sympathetic tone is insufficient to maintain cardiac output, ventricular dilatation ensues in an attempt to maintain output by the use of the Frank-Starling mechanism. Left ventricular enlargement can often be detected by precordial palpation of lateral displacement of the apical impulse or an increase in its size. Extensive dyskinesis of the apex can mimic left ventricular enlargement but usually the two conditions coincide. Dyskinesis of other parts of the left ventricle may be appreciated as *abnormal outward impulses* during systole on the anterior chest wall. A persistent dyskinetic area may represent a ventricular aneurysm. Occasionally surgical excision of a left ventricular aneurysm can ameliorate chronic congestive failure which has been refractory to adequate medical therapy.

Ventricular dilatation may lead to enlargement of the atrioventricular valve annuli, altered geometry of the papillary muscles, and malfunction of the valve apparatus resulting in *regurgitant murmurs*. Atrioventricular valve regurgitation can also be due to damage of the papillary muscles or their supporting ventricular wall. Since left ventricular damage predominates in most myocardial infarctions, mitral regurgitation occurs much more frequently than tricuspid regurgitation and will be discussed more fully below.

CARDIAC RUPTURE

Rupture of the free wall of the left ventricle is the third most common cause of death from myocardial infarction and accounts for approximately nine percent of fatal infarctions[6]. There are no specific clinical features that predict who will suffer this complication. However, rupture of the free wall of the heart is statistically more common in elderly female patients with hypertension without prior infarctions. A second high risk group is patients in whom hospital admission and identification of infarction were delayed. Occasionally myocardial rupture is associated with early overexertion, such as straining with bowel movements[7].

Cardiac rupture usually occurs in patients with extensive transmural myocardial infarction who have repeated and prolonged bouts of pain in the first few days after the onset of infarction[8]. One of these bouts of pain usually leads to sudden dyspnea, hypotension, bradycardia, and finally electromechanical dissociation. Rarely, the presentation is slower with signs of developing cardiac tamponade (increased jugular venous pressure, pulsus paradoxus, pericardial friction rub, and increased cardiac size), followed by the development of signs of congestive heart failure or cardiogenic shock. Under rare circumstances the resulting hematoma may seal the rupture, allowing the patient to survive. The hematoma may develop into a false aneurysm of the left ventricular wall which may be associated with a low pitched rumbling systolic and diastolic murmur as blood flows in and out of the narrow necked aneurysm. In contrast to true aneurysms of the ventricular wall (saccular transformation of thinned myocardium), false aneurysms have a greater tendency to rupture[9]. Whenever a false aneurysm of the ventricle is suspected, cardiac catheterization should be performed with a view towards early surgical correction. An emergency operation also may be indicated in some patients with the slower onset of cardiac rupture since successful results have been reported in a few patients[10].

VENTRICULAR SEPTAL RUPTURE

Rupture of the interventricular septum (VSR) is less common than rupture of the free wall of the ventricle, because of the dual coronary artery blood supply to the septum. VSR accounts for one to three percent of fatal acute myocardial infarctions and often is more amenable to medical or surgical therapy than rupture of the free wall[11]. Thus, it is an important complication to recognize early in the course of acute myocardial infarction prior to the development of irreversible heart failure.

The clinical presentation of VSR is punctuated by a sudden change in the status of the patient. Dyspnea is a frequent complaint but pain is rare, in contrast to rupture of the free wall. Physical exam shows an increase in heart rate, a decrease in systemic blood pressure and a new systolic murmur. Typically this *loud, harsh, holosystolic murmur* is located along the lower left sternal border and is associated with a thrill; however, the murmur may be soft in a patient with systemic hypotension and a small difference between the left and right ventricular systolic pressures. A loud VSR murmur can be heard to the right of the sternum and at the apex, and is frequently associated with a third heart sound. A systolic parasternal lift of right ventricular overload and a diastolic flow rumble across the mitral valve due to the left to right shunt are rare early after rupture, but develop with time in some survivors. Signs of right ventricular failure are also unusual early after rupture but develop progressively with time. Signs of pulmonary congestion almost always develop and audible bibasilar rales are the most frequent finding.

RUPTURED PAPILLARY MUSCLE HEAD

Papillary muscle rupture (PMR) is a rare complication of myocardial infarction and accounts for less than one percent of fatal myocardial infarctions[12]. If the entire muscle ruptures, death rapidly ensures without time for therapeutic intervention. If a single head of the papillary muscle ruptures (Figure 1), survival with or without surgery is possible depending on the extent of the accompanying left ventricular damage[13].

The typical presentation of a patient with a ruptured papillary muscle head is the sudden onset of acute pulmonary edema associated with a new

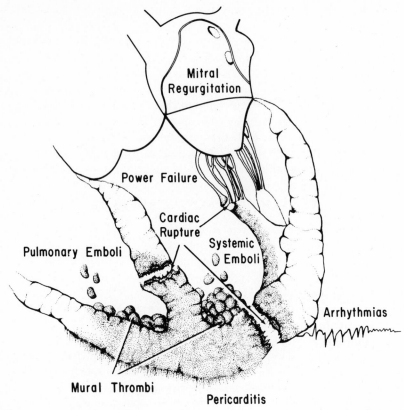

Figure 1 Schematic representation of the major complications of myocardial infarction. Note that only one head of the papillary muscle has reptured.

systolic murmur[14]. Characteristically the murmur is heard best at the apex and radiates to the axilla. Depending on the direction of the regurgitant jet in the left atrium, the murmur may also be heard along the left sternal border and in the aortic area, or it may radiate back to the axial skeleton. It is usually *a high pitched holosystolic murmur*; however, the murmur may not always extend to the second heart sound because the large regurgitant "v" wave in the left atrial pressure may equal left ventricular pressure in late systole. It is occasionally *musical* in quality, but associated thrills are unusual. The murmur is almost always accompanied by *a third heart sound* and often a short *diastolic rumble* can be heard.

DIFFERENTIAL DIAGNOSIS OF VSR AND PMR

The bedside differentiation between the murmurs of VSR and PMR is often difficult. Ventricular septal defects associated with myocardial infarction are in the muscular septum near the apex of the heart, in contrast to the usual congenital variety which occur higher in the septum. Thus, the murmur of VSR is often heard well at the apex and may mimic the murmur of mitral regurgitation. The murmur of PMR can mimic the murmur of VSR if it radiates medially and both murmurs can be associated with a *thrill*, although thrills are more common with VSR[15]. Also, signs of right ventricular overload and diastolic sounds can occur with either condition. Echocardiographic differentiation is discussed in Chapter 8.

Some believe that the best way to differentiate between the two conditions is by assessing the magnitude of left ventricular failure. Patients with rupture of a papillary muscle head usually develop severe pulmonary edema and do very poorly. Patients with VSR tend to have less severe pulmonary congestion and do better[16]. However, there are many exceptions to this and the only definitive way to establish the diagnosis is by bedside right heart catheterization using balloon-tipped flow-directed catheters. VSR is characterized by an oxygen step-up of greater than 0.9 volume percent (3-5 percent saturation) in the right ventricle and PMR usually can be diagnosed by noting the *large "v" wave* in the pulmonary capillary wedge tracing[17]. Rarely, severe mitral regurgitation can lead to an oxygen step-up in the pulmonary artery which may cause confusion[18]. In such cases, left heart catheterization and angiography are diagnostic.

PAPILLARY MUSCLE DYSFUNCTION

Myocardial infarction frequently results in papillary muscle dysfunction (PMD) due to ischemic damage to the papillary muscles or their supporting ventricular wall[19]. PMD often causes mild to moderate mitral or tricuspid regurgitation which occasionally is severe enough to be confused with VSR or PMR. Characteristically the murmur of PMD, which usually involves the mitral valve, develops gradually during the first few days of myocardial infarction and may vary in intensity. Classically this mitral regurgitant murmur begins after the first heart sound and is *diamond shaped*, peaking in the latter part of systole. It is usually best heard at the apex and often radiates to the axilla or occasionally to the base. The murmur almost never is loud enough to have an associated thrill[20]. Although the above description is the most common characterization of the murmur of PMD, considerable variability exists. The exact character of the murmur depends upon the type and degree of papillary muscle damage, the time course of papillary muscle activation, and the functional state of the adjacent left ventricular wall. Thus, the shape of the murmur can vary from pansystolic to late systolic[21].

Pulmonary edema due to PMD is unusual, but lesser degrees of left ventricular failure are not uncommon. Ordinarily, PMD is readily distinguished from PMR or VSR clinically, but occasionally cardiac catheterization is required to confirm the diagnosis (Table II). In PMD the pulmonary artery wedge pressure may be normal or exhibit mild to moderate elevation in contrast to the giant "v" wave usually seen in PMR. However, if the cardiac output is low, these two conditions may be difficult to distinguish and left ventricular angiography will be required.

PERICARDITIS

Pericarditis is common post infarction and various studies have reported a

TABLE II

	VENTRICULAR SEPTAL RUPTURE	PAPILLARY MUSCLE RUPTURE	PAPILLARY MUSCLE DYSFUNCTION
INCIDENCE	UNUSUAL	RARE	COMMON
MURMUR: TYPE LOCATION THRILL	PANSYSTOLIC LEFT STERNAL BORDER 95% > 50%	EARLY TO PANSYSTOLIC APEX→AXILLA 50% RARE	VARIABLE APEX NO
CLINICAL PRESENTATION	LEFT & RIGHT VENTRICULAR FAILURE	PROFOUND PULMONARY EDEMA	NONE TO MODERATE LEFT VENTRICULAR FAILURE
CATHETERIZATION DATA	O$_2$ STEP-UP IN RIGHT VENTRICLE	LARGE LEFT ATRIAL "V" WAVE	MILD TO MODERATE ELEVATION OF LEFT ATRIAL PRESSURE

seven to forty-two percent incidence of pericardial *friction rubs* early in the course of myocardial infarction[22]. However, the frequency with which clinical evidence of pericarditis occurs early after myocardial infarction probably depends largely on the frequency of auscultation. Ordinarily, it is a benign complication which must be distinguished from other more serious complications, such as infarct extension, pulmonary embolus, and papillary muscle dysfunction. Pericarditis is usually associated with larger trans-mural myocardial infarctions; however, pericarditis *per se* does not herald a worse prognosis[23].

Approximately half of the patients with post-infarction pericarditis complain of chest pain which may be pleuritic in nature or associated with changes in position. Dyspnea may also present which may be related to hyperventilation in association with the pain. Occasionally the ECG shows diffuse *ST elevation* consistent with pericarditis, but such changes can also represent infarct extension or aneurysm development. In our experience a second increase in the amount of ST segment elevation when it has begun to decrease 24 or more hours after the acute myocardial infarction is more commonly due to pericarditis than to extension of the infarct. Frequently *atrial tachyarrhythmias* occur with the development of pericarditis. Also, *fever* is more common with myocardial infarction when pericarditis is present. Since the preceding findings are all nonspecific, a pericardial friction rub is required for the bedside diagnosis of pericarditis. Pericardial friction rubs are best heard along the left sternal border with the patient sitting up and leaning forward. They usually have three components: the loudest and longest is in systole and there are often two softer components in diastole, one during rapid filling and one during atrial systole. Pericardial friction rubs tend to be very evanescent. They may vary with position and various components may be missing at any time. However, they are usually easily distinguished from murmurs by their higher frequency, scratchy sound, and transient nature.

Pericardial friction rubs post-infarction rarely last longer than six days. If a rub persists longer than three days it may be a poor prognostic sign because it implies further extension of myocardial damage. Infarct extension can usually be confirmed by serum enzyme studies. An occasional patient will have a persistent rub and fever associated with the development of pericardial and pleural effusion which resembles the post-myocardial infarction (Dressler's) syndrome. This syndrome usually occurs later (2-6 weeks) in the course of myocardial infarction but occasionally begins within the first week[24]. The post-myocardial infarction syndrome is thought to be due to autoimmune phenomena, whereas early pericarditis is felt to be due to pericardial inflammation caused by the adjacent necrotic myocardium. Early pericarditis almost never results in pericardial tamponade and it is not necessary to discontinue anticoagulant therapy. However, anticoagulant therapy should be discontinued if Dressler's syndrome is suspected since hemorrhagic effusions are not uncommon with this disease.

EMBOLI

Pulmonary emboli are not uncommon during the course of acute myocardial infarction. Venous thrombi in the calves of the legs are probably the most common source of pulmonary emboli in postinfarction patients[25]. Patients with congestive heart failure, low output states, and those with complicated myocardial infarction who require prolonged bed rest are especially susceptible to venous thrombosis and should be treated prophylactically with anticoagulants. In addition, extensive *right ventricular infarction* may lead to the formation of mural thrombi in this chamber which can dislodge and cause pulmonary emboli. Right ventricular infarction may be suspected in anteroseptal infarctions when signs of right ventricular failure are out of proportion to left ventricular failure. Such patients should also receive prophylactic anticoagulants.

Pulmonary emboli usually present as sudden unexplained dyspnea. If greater than 60 percent of the pulmonary circulation is occluded there may be signs of acute right heart decompensation which may be difficult to distinguish from right ventricular infarction. *Pulmonary infarction* as a result of emboli is relatively more common in the setting of myocardial infarction because the bronchial collateral circulation is often compromised by pulmonary venous hypertension or systemic hypotension. Also in-dwelling right heart catheters may occlude pulmonary arteries or be the source of thrombi[26]. The classic *triad* of a rise in temperature, pulse, and respiration should alert the physician to the possibility of pulmonary infarction, especially if there is associated pleuritic pain, cough, and hemoptysis. A *pleural friction rub* may be heard over the area of the infarction and can usually be distinguished from pericardial rubs by its location, its augmentation by breathing, and its lack of relationship to various components of the cardiac cycle. Later (12-24 hr) there may be elevations in the serum LDH and the chest x-ray may show a consolidated segment of lung associated with a pleural effusion. Although arterial PO_2 is invariably depressed by pulmonary emboli, this finding is of little value in the setting of an acute myocardial infarction where PO_2 may be decreased for a variety of reasons (left ventricular failure, sedation, etc.). Massive embolization may produce severe chest pain, syncope, and shock.

The diagnosis of pulmonary embolism in the setting of acute myocardial infarction is difficult. Pulmonary infarction may be confused with pneumonia and it may be difficult to distinguish acute right heart decompensation due to pulmonary emboli from other causes of right heart failure. Pulmonary embolus should always be considered during the course of myocardial infarction if there is: (1) unexplained dyspnea and tachypnea, (2) persistent fever or tachycardia, (3) disproportionate right heart failure, (4) pleuritic pain, (5) sudden circulatory decompensation, (6) hemoptysis. Whenever pulmonary embolus is considered a lung scan should be obtained since this is the least traumatic test which is useful for making the diagnosis[27].

Large *transmural myocardial infarctions*, especially those with large dyskinetic areas, are subject to the formation of endocardial thrombosis. The clot may be dislodged at any time during the course of myocardial infarction and travel to peripheral arteries giving rise to a variety of signs and symptoms depending on the artery occluded. Occasionally, such a peripheral occlusive event (stroke, cold extremity) may be the presenting manifestation of an otherwise silent myocardial infarction. When such events occur, it is important to exclude other causes of systemic emboli, such as cardiac tumors and endocarditis.

A low cardiac output can lead to *cerebral ischemia*, especially in patients with cerebral vascular disease. This situation usually can be distinguished from embolic stroke because the central nervous system dysfunction is more diffuse. Occasionally central nervous system complications of a lidocaine infusion may simulate low output states or focal defects, but stopping the infusion should rapidly correct the situation.

References

1. Mitchell, J.H., Sarnoff, S.J., and Sonnenblick, E.H.: The dynamics of pulsus alternans: alternating end-diastolic fiber length as a causative factor. *J. Clin. Inves.*, **42**: 55, 1963.
2. Guntheroth, W.G., Morgan, B.C., McGough, G.A., and Scher, A.M.: Alternate deletion and potentiation as the cause of pulsus alternans. *Am. Heart. J.*, **78**: 669, 1969.
3. Cohn, J.N., Guiha, N.H., Broder, M.I., and Limas, C.J.: Right ventricular infarction. Clinical and hemodynamic features. *Am. J. Cardiol.*, **33**: 209, 1974.
4. Forrester, J., Diamond, G., McHugh, T.J., and Swan, H.J.C.: Filling pressures in the right and left sides of the heart in acute myocardial infarction. *N. Engl. J. Med.*, **285**: 190, 1971.
5. Hill, J.C., O'Rourke, R.A., Lewis, R.P., and McGranahan, G.M.: The diagnostic value of the atrial gallop in acute myocardial infarction. *Am. Heart J.*, **78**: 194, 1969.
6. Mundth, E.: Rupture of the heart complicating myocardial infarction. *Circulation*, **46**: 427, 1972.
7. Friedman, H.S., Kuhn, L.A., and Katz, A.M.: Clinical and electrocardiographic features of cardiac rupture following acute myocardial infarction. *Am. J. Med.*, **50**: 709, 1971.
8. Lewis, A.J., Burchell, H.B., and Titus, J.L.: Clinical and pathological features of postinfarction cardiac rupture. *Am. J. Cardiol.*, **23**: 43, 1969.

9. Vlodaver, A., Coe, J.I., and Edwards, J.E.: True and false left ventricular aneurysms. Propensity for the latter to rupture. *Circulation*, **51**: 567, 1975.
10. FitzGibbon, G.M., Hooper, G.D., and Heggtveit, A.: Successful surgical treatment of postinfarction external cardiac rupture. *J. Thorac. Cardiovasc. Surg.*, **63**: 622, 1972.
11. Campion, B.C., Harrison, C.E., Jr., Guilaiani, E.R., Schattenberg, T.T., and Ellis, F.H.: Ventricular septal defect after myocardial infarction. *Ann. Intern. Med.*, **70**: 251, 1969.
12. Craddock, W.L. and Mahe, G.A.: Rupture of papillary muscle of heart following myocardial infarction. *JAMA*, **151**: 884, 1953.
13. Perloff, J.K. and Roberts, W.C.: The mitral apparatus. *Ciculation*, **46**: 227, 1972.
14. Breneman, G.M. and Drake, E.H.: Ruptured papillary muscle following myocardial infarction with long survival. *Circulation*, **25**: 862, 1962.
15. Selzer, A., Gerbode, F., and Kerth, W.J.: Clinical, hemodynamic, and surgical considerations of rupture of the ventricular septum after myocardial infarction. *Am. Heart J.*, **78**: 598, 1969.
16. Sanders, R.J., Kern, W.H., and Blount, S.G.: Perforation of the interventricular septum complicating myocardial infarction. *Am. Heart J.*, **51**: 736, 1956.
17. Meister, S.G. and Helfant, R.H.: Rapid bedside differentiation of ruptured interventricular septum from acute mitral insufficiency. *N. Engl. J. Med.*, **287**: 1024, 1972.
18. Tatooles, C.J., Gault, J.H., Mason, D.T., and Ross, J., Jr.: Reflux of oxygenated blood into the pulmonary artery in severe mitral regurgitation. *Am. Heart J.*, **75**: 102, 1968.
19. Heikkila, J.: Mitral incompetence as a complication of acute myocardial infarction. *Acta Medica Scand.*, (suppl) **475**: 1, 1967.
20. Phillips, J.H., Burch, G.E., and DePasquale, N.P.: The syndrome of papillary muscle dysfunction. *Ann. Intern. Med.*, **59**: 508, 1963.
21. Cheng, T.O.: Some new observations on the syndrome of papillary muscle dysfunction. *Am. J. Med.*, **47**: 924, 1969.
22. Thadani, U., Chopra, M.P., Aber, C.P., and Portal, R.W.: Pericarditis after acute myocardial infarction. *Brit. Med. J.*, **2**: 135, 1971.
23. Niarchos, A.P. and McKendrick, C.S.: Prognosis of pericarditis after acute myocardial infarction. *Brit. Heart J.*, **35**: 49, 1973.
24. Kossowsky, W.A., Epstein, P.J., and Levine, R.S.: Post myocardial infarction syndrome: an early complication of acute myocardial infarction. *Chest*, **63**: 35, 1973.
25. Dexter, L. and Dalen, J.E.: Pulmonary embolism and acute cor pulmonale. In J.W. Hurst (Ed.): *The Heart*. McGraw Hill Book Co., New York, 1974, p. 1264.
26. Foote, G.A., Schabel, S.J., and Hodges, M.: Pulmonary complications of the flow-directed balloon-tipped catheter. *N. Engl. J. Med.*, **290**: 927, 1974.
27. Moses, D.C., Silver, T.M., and Bookstein, J.J.: The complementary roles of chest radiography, lung scanning, and selective pulmonary angiography in the diagnosis of pulmonary embolism. *Circulation*, **49**: 179, 1974.

CHAPTER 6
Syncope

Marvin I. Dunn, M.D.; James E. Carley, M.D.

Syncope and low back pain are equally frequent in clinical practice. This chapter depicts a scientific approach to the selection of the correct pathophysiologic mechanism in syncope. A neurological, endocrine, or cardiovascular abnormality may be responsible for syncope. The clinical approach to the many etiologic possibilities is reviewed herein.

Syncope is any nontraumatic loss of consciousness, and includes neurologic disorders such as epilepsy, metabolic disorders such as hypoglycemia, and cardiovascular disorders such as arrhythmias[1-3]. In this chapter we will limit discussion to the cardiovascular causes of syncope, but one should remember that the clinical presentation of syncope is essentially the same regardless of the etiology. It is characterized by a sudden, but transient, loss of consciousness. Associated clinical findings may include profuse perspiration, urinary and fecal incontinence, convulsions, and amnesia. A classification of cardiovascular causes of syncope and a differential diagnosis is presented in Table I.

A meticulous account of the syncopal attack must be obtained with special regard to circumstances leading up to the episode. Deliberate questioning must include exacerbating or alleviating factors, medications, duration of loss of consciousness, associated medical illnesses, familial occurrence, postural association, palpitations, hemoptysis, and history of heart murmurs. The physical examination should include blood pressure and pulse measurements supine and standing. Auscultation of the heart and great vessels should take place in a quiet room. Laboratory evaluation should include electrolyte determinations, arterial blood gases, chest x-ray, electrocardiogram, echocardiogram, a twenty-four hour monitor of the cardiac rhythm, and an exercise electrocardiogram.

A comprehensive approach to cardiovascular causes of syncope follows. It is necessary to include or exclude diagnoses which may seem remote. It is helpful in the workup of the patient with syncope to think in terms of pathophysiological mechanisms in order to ensure that the etiology is determined since appropriate treatment is entirely dependent on an accurate diagnosis.

TABLE I

CARDIOVASCULAR CAUSES OF SYNCOPE

I.   Impaired cardiac filling
   A. Orthostatic hypotension
   B. Cardiac tamponade
II. Impaired cardiac ejection
   A. Arrhythmias
      1. Tachyarrhythmias
         a. Atrial
            1) Fibrillation
            2) Flutter
            3) Paroxysmal atrial tachycardia
            4) Wolff-Parkinson-White Syndrome
            5) Sick sinus syndrome
            6) Hyperkalemia
         b. Ventricular
            1) Tachycardia
            2) Fibrillation
            3) Syndromes associated with prolonged Q-T interval
               (Jervell and Lange-Nielson and Romano-Ward syndromes)
            4) Artificial pacemaker failure
      2. Bradyarrhythmias
         a. Complete heart block
         b. Artificial pacemaker failure
         c. Sick sinus syndrome
         d. Hypersensitive carotid sinus syndrome
         e. Sinus bradycardia with myocardial ischemia
   B. Valve and vessel obstruction
      1. Atrial outflow obstruction
         a. Right and left atrial myxomas
         b. Obstruction of valvular prosthesis
      2. Ventricular outflow obstruction
         a. Left ventricle
             1) Supravalvular stenosis
            2) Valvular stenosis
            3) Subvalvular stenosis
         b. Right ventricle
             1) Pulmonary stenosis
            2) Tetralogy of Fallot
      3. Pulmonary vascular obstruction
         a. Pulmonary embolism
         b. Primary pulmonary hypertension
         c. Eisenmenger's complex
III. Interference with quantity or quality of cerebral blood flow
   A. Extracranial large artery obstruction
      1. Carotid and vertebral artery stenosis
      2. Pulseless disease
      3. Subclavian steal syndrome
   B. Hyperventilation syndrome
   C. Acceleration

IV.   Combinations—Miscellaneous
   A.   Vasomotor syncope
   B.   Carotid sinus syncope
   C.   Cough syncope
   D.   Weight-lifter's syncope
   E.   Micturition syncope
   F.   Swallowing syncope and glossopharyngeal neuralgia
   G.   Pacemaker syncope
   H.   Drug syncope

IMPAIRED CARDIAC FILLING

Man is unique in the animal world since he stands, walks, and works in the upright position. In order to accomplish this evolutionary feat, a number of physiologic mechanisms have evolved which prevent venous pooling, regulate the blood pressure, and maintain cerebral flow when a person changes from the supine to the upright position, as well as when he remains in the upright position. When a person stands, there is pooling of blood in the venous capacitance vessels of the lower extremities. This is partially prevented by tissue pressure, the pumping action of skeletal muscles, and the inhibition of retrograde venous flow by venous valves. The net effect, however, is diminished venous return resulting in diminished stroke volume, decreased cardiac output, and a fall in systolic blood pressure.

The drop in pressure stimulates the baroreceptors in the sinus and aorta, initiating the afferent limb of a reflex arc to the vasomotor center of the brain. The efferent limb is mediated through sympathetic pathways causing peripheral vasoconstriction, an increase in heart rate, and a rise in catecholamine and renin levels. As a result of these mechanisms, there is increased venous return to the heart, augmented ventricular stroke volume (due to increased venous return and increased inotropic effect), increased cardiac output, and a rise in systolic blood pressure (Figure 1)[4].

Orthostatic Hypotension

When this orthostatic blood pressure regulating mechanism referred to above fails, syncope occurs, characterized by a drop in systolic pressure, an initial rise in diastolic pressure, tachycardia, pallor, perspiration, nausea, and then a drop in diastolic pressure. In this form of syncope, there is an initial lack of venous return, but the cardiac output remains normal until the veins in the skeletal muscle and splanchnic bed dilate. This is followed by a decrease in venous return, diminished cardiac output, and a decrease in cerebral perfusion. The secondary symptoms of tachycardia, pallor and sweating, are due to sympathetic stimulation and are absent in asympathetic forms of orthostatic hypotension, such as the idiopathic orthostatic hypotension syndrome.

Orthostatic hypotension may be acute or chronic. The common causes are listed in Table II, and a few deserve special comment:

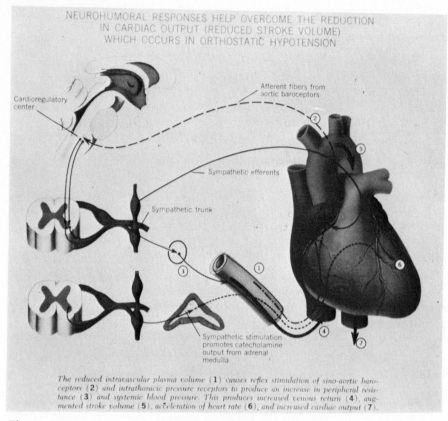

NEUROHUMORAL RESPONSES HELP OVERCOME THE REDUCTION
IN CARDIAC OUTPUT (REDUCED STROKE VOLUME)
WHICH OCCURS IN ORTHOSTATIC HYPOTENSION

The reduced intravascular plasma volume (1) causes reflex stimulation of sino-aortic baroceptors (2) and intrathoracic pressure receptors to produce an increase in peripheral resistance (3) and systemic blood pressure. This produces increased venous return (4), augmented stroke volume (5), acceleration of heart rate (6), and increased cardiac output (7).

Figure 1
Blood loss syncope

It is sometimes difficult to estimate the volume of blood loss due to external or internal bleeding. Initially, the hemoglobin and hematocrit are poor indicators of blood loss because hemodilution has not yet taken place. Under these circumstances, a reliable method of determining the hemodynamic importance of the blood loss is the observation of the integrity of the orthostatic blood pressure regulatory mechanism. Take the blood pressure and pulse with the patient supine and repeat with the patient tilted 60° in the head-up position. If there has been a significant blood loss, the systolic blood pressure will decreasse at least 16 mm Hg, the diastolic will decrease at least 8 mm Hg, and the pulse rate will increase more than 10 beats per minute[5].

Post-exercise syncope

Post-exercise syncope occurs primarily in teenagers who have engaged in vigorous, strenuous activity in a warm environment. With exercise, there is a marked increase in cardiac output and maximum vasodilatation occurs. When the exercise is terminated, the cardiac output decreases rapidly, but

TABLE II
CAUSES OF ORTHOSTATIC HYPOTENSION

I. Acute problems causing orthostatic hypotension
   A. Volume depletion
      1. Blood loss
      2. Massive diuresis
      3. Post-gastrectomy dumping syndrome
   B. Venous obstruction or pooling
      1. Pregnancy
      2. Prolonged standing
      3. Prolonged bed rest
      4. Post-exercise vasodilatation
      5. Spinal anesthesia
      6. Drug-induced
         a. Antihypertensive drugs
         b. Diuretics
         c. Nitrates
         d. Phenothiazines
         e. L-dopa
II. Chronic problems causing orthostatic hypotension
   A. Neurologic disease
      1. Diabetic neuropathy
      2. Alcoholic neuropathy
      3. Pernicious anemia
      4. Tabes dorsalis
      5. Amyloid disease
      6. Guillain-Barré syndrome
      7. Syringomyelia
      8. Post-sympathectomy syndrome
      9. Porphyria
   B. Endocrine disease
      1. Hyperaldosteronism
      2. Addison's disease
      3. Pheochromocytoma
      4. Simmond's disease
   C. Idiopathic

the vasodilatation persists, resulting in a disparity between the expanded vascular bed and the decreased cardiac output, which causes hypotension and syncope.

Hypotension of pregnancy

Pregnant women often have marked fluctuations in cardiac output which may depend on body position. In Metcalfe's studies[6] when women in their third trimester were placed in the supine position, they experienced a decrease in cardiac output and stroke volume, but an increase in heart rate. He attributed the abrupt decrease in cardiac output and stroke volume to vena caval obstruction with a subsequent decrease in venous return to the heart. As the venous return diminishes, the heart rate increases in an attempt to maintain cardiac output. All of these findings were reversed when these women assumed a lateral decubitus position.

Many of the common causes of syncope listed in Table II are due to neurologic disorders which affect the afferent limb, synapse, or efferent limb of the vasoconstrictive reflex arc. Although most of these diseases are irreversible, the neuropathy associated with pernicious anemia, diabetes, and alcoholism may be corrected. The skeletal muscular contribution to venous return may be impaired due to muscle wasting or disuse; when severe, syncope may result.

Most of the medications which cause orthostatic hypotension have a direct effect on the vascular smooth muscle, causing vasodilatation. Some antihypertensive medications such as guanethedine and alphamethyldopa interfere with sympathetic nerve transmission at the nerve-end organ interface.

Idiopathic orthostatic hypotension

The idiopathic orthostatic hypotension syndrome is characterized by the triad of orthostatic hypotension, anhidrosis, and impotence[7]. It occurs more frequently in men than women, usually in their fifth to sixth decades. Other associated symptoms are listed in Table III. Although the exact pathologic mechanism of this interesting disorder has not been defined, Shy and Drager feel it is part of a generalized neurologic degenerative disease, and they have demonstrated specific pathologic lesions[8]. In the initial stage of the disease, the primary defect appears to be in the afferent limb of the reflex arc, since vasoconstriction can occur when catecholamines are injected intravenously, and when reflexes are stimulated at the cerebral level, by producing unpleasant situations or through the cold pressor mechanism.

This form of orthostatic hypotension differs from most others since there is no reflex tachycardia. The blood pressure falls precipitously without a compensatory rise in heart rate. The patient usually has total amnesia during the event. We have observed patients awaken and continue with the same sentence interrupted by the syncopal spell. Due to the impairment of heat regulation, syncopal spells are more likely to occur during the summer.

TABLE III

SIGNS AND SYMPTOMS OF IDIOPATHIC ORTHOSTATIC HYPOTENSION

1. Orthostatic hypotension
2. Anhidrosis
3. Impotence
4. Reversed diurnal urinary output
5. Heat intolerance
6. Diarrhea
7. Loss of temperature regulation
8. Tremor
9. Loss of muscle tone
10. Drowsiness
11. Square wave response of blood pressure to valsalva maneuver
12. Absence of blood pressure rise with supine exercise
13. Increased urinary output and renal blood flow in supine position

Patients who have syncope from orthostatic hypotension should be placed in the horizontal position and care taken to avoid aspiration. When the patient has recovered consciousness, attention must be directed to prevent recurrence by establishing the specific cause for the orthostatic hypotension.

For the management of idiopathic orthostatic hypotension, Florinef® (9α fluorohydrocortisone) in doses of 1 to 16 mg per day has been helpful. If the patients do not have severe hypertension when horizontal, this can be supplemented with 10 grams of sodium chloride[9]. If this does not produce adequate volume expansion, the Jobst® leotard is usually successful in supporting venous return and preventing venous pooling (Figure 2). Although we have had no experience with tyramine and monomine oxidase inhibitors in combination, these have been used to produce prolonged vasoconstriction[3].

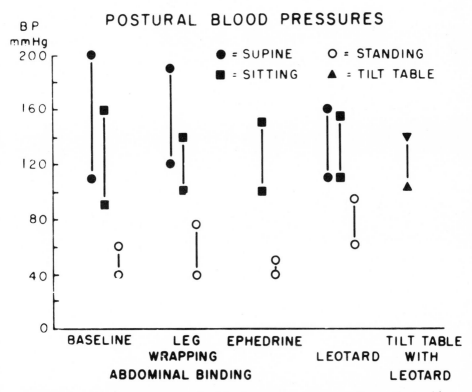

Figure 2 This figure shows the blood pressure response of a patient with idiopathic orthostatic hypotension whose blood pressure could not be maintained by medication. He was successfully managed by using a Jobst® leotard.

Cardiac Tamponade

Another form of syncope caused by inadequate cardiac filling is that due to cardiac tamponade. With the rapid accumulation of a small amount of pericardial fluid or the gradual accumulation of a large amount of fluid, cardiac tamponade and syncope may occur. The high intrapericardial pressure impairs venous return by compressing the heart, causing marked reduction in stroke volume, cardiac output, and cerebral perfusion (Figure 3).

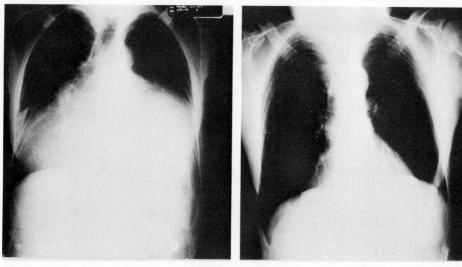

Figure 3 These chest x-rays were obtained from a 46 year old male plant foreman with ankylosing spondylitis. He experienced exertional syncope for one week prior to admission to the hospital. The x-ray on the left was taken at the time of admission and the one on the right was taken about four weeks after removing 2.5 liters of serosanguineous fluid from his pericardial sac.

IMPAIRED EJECTION OF BLOOD

Arrhythmias

Cerebral perfusion may be profoundly reduced by cardiac arrhythmias due to the reduction in cardiac output. The cardiac output is a product of stroke volume and heart rate, increasing as the stroke volume and heart rate increase and decreasing as the heart rate and stroke volume diminish. It is easy to understand how a profound reduction in heart rate will result in decreased cardiac output; however, if the heart rate increases and the cardiac output diminishes, there must be an associated reduction in stroke volume. This reduction is in turn the result of both diminished ventricular filling and impaired ventricular contraction. To understand this chain of events, it is necessary to review the mechanisms of ventricular filling.

Ordinarily, ventricular filling occurs in two phases. The initial passive phase occurs with the opening of the mitral valve and, under normal circumstances, 75 to 85 percent of the ventricular diastolic filling occurs during this interval. Late in diastole, ventricular filling is completed by the atrial contraction. At usual heart rates, 15 to 25 percent of the ventricular filling occurs at this time. As the heart rate increases, a larger percentage of ventricular filling occurs with the atrial contraction. If the atrial contribution to ventricular filling is absent (as in atrial fibrillation) or is asynchronous (as in paroxysmal atrial tachycardia), a serious reduction in ventricular filling occurs which is associated with a marked reduction in stroke volume.

This derangement of function is even more severe in the presence of ventricular tachycardia. Not only is there atrial and ventricular asynchrony, but also asynchronous ventricular contraction which further diminishes stroke volume. If in addition the ventricle is diseased, there will be even more serious impairment of stroke volume.

Although syncope can result from any of the supraventricular arrhythmias, it is most likely to occur with atrial fibrillation with a very rapid ventricular response, and with atrial flutter when there is a 1:1 response. It is important to check the heart rate in the erect as well as the supine position. In the erect position, there is an increase in the sympathetic stimuli to the heart and a decrease in the vagal stimuli, which may decrease the A-V block in atrial flutter as illustrated in Figure 4.

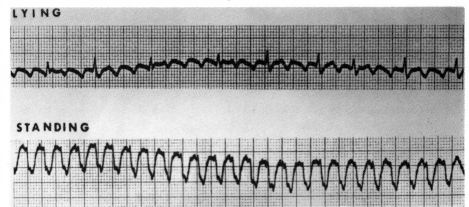

Figure 4 These electrocardiographic tracings were obtained from a 46 year old roofer who had a four month history of syncope. He did not have organic heart disease but did have paroxysmal atrial flutter. The upper tracing was obtained when the patient was lying down and shows atrial flutter with 3:1 and 4:1 AV block. The lower tracing was recorded when the patient stood and shows 1:1 conduction.

Although ventricular arrhythmias usually occur in the setting of an acute myocardial infarction, they are also found in the absence of organic heart disease and should be considered in the differential diagnosis of syncope (Figure 5).

In 1957, Jervell and Lange-Nielsen[10] described a syndrome of syncope,

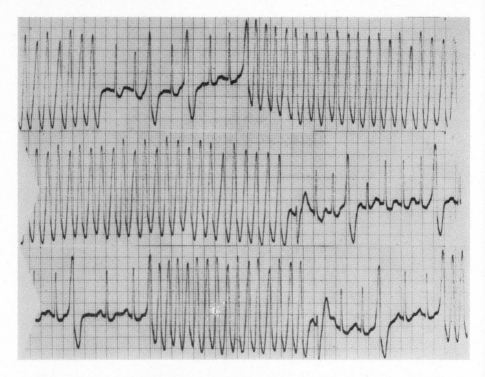

Figure 5   This electrocardiographic tracing was recorded from a 42 year old male school teacher who was under psychiatric care. He began having syncopal spells in class and on one occasion was seen by the school nurse who could not find a pulse. He was thought to have intermittent heart block or hyperventilation syndrome until this electrocardiogram showing paroxysmal ventricular tachycardia was recorded.

congenital deafness, hereditary prolongation of the Q-T interval of the electrocardiogram, and sudden death. Romano et al[11] and Ward[12] in 1963 separately described the same constellation of findings in patients with normal hearing. These syncopal episodes have been documented to be due to ventricular tachycardia, fibrillation, and, less often, to cardiac standstill. Most patients with this disorder who have received propranolol have experienced fewer syncopal attacks, but the medication has not altered the Q-T interval. These patients are most susceptible to arrhythmias from infancy to adolescence, but may have a symptom-free period until adulthood when syncopal episodes recur. The Q-T prolongation is not due to an abnormality of potassium, calcium, magnesium, or antiarrhythmic drugs. The true etiology of the Q-T prolongation is not completely understood, but may represent abnormal autonomic influence on the myocardium[13-17].

Bradyarrhythmias are common causes of syncope. Reduced cardiac output and cerebral flow are the consequence of the slow rate in spite of the compensatory increase in stroke volume. Syncope is more likely to occur when there is a sudden reduction in rate, as opposed to a gradual reduction.

In the latter situation, compensatory mechanisms are more likely to be effective.

There are many etiologic causes for complete heart block. These are listed in Table IV. Rosenbaum et al[18], Pryor and Blount[19], and Lasser et al[20] have defined the clinical significance of bifasicular and trifasicular blocks, and have identified potential candidates for complete block. Indeed, patients who are known to have right bundle branch block with anterior or posterior fasicular block are now considered candidates for pacemaker implantation if they have had a syncopal episode even though the event was not documented. Occasionally, complete block can be induced by exercise in patients with bifasicular block even though the resting cardiogram shows normal A-V conduction (Figure 6).

TABLE IV
CAUSES OF HEART BLOCK

I.   Congenital
II.   Degenerative
    A.   Ischemic heart disease
    B.   Amyloid disease
    C.   Paget's disease
    D.   Lev's disease
    E.   Lenegre's disease
    F.   Calcific aortic stenosis
    G.   Calcification of mitral annulus
III. Infectious
    A.   Syphilis
    B.   Diphtheria
    C.   Sarcoidosis
IV. Endocrine
    A.   Myxedema
    B.   Hyperthyroidism
V.   Neoplastic
    A.   Multiple myeloma
    B.   Hodgkin's disease
    C.   Tumors of the heart
VI. Collagen
    A.   Dermatomyositis
    B.   Rheumatoid arthritis
    C.   Rheumatic fever
VII. Neuromuscular
    A.   Progressive muscular dystrophy
    B.   Myotonia dystrophica
VIII. Drug-induced
    A.   Digitalis
    B.   Potassium
IX. Trauma
X.   Idiopathic

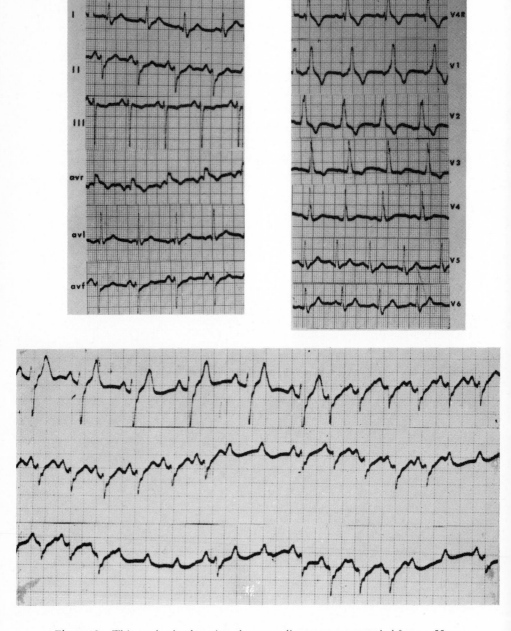

Figure 6 This twelve lead resting electrocardiogram was recorded from a 55 year old male with a six month history of exertional syncope and demonstrates complete right bundle branch block and left anterior superior fascicular block. The lower electrocardiographic tracings were recorded on initiation of exercise and show the abrupt onset of intermittent heart block.

Sick sinus syndrome

Another recently described entity which is associated with either tachycardia or bradycardia is the sick sinus syndrome. This entity includes many tachy- and bradyarrhythmias as listed in Table V[21]. The recognition of some of these disturbances can be accomplished only by continuous monitoring of the heart rhythm with a Holter monitor. The precise method of management depends on the exact mechanism of the arrhythmia. As a general plan, we use pacemakers to control the slow rhythms so that antiarrhythmic medication can be given for the fast rhythms.

TABLE V
SICK SINUS SYNDROME

I. Bradyarrhythmias
    A. Sinus bradycardia
    B. Sinus node exit block
    C. Intermittent sinus arrest
    D. Temporary asystole following tachycardia
II. Tachyarrhythmias
    A. Atrial fibrillation
    B. Atrial flutter
    C. Supraventricular tachycardia and PAT
    D. Ventricular tachycardia and/or fibrillation

Hyperkalemia

Hyperkalemia may cause sinus arrest and a nodal bradycardia with or without aberrant ventricular conduction. The high potassium levels also adversely affect myocardial contractility. The resultant slow rate and impaired contractility can cause syncope. A less common cause is sino-ventricular rhythm (Figures 7 and 8), which is often mistaken for ventricular tachycardia, an error that can have serious complications. If anti-arrhythmic drugs such as quinidine, procainamide or Dilantin® are given, they may potentiate the effect of the hyperkalemia, resulting in severe aberrancy (Figures 9 and 10) and decreased cardiac output, cerebral flow, and syncope.

Hypersensitive carotid sinus syndrome

There are three forms of carotid syncope: (a) hypersensitive carotid sinus syndrome, (b) vasodepressor type, and (c) cerebral type. The vasodepressor and cerebral forms of carotid sinus syncope will be discussed with the miscellaneous causes. The hypersensitive carotid sinus syndrome is characterized by sudden exaggerated slowing of the heart rate due to carotid sinus stimulation. This occurs predominantly in older persons, many with concomitant arteriosclerotic heart disease or diffuse atherosclerosis. The reflex cardiac slowing is often a sinus bradycardia but may be sinus arrest

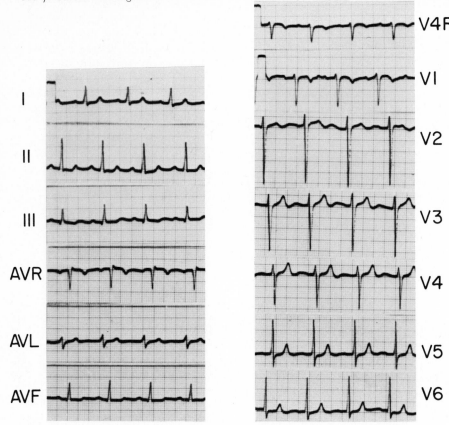

Figure 7 This twelve lead electrocardiogram was recorded from a 19 year old girl with chronic glomerulonephritis and shows left ventricular hypertrophy and a normal QT interval.

with nodal or ventricular escape, atrioventricular block, or even asystole. It is precipitated by pressure over the carotid sinus which might result from gazing upward with the extremities extended, shaving, or wearing a tight collar (Figure 11)[22-24].

VALVE AND VESSEL OBSTRUCTION

Atrial Obstruction

Myxoma of the left atrium can produce syncope by obstructing the flow of blood from left atrium to left ventricle. The physical findings of atrial myxoma frequently mimic mitral stenosis. Peripheral embolization in the presence of normal sinus rhythm, fast sedimentation rate, and increased gamma globulin are helpful laboratory findings, but the diagnosis can be established by echocardiography. Atrial thrombus may mimic a myxoma.

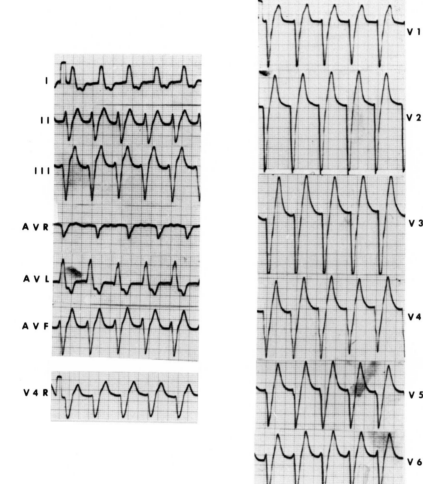

Figure 8 This electrocardiogram was recorded from the same girl immediately after she had a syncopal spell. Although on superficial examination this is suggestive of ventricular tachycardia, on more careful examination there are a number of discrepancies: (1) no P waves are seen, (2) the rhythm is completely regular, (3) the QRS complexes have the morphology of left bundle branch block rather than right bundle branch block, (4) the QT interval is short in the face of a wide QRS complex, (5) the T waves are tall and peaked. This is a sinoventricular rhythm produced by potassium intoxication (serum potassium was 7.5 mEq/L).

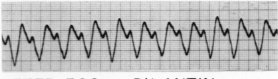

AFTER 300mg DILANTIN

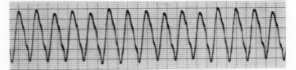

AFTER 500mg PRONESTYL

Figure 9   The upper panel is an electrocardiographic tracing obtained from the same girl after she received 300 mg of Dilantin® intravenously for treatment of presumed ventricular tachycardia. The additive effect of the Dilantin® was responsible for the increased heart rate and widened QRS complex. The lower panel demonstrates the same adverse reaction when Pronestyl® was given intravenously.

AFTER GLUCOSE AND INSULIN

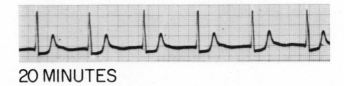

20 MINUTES

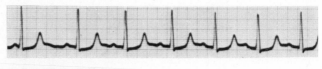

90 MINUTES

Figure 10   This shows restoration of a normal sinus rhythm after the intravenous administration of glucose and insulin which brought the serum potassium to normal.

Mitral obstruction may also result from thrombus formation on a prosthetic valve.

Ventricular Obstruction

Left ventricular outflow obstruction is associated with syncope which can

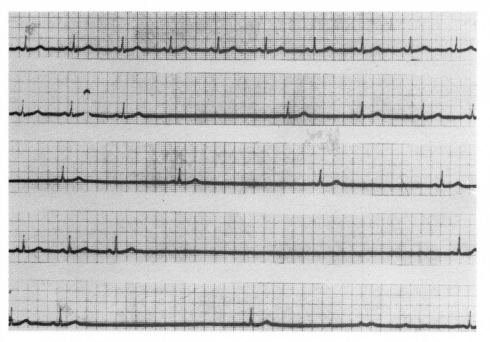

Figure 11 This electrocardiogram was recorded from a 74 year old retired farmer who had a syncopal episode while shaving. He fractured his left humerus when he fell and was admitted to the orthopedic service. This electrocardiogram was recorded the morning after he was hospitalized. He was shaving his neck with an electric razor. The tracing shows sinus bradycardia and sinus arrest resulting from carotid sinus stimulation by the razor.

occur at rest or with exertion. The syncope may be due to arrhythmias resulting from impaired coronary flow and is most likely to occur in patients with severe obstruction[25].

In patients with idiopathic hypertrophic subaortic stenosis[26], relatively insignificant arrhythmias may have dire hemodynamic consequences. For example, bigeminy is ordinarily a benign arrhythmia; however, post-extrasystolic potentiation produces increased obstruction and diminished stroke volume. Under these circumstances bigeminy can cause a marked decrease in cardiac output and cerebral flow (Figures 12 and 13). Frequently the syncope associated with idiopathic hypertrophic subaortic stenosis occurs after exercise, whereas the syncope of valvular stenosis occurs with exercise.

Pulmonary Vascular Obstruction[27-29]

Syncope may be a presenting symptom of pulmonary embolism. This may be due to an arrhythmia when there are multiple small pulmonary emboli, or reduced pulmonary flow when there is a massive pulmonary embolus.

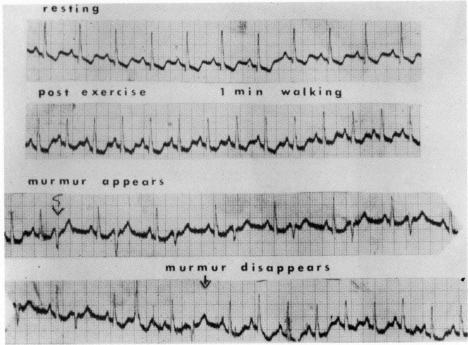

resting

post exercise   1 min walking

murmur appears

murmur disappears

Figure 12   This electrocardiogram was recorded from a 64 year old housewife with exertional syncope who was admitted to the neurology service. She had no heart murmur at rest but developed a grade IV systolic ejection murmur when she developed bigeminy. She also became lightheaded and dizzy at this time. The murmur and her symptoms disappeared when sinus rhythm was restored. These findings are diagnostic of idiopathic hypertrophic subaortic stenosis. (See text for explanation.)

INTERFERENCE WITH QUANTITY OR QUALITY OF CEREBRAL BLOOD FLOW

Extracranial Large Vessel Disease

Although rarely a cause of syncope by itself, severe atherosclerosis of the aortic arch and its main branches may produce unconsciousness if there is vigorous carotid massage or an arrhythmia. Transient ischemic attacks, vertigo, amaurosis fugax, paresthesias, and other neurologic symptoms frequently accompany carotid artery stenosis and pulseless disease. Fainting may result from exercise of an upper extremity when there is marked proximal obstruction of the ipsilateral subclavian artery. This occurs because of retrograde flow down the vertebral artery into the subclavian artery distal to the obstruction (subclavian steal syndrome)[30]. The retrograde flow occurs at the expense of the cerebral circulation.

Hyperventilation Syndrome

Probably the most common cause of syncope is the hyperventilation syn-

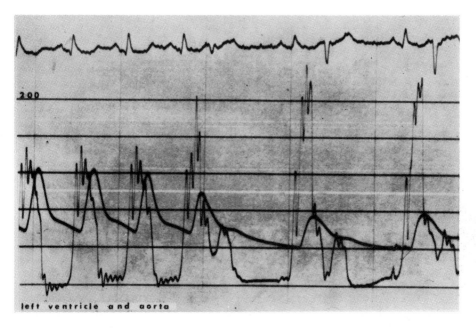

left ventricle and aorta

Figure 13 This is a left ventricular and aortic pressure recording from the same patient. When bigeminy is induced the left ventricular pressure increases from 120 mm Hg to 200 mm Hg and the aortic pressure decreases from 120 mm Hg to 80 mm Hg. These findings are pathognomonic of idiopathic hypertrophic subaortic stenosis.

drome. The overbreathing is usually the result of an underlying anxiety but may be due to central stimulation from drugs. The symptoms are giddiness, circumoral and extremity paresthesias, tetany, a feeling of suffocation, and dyspnea. The hyperventilation results in hypocapnia and alkalosis which in turn leads to cerebral arterial vasoconstriction and diminished flow. With diminished cerebral perfusion there is a progressive decrease in oxygen delivery to the brain as evidenced by diffuse slowing of brain wave activity on the electroencephalogram. This is one syncopal attack which may have its onset in the recumbent position. Treatment consists of restoring the pCO$_2$ to normal levels by letting the patient rebreathe his own expired air and attempting to allay his anxiety.

Acceleration

Acceleration may produce syncope in airplane pilots by overcoming the normal force of blood returning to the right side of the heart. This rapidly leads to venous pooling with a marked fall in cardiac output.

MISCELLANEOUS

The causes of syncope grouped under this heading generally are not related to a primary defect, but rather are the results of a *combination* of factors that result in decreased cerebral perfusion.

Vasomotor Syncope

The common faint is one of the easiest syndromes to recognize, usually occurring in normal people who have experienced a noxious afferent stimulus such as an unpleasant sight or shocking news (Figure 14). Often it occurs in a crowded or warm environment, and there are premonitory symptoms of nausea, flushing, lightheadedness, weakness, yawning, and confusion. Pathophysiologically, there is initially a phase of vasodilatation with decrease in peripheral resistance and hypotension quickly followed by a bradycardia, usually in the range of 40 to 50 beats per minute, with a further reduction in cardiac output and then unconsciousness. The patient regains consciousness quickly after he assumes a more horizontal position which increases venous return from the extremities. If possible, the inciting stimulus should be removed to prevent recurrence.

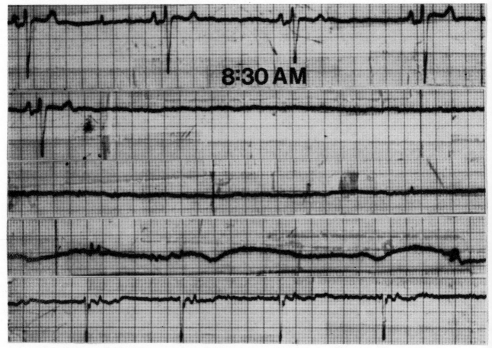

Figure 14 This electrocardiogram was recorded from a 42 year old male janitor and lay preacher who had experienced multiple syncopal episodes. He was in the coronary care unit under observation. The electrocardiogram was recorded in the morning when blood was drawn for laboratory tests. The patient experienced 17 seconds of asystole due to a vasovagal reaction. The asystole was terminated by a blow to the chest.

Carotid Sinus Syncope

The hypersensitive carotid sinus syndrome associated with bradycardia has already been discussed earlier in the chapter. The vasodepressor carotid sinus syncope is manifested by progressive hypotension without change in heart rate. The fall in blood pressure is secondary to peripheral vaso-dilatation with inhibition of sympathetic vasoconstriction. Atropine will not prevent the fall in blood pressure. In cerebral carotid sinus syncope a loss of consciousness is unaccompanied by a decrease in heart rate or hypotension. The true nature of this form of syncope is not known.

Cough Syncope

This syndrome can be defined as a loss of consciousness which is preceded by a paroxysm of coughing. The clinical spectrum has been characterized by Kerr and Derbes in a study of 25 patients[31]. Typically, these patients are middle-aged males, usually obese, often heavy smokers, and frequently have a history of chronic bronchitis, asthma, or emphysema. The cough is dry and nonproductive, and syncope occurs after a paroxysm of violent coughing. The syncope is sudden and may occur in any position. Following a coughing paroxysm, there is a period of marked arterial hypotension and syncope. When patients are monitored during these spells, the intrathoracic pressure has been recorded near 300 mm Hg[32]. Under these circumstances there is marked reduction in venous return to the heart and a marked decrease in cardiac output. In a study of twenty patients, McIntosh et al discovered that the cerebrospinal fluid pressure rose to the same level as the intrathoracic pressure[33]. In addition to the arterial hypotension, they concluded that the syncope resulted from blood being "squeezed" from the brain by the high extravascular pressure around the cranial vessels. Under these circumstances the brain was relatively bloodless and the hypoxia contributed to the fainting.

Weight-Lifter's Syncope

Loss of consciousness during weight lifting is not uncommon. In addition to extremely high intrathoracic pressures produced with a Valsalva maneuver during lifting, Compton et al[34] also noted a pre-lift hyper-ventilation period, and postulated that hypocapnia associated with the hyperventilation caused cerebral artery vasoconstriction and systemic arterial dilatation. The net effect was a rapid fall in venous return, stroke volume, and cardiac output. If the lift is prolonged, there is more time for reflex vasodilatation to occur in response to the parallel rise in arterial pressure. Following the lift, there is a release of intrathoracic pressure and sudden expansion of previously compressed great veins and splanchnic vessels. When these vessels fill, there is a lag period in which venous return to the left ventricle and stroke volume are markedly reduced. Squatting seems to aggravate the problem, as it causes further dilatation of systemic arteries.

Micturition Syncope

This form of syncope usually occurs in young to middle-aged men who rise to void after being asleep or recumbent for several hours[35-37]. The patient feels dizzy or lightheaded while voiding or shortly thereafter, and there is a transient loss of consciousness. Consciousness is soon regained, and no abnormality of the physical examination can be detected. The true pathogenesis of this condition has not been elucidated but speculations have included postural hypotension, effects of the Valsalva maneuver, and vagal slowing of the heart.

Swallow Syncope

Swallowing has been presumed to cause syncope, and the mechanism responsible seems to be a cardiac arrhythmia. Sino-atrial block, atrio-ventricular block, complete heart block, sinus and junctional bradycardias, premature ventricular contractions, as well as asystole have been documented to occur with swallowing[38-40]. Most of these arrhythmias are prevented by using atropine, suggesting a vagal reflex. Several individuals have had esophagael diverticuli, and syncope has been induced by balloon inflation at the site of the diverticuli. Other esophageal diseases associated with swallowing and arrhythmias have included esophageal spasm, peptic strictures, and achalasia. Observations of individuals with glossopharyn-geal neuralgia have shown that soon after pain begins, there is a brady-cardia and syncope ensues. This is also a vagal reflex, for the arrhythmia and syncope can be prevented with atropine.

Pacemaker-Induced Syncope

Inhibition of impulse signals from permanent pacemakers have been observed to occur near certain electrical appliances, electric razors, micro-wave ovens, diathermy machines, electrical mixers, vacuum cleaners, hair dryers, automobile engines, or even television transmitters[41]. Some pulse generators are covered with titanium to prevent outside interference while others will convert to a fixed-rate mode.

Drug-Induced Syncope

Several categories of medication produce syncope. The mechanism is either vasodilatation or cardiac arrhythmia. Vasodilators include nitro-glycerine, long-acting nitrates, antihypertensive medications, diuretics, phenothiazine derivatives, and quinidine. Digitalis and quinidine[42,43] are medications most likely to produce ventricular arrhythmias, but overdosage of tricyclic antidepressants may also have this effect.

CONCLUSION

This has been an attempt to present an extensive evaluation for cardiovascular causes of syncope. We have arbitrarily excluded psychologic, endocrine, and neurologic etiologies from consideration. The differential diagnosis of syncope is a frequent challenge, but puzzling cases can lead to gratifying treatment results when the etiology is determined.

References

1. Wayne, H.H.: Syncope: physiological considerations and an analysis of the clinical characteristics in 510 patients. *Am. J. Med.*, **30**: 418, 1961.
2. Wright, Jr., K.E. and McIntosh, H.D.: Syncope: a review of pathophysiological mechanisms. *Prog. Cardiovasc. Dis.*, **13 (6)**: 580, 1971.
3. Friedberg, C.K.: Syncope: pathological physiology: differential diagnosis and treatment, Parts I and II. *Mod. Concepts Cardiovasc. Dis.*, **40**: 55 and 61, 1971.
4. Dunn, M.: Orthostatic hypotension. *Hosp. Med.*, **7**: 119, 1971.
5. Wechsler, R.L., Roth, J.L.A., and Bockus, H.: The use of serial blood volumes and head-up tilts as important indicators of therapy in patients with bleeding from the gastrointestinal tract. *Gastroenterology*, **30**: 221, 1956.
6. Metcalfe, J. and Ueland, K.: Maternal cardiovascular adjustments to pregnancy. *Prog. Cardiovasc. Dis.*, **16 (4)**: 363, 1974.
7. Lewis, Jr., H.D. and Dunn, M.: Orthostatic hypotension syndrome: a case report. *Am. Heart J.*, **74 (3)**: 396, 1967.
8. Shy, G.M. and Drager, G.A.: A neurological syndrome associated with orthostatic hypotension: a clinico-pathologic study. *Arch. Neurol.*, **2**: 511, 1960.
9. Bannister, R., Ardill, L., and Fentem, P.: An assessment of various methods of treatment of idiopathic orthostatic hypotension. *Quarterly J. Med.*, New Series, **38 (152)**: 377, 1969.
10. Jervell, A. and Lange-Nielsen, F.: Congenital deaf mutism, functional heart disease, with prolongation of the Q-T interval and sudden death. *Am. Heart J.*, **54**: 59, 1957.
11. Romano, C., Genrme, G., and Pongiglione, R.: Aritmic cardiache rare dell'etta pediatrica, II. Accessi pincopali per fibrillozione ventricolare porossisties. (Presentazione del primo case della letteratura pediatrica italiana.) *Clinic Paediate*, **45**: 656, 1963.
12. Ward, O.: Report Council Royal Academy of Medicine in Ireland. 1963.
13. Vincent, G.M., Abildskov, J.A., and Burgess, M.J.: Q-T interval syndromes. *Prog. Cardiovasc. Dis.*, **16 (6)**: 523, 1974.
14. Mathews, Jr., E.C., Blount, Jr., A.W., and Townsend, J.I.: Q-T prolongation and ventricular arrhythmias, with and without deafness, in the same family. *Am. J. Cardiol.*, **29**: 702, 1972.
15. Furlanello, F., Macca, F., and Palu, C.: Observation on a case of Jervell and Lange-Neilsen syndrome in an adult. *Brit. Heart J.*, **34**: 648, 1972.
16. Csanady, M. and Kiss, Z.: Heritable Q-T prolongation without congenital deafness (Romano-Ward syndrome). *Chest*, **64 (3)**: 359, 1973.
17. James, T.N.: QT prolongation and sudden death. *Mod. Concepts Cardiovas. Dis.*, **38**: 35, 1969.
18. Rosenbaum, M., Elizari, M., and Lazzari, J.: The hemiblocks. *Tampa Tracings.* 1970.
19. Pryor, R. and Blount, S.G.: The clinical significance of true left axis deviation. *Am. Heart J.*, **72**: 391, 1966.
20. Lasser, R.P., Haft, J.I., and Friedberg, C.K.: Relationship of right bundle branch block and marked left axis deviation (with left parietal or peri-infarction block) to complete heart block and syncope. *Circulation*, **37**: 429, 1968.

21. Moss, A.J. and Davis, R.J.: Brady-tachy syndrome. *Prog. Cardiovasc. Dis.*, **16** (5): 439, 1974.
22. Weiss, S. and Baker, J.P.: The carotid sinus reflex in health and disease: its role in the causation of fainting and convulsions. *Medicine*, **12**: 297, 1933.
23. Thomas, J.E.: Hyperactive carotid sinus reflex and carotid sinus syncope. *Mayo Clin. Proc.*, **44**: 127, 1969.
24. von Maur, K., Nelson, E.W., Holsinger, Jr., J.W., and Eliot, R.S.: Hypersensitive carotid sinus syncope treated by implantable demand cardiac pacemaker. *Am. J. Cardiol.*, **29**: 109, 1972.
25. Schwartz, L.S., Goldfischer, J., Sprague, G.J., and Schwartz, S.P.: Syncope and sudden death in aortic stenosis. *Am. J. Cardiol.*, **23**: 647, 1969.
26. Joseph, S., Balcon, R., and McDonald, L.: Syncope in hypertrophic obstructive cardiomyopathy due to asystole. *Brit. Heart J.*, **34**: 974, 1972.
27. Soloff, L.A. and Rodman, T.: Acute pulmonary embolism. II. Clinical. *Am. Heart J.*, **74** (6): 829, 1967.
28. Oster, M.W. and Leslie, B.: Syncope and pulmonary embolism. *JAMA*, **224** (5): 630, 1973.
29. Dressler, W.: Effort syncope as an early manifestation of primary pulmonary hypertension. *Am. J. Med. Sci.*, **223**: 131, 1952.
30. Reivich, M., Holling, H.E., Roberts, B., and Toole, J.F.: Reversal of blood flow through the vertebral artery and its effect on cerebral circulation. *N. Engl. J. Med.*, **265**: 878, 1961.
31. Kerr, Jr., A. and Derbes, V.J.: The syndrome of cough syncope. *Ann. Intern. Med.*, **39**: 1240, 1953.
32. Sharpey-Schafer, E.P.: The mechanism of syncope after coughing. *Brit. Heart J.*, **2**: 860, 1953.
33. McIntosh, H.D., Estes, E.H., and Warren, J.V.: The mechanism of cough syncope. *Am. Heart J.*, **52** (1): 70, 1956.
34. Compton, D., Hill, P. McN., and Sinclair, J.D.: Weight-lifter's blackout. *Lancet*, **2**: 1234, 1973.
35. Proudfit, W.L. and Forteza, M.E.: Micturition syncope. *N. Engl. J. Med.*, **260** (7): 328, 1959.
36. Haldane, J.H.: Micturition syncope: Two case reports and a review of the literature. *Can. Med. Assoc. J.*, **101**: 712, 1969.
37. Schoenberg, B.S., Kuglitsch, J.F., and Karnes, W.E.: Micturition syncope—not a single entity. *JAMA*, **229** (12): 1631, 1974.
38. Levin, B. and Posner, J.B.: Swallow syncope. Report of a case and review of the literature. *Neurol.*, **22**: 1086, 1972.
39. Lichstein, E. and Chadda, K.D.: Atrioventricular block produced by swallowing, with documentation by His bundle recordings. *Am. J. Cardiol.*, **29**: 561, 1972.
40. Alstrup, P. and Pedersen, S.A.: A case of syncope on swallowing secondary to diffuse Oesophageal spasm. *Acta Med. Scand.*, **193**: 365, 1973.
41. D'Cunha, G.F., Nicoud, T., Pemberton, A.H., Rosenbaum, F.F., and Boticceli, J.T.: Syncopal attacks arising from erratic demand pacemaker function in the vicinity of a television transmitter. *Am. J. Cardiol.*, **31**: 789, 1973.
42. Selzer, A. and Wray, H.W.: Quinidine syncope: paroxysmal ventricular fibrillation occurring during treatment of chronic atrial arrhythmias. *Circulation*, **30**: 17, 1964.
43. Selzer, A. and Wray, H.W.: Lidocaine for quinidine syncope. *Chest*, **66**: 463, 1974.

CHAPTER 7

The Use of Chest Roentgenograms in Cardiac Emergencies

James J. Phalen, M.D.; Charles A. Dobry, M.D.;
Harold A. Baltaxe, M.D.

This chapter presents guidelines for the use of radiologic investigations in patients with an apparent cardiac emergency. Presented are the appropriate pathophysiologic bases for radiographic changes, discussions of those conditions most amenable to radiologic detection, precautions regarding the interpretation of various techniques, and a discussion of the type of techniques available and appropriate.

INTRODUCTION

The radiographic evaluation of the heart during cardiac emergencies, although not a perfect tool, can give valuable information which will affect the management of the patient. Positive and negative information can be obtained which may be of great assistance both diagnostically and prognostically. Radiographic signs may precede clinical manifestations, as in the case of congestive heart failure.

The value of the chest radiograph in cardiac emergencies lies chiefly in the diagnosis of the disease state, in estimating its severity, and in the followup of the efficacy and/or complications of the treatment program. In addition, the detection of conditions or complications coincidental to the primary disease can be greatly facilitated by chest roentgenography.

ACUTE CONGESTIVE HEART FAILURE

Congestive heart failure (CHF) is one of the presenting signs common to many cardiac emergencies. Recognition of the radiographic manifestations and progression of CHF is of prime importance. Cardiac enlargement may or may not be present in CHF and is an unreliable indicator of the presence of this condition. Emphasis must be placed on the evaluation of the pulmonary circulation and the abnormal accumulation of intrapulmonary and intrathoracic fluid. Radiographic observations reflect changing hemodynamic events and allow the clinician to gauge both progression and response to therapy.

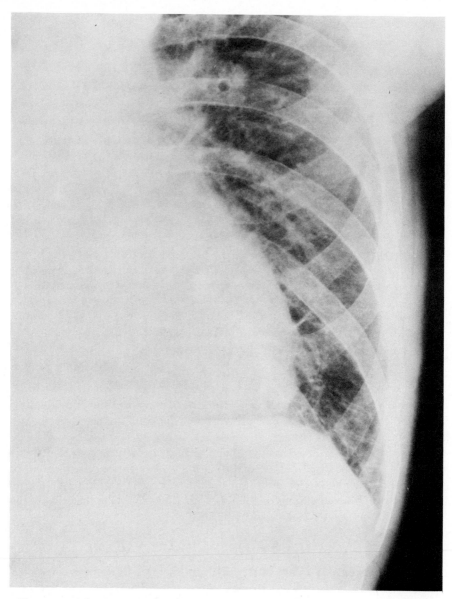

Figure 1 Edema of interlobular septa (Kerley B Lines) presents as short (1-3 cm) usually fine lines perpendicular to and reaching the pleural surface in the lower lung fields. Several septal lines can be seen in this close-up view of the left lower lobe. These lines commonly appear whenever there is elevated pulmonary venous pressure—most notably in case of mitral valve disease or left heart failure. The septal lines commonly disappear as the pulmonary venous pressure returns to normal. Similar lines may appear and may become fixed in interstitial disease processes of the lung and may be the result of inflammatory infiltration and collagen proliferation of the interlobular septa as well as edema. These lines may also become permanent in chronic congestive heart failure.

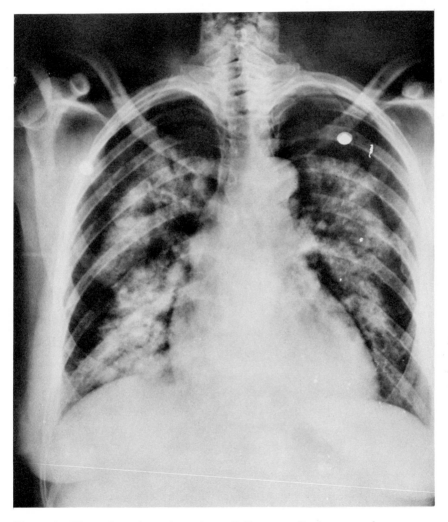

Figure 2 This "classic bat-wing or butterfly" pattern of pulmonary edema occurs in about 5% of cases.

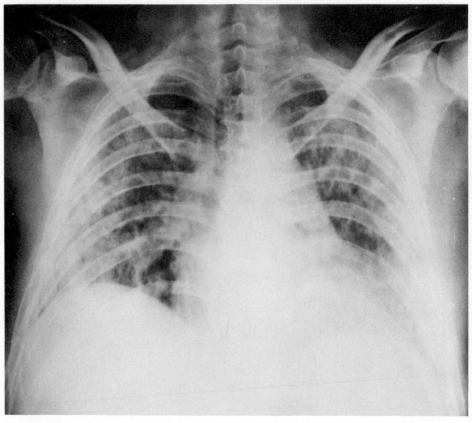

Figure 3 Patchy inhomogenous diffuse distribution of the alveolar fluid is a more common appearance of pulmonary edema, especially in the early phases.

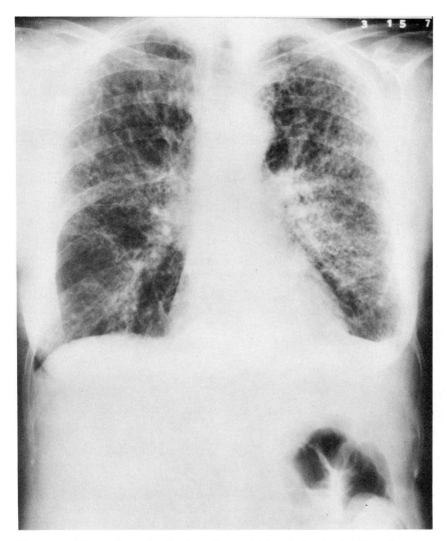

Figure 4 Non-uniform distribution of interstitial and alveolar fluid in pulmonary edema may occur, especially in patients with chronic inflammatory or obstructive lung disease. Areas of the lung with the more normal pulmonary circulation or in areas where lymphatic obstruction has occurred will accumulate edema fluid to a larger extent. The resultant radiographic appearance can be confusing and comparison with prior films and correlation with clinical findings is necessary for most precise interpretaton.

This example demonstrates early pulmonary edema with interval increase in interstitial density in the left and right upper lungs with increased blurring of the vessel margins in a patient with both COPD and old inflammatory disease. The blunting of the left pleural sulcus resulted from old inflammatory scarring.

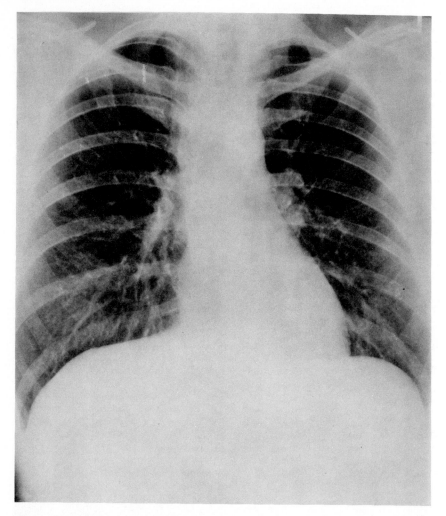

Figure 5 The pleuropericarditis of the postmyocardial infarction syndrome (Dressler's syndrome) may be recognized radiographically by the presence of pericardial and/or pleural effusion, as in this case (Dr. Eliot has really put his heart into this book).

Panel a is the premorbid control study.

Panel b was obtained 15 days after myocardial infarction and reveals a small left pleural effusion and mild increase in heart size.

Panel c, a close-up view of the lateral film, again reveals the left pleural effusion.

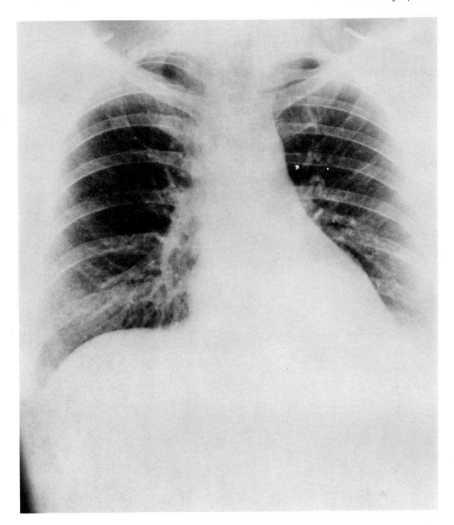

The pericardial effusion (*) indicates that at least part of the apparent increase in heart size is due to the effusion. The radiodensity of the heart (+) is more posterior.

Panel d is a line tracing of Panel c. The (*) represents the pericardial effusion, bounded in front by the slightly radiolucent retrosternal fat (A) and posteriorly by the radiolucent epicardial fat (B). The pericardium can often be seen in normal people but should never be greater than 2 millimeters thick. Excessive thickness indicates pericardial effusion or pericardial thickening.

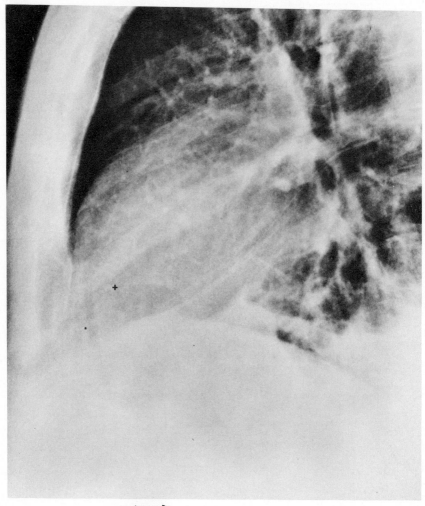

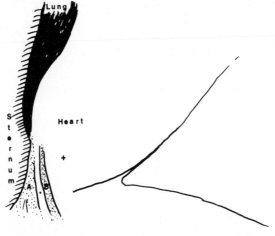

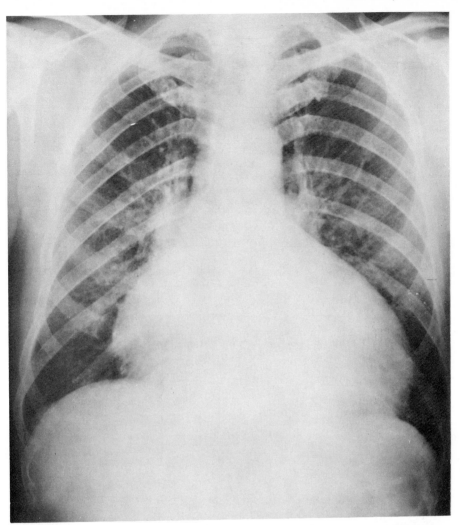

Figure 6 Large pericardial effusions such as this cause the lower part of the cardiac silhouette to be disproportionately wide—the so called "water bottle" contour—when the patient is erect. The silhouette assumes a globular contour when the patient is supine. This change in contour can be of diagnostic assistance in some cases when attempting to differentiate between large pericardial effusion and cardiac dilatation.

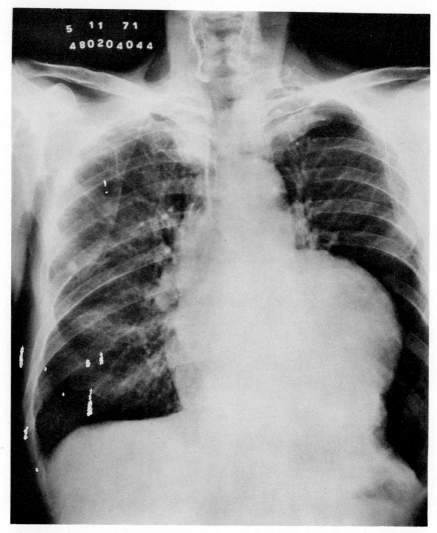

Figure 7 Ventricular aneurysms, when evident on the chest x-ray, alter the cardiac contour by the addition of a second convexity above the cardiac apex or by accentuating the convexity of the apex. They seldom reach the magnitude of the large left ventricular aneurysm above the cardiac apex illustrated in this case.

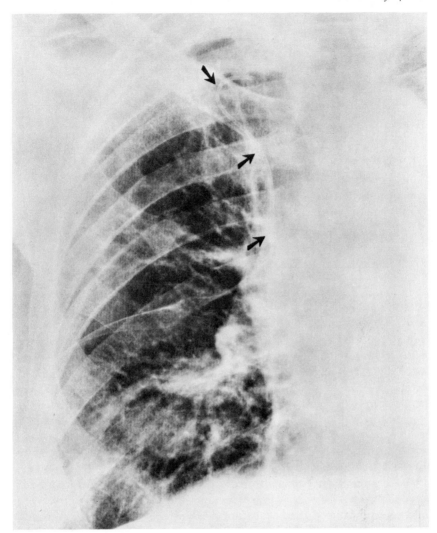

Figure 8 The course, location and possible complications attendant to the use of therapeutic and monitoring devices introduced into natural or created body spaces can be checked radiographically. Retained intravascular fragments, as seen in this case, can commonly be removed non-operatively by physicians expert in vascular catheterization techniques.

As the left ventricle fails, whatever the reason may be, the left ventricular end diastolic pressure (LVEDP) increases with more or less concomitant dilatation of the left ventricle. The left atrial pressure rises in concert with the LVEDP and enlarges more or less rapidly depending on its compliance. As the left atrial pressure rises in turn it produces pulmonary venous hypertension and eventually pulmonary arterial hypertension. In the acute condition when the pulmonary venous pressure rises beyond 15 to 18 mm of mercury, the first recognizable radiographic changes become evident[26].

Dilatation of the upper lobe veins heralds the first apparent radiographic changes of CHF[23,30,34,35]. The engorgement of these veins is due to increased pulmonary venous pressure. Redistribution of blood to the upper lobes is thought to be due to perivascular edema in the lower lobes which is caused by the upright position of the patient and which results in localized arterial hypertension[40]. This produces shunting to areas of less resistance which are located in the upper lobes. The exact pathogenesis, however, of this redistribution has not been fully elucidated[8,12,15,26,29,31,34,36,37,40]. The changes of redistribution become more obvious with increased constriction of lower lobe vessels and with increased shunting of blood to the upper lungs.

As the pulmonary venous pressure rises above 18 to 20 mm of mercury, there is accumulation of fluid in extravascular areas which may be visualized radiographically. Initially, there are faint non-uniform patchy or reticular densities in the lung bases which blur the edges of the pulmonary vessels[15,26,30,35]. This collection is largely interstitial (localized in the interalveolar septal wall and in the perivascular interstitial space)[36]. As the fluid increases in extent and volume, interstitial structures not normally visible become apparent on the chest radiograph. Thus, the interlobular septa may become thickened by edema and visible radiographically as short lines perpendicular to and reaching the pleural surface in the lower lungs (Kerley's B Lines)[10]

When the pulmonary venous pressure rises above 25 mm of mercury and certainly when it exceeds 30 mm of mercury, the acinus becomes filled with fluid resulting in the roentgenographic changes of pulmonary edema[26,30]. The alveolar pulmonary edema may appear in the classic "bat wing" perihilar radiating pattern[9], with relative sparing of the periphery of the lung. Atypical patterns such as unilateral, lobar, or patchy edema are not uncommon, especially in chronic obstructive pulmonary disease. The edema usually has a confluent tendency, ill-defined edges, and tends not to follow lobar or a segmental anatomy. It often results in the demonstration of the air filled bronchi seen through a consolidated lung ("air bronchogram").

As failure progresses pulmonary arterial dilatation ensues reflecting the increased pulmonary artery pressure. As the pulmonary artery pressure rises, it puts a greater load on the right ventricle which eventually results in right heart failure and dilatation of this chamber. Right ventricular dilatation is diagnosed radiographically by the filling in of the retrosternal space on the lateral chest film. It produces cardiac enlargement and on the left anterior oblique projection is detected by the pushing back of the left ventricle beyond the spine and the elevation of the apex above the diaphragm. The azygous vein and superior vena cava also may dilate and this can be easily detected on the chest x-ray. The normal azygous vein measures less than 8 mm on the PA, upright chest film[19]. Pleural effusion may make its appearance together with right ventricular failure, because the lymphatics of the parietal pleura (which drain into the systemic venous system) are usually able to keep the pleural space relatively dry until the systemic venous pressure rises[6,28].

The coexistence of COPD may significantly alter the radiographic manifestations of congestive heart failure. The chest roentgen findings vary and are related to the degree and form of the underlying lung disease[17,18]. Infiltrates are usually patchy in distribution as the lesser affected portions of the lungs tend to show changes of cardiac heart failure sooner and to a greater degree than the more severely damaged areas[18,30].

The chest x-ray during uncomplicated myocardial infarction is usually normal. More complicated myocardial infarctions may result in CHF with corresponding x-ray findings. Those patients who have such radiographic findings have a worse prognosis than those with normal chest x-rays[11,32,39].

COMPLICATIONS OF MYOCARDIAL INFARCTION

The complications of myocardial infarction can be summarized as follows:

1. Rupture of the interventricular septum.
2. Papillary muscle dysfunction, ruptured cordi, or papillary muscle necrosis.
3. Hemopericardium and pericardial effusion.
4. Rupture of the left ventricle.
5. Ventricular aneurysms.

1.*Rupture of the interventricular septum* occurs in 0.1 to 2% of patients with myocardial infarction[14,25]. The rupture is caused by a lesion of the left anterior descending coronary artery or a lesion of the posterior descending artery which both give rise to septal branches. The time of rupture varies, but averages 7 days post-myocardial infarction[25]. Fifty percent of patients with ventricular septal defect due to post-myocardial infarction will die within the first week[25]. Some patients, however, can survive for years. The radiographic findings of a rupture of the interventricular septum will be caused by the hemodynamic effects of the rupture. A left to right shunt will be established and this will produce an overcirculation of the pulmonary arteries. The main pulmonary artery as well as the pulmonary artery branches will dilate. These findings, however, may not be easily detectable due to the associated pulmonary edema which often obscures the dilated vessels. Clinically, the rupture of the interventricular septum is difficult to distinguish from mitral insufficiency caused by either papillary muscle dysfunction or a papillary muscle rupture. The appearance of a systolic murmur with the above described radiographic findings may alert one to the possibility of either a rupture of the interventricular septum or mitral insufficiency. The diagnosis can be made either angiographically via left ventriculography or by floating a balloon catheter into the pulmonary artery and sampling the blood for oxygen saturation.

2. *Mitral insufficiency caused by papillary muscle dysfunction or a ruptured papillary muscle.* Myocardial infarction of the base of the heart may produce papillary muscle dysfunction or rupture. As mentioned above, the clinical presentation of this condition is very similar to that of the rupture of the interventricular septum. Radiographically, one may be able to detect tremendous enlargement of the left atrium and severe pulmonary venous congestion. The patients may go into pulmonary edema and massive cardiac enlargement. This diagnosis can also be made angiographically, but with the new advent of echocardiography an invasive procedure may not be necessary (see Chapter 8).

3. *Hemopericardium and pericardial effusion.* A number of patients with acute myocardial infarction may present with a pericardial effusion or a hemopericardium. The radiographic changes of pericardial effusion range from apparently normal to the grossly "dilated" and globular appearing heart[3,19,22,28]. Fluoroscopically, the pulsations of the heart may be decreased. They may or may not be associated with changes of pulmonary venous hypertension. The most reliable radiographic sign for pericardial effusion is the displaced epicardial fat[21]. The pericardial space may occasionally be seen on a normal lateral chest x-ray as a lucent line in the retrosternal region contrasted by retrosternal fat anteriorly and epicardial fat posteriorly. When fluid is present in the pericardial space there is apparent thickening of this pericardial line as the fluid separates the pericardium from the epicardial fat, the apparent separation depending on the volume of fluid present. Large effusions result in broadening of the lower heart contour, obliteration of the cardiophrenic angles, and changing of the usual concave upper heart border to a convex configuration[3]. In the past the most reliable diagnostic tool for pericardial effusion was injection of either contrast or CO_2 into the right atrium. Recently, ultrasonography has replaced the invasive techniques and can reliably demonstrate pericardial effusion (see Chapter 8). Computerized axial tomography will likely be very useful in diagnosing pericardial effusion.

Chronic pericarditis following myocardial infarction or Dressler's syndrome can be diagnosed radiographically by noting the sudden cardiac enlargement in a patient who had a normal cardiac contour 3 to 6 weeks following a myocardial infarction.

4. *Left ventricular rupture.* This is a catastrophic advent during a myocardial infarction and results in cardiogenic shock and sudden death of the patient. The roentgenographic diagnosis is non-contributory in this condition.

5. *Ventricular aneurysms.* The formation of ventricular aneurysms is not really a cardiac emergency. These aneurysms develop weeks after the advent of the acute myocardial infarction[1]. The infarcted muscle is replaced by

fibrotic tissue and produces an area of dyskinesia. If the aneurysm is totally fibrotic, it may result in paradoxical motion in the left ventricle. Thus, during ventricular systole the aneurysm will dilate instead of contracting. This observation can often be made fluoroscopically. When the myocardial infarction only produces partial fibrosis, the area affected will become akinetic. This means that the infarcted portion does not contract during systole. This finding cannot be made by chest fluoroscopy and can only be seen by left ventriculography. Old aneurysms sometimes calcify, and this may be detected on the plain chest roentgenogram.

Left ventricular aneuryms rarely rupture. The main hemodynamic difficulty caused by the left ventricular aneurysm is left ventricular dysfunction resulting in left ventricular failure. Furthermore, left ventricular aneurysms may contain clots which can break up and shower into the systemic circulation, resulting in strokes, myocardial infarctions, and other vascular accidents.

Following an acute myocardial infarction, the patient should be examined periodically by chest roentgenograms since any sudden change in size or configuration of the heart should be suspected as representing a left ventricular aneurysm.

TRAUMA TO THE HEART AND GREAT VESSELS

Trauma to the heart can be either caused by a penetrating object or by compression of the chest[7,14,33]. Trauma by a penetrating object such as a knife or a bullet will often produce a hemopericardium and may result in the formation of a pseudoaneurysm. The radiographic appearance of the pseudoaneurysm is similar to that described in the previous portion on cardiac aneurysms. Such pseudoaneurysms may remain stagnant, but may rupture and require immediate surgery. If the penetrating object injures a major coronary artery, the result is catastrophic.

Compression of the chest may injure a major coronary artery and result in a myocardial infarction. Rupture of the interventricular septum may result from this. If a patient develops a myocardial infarction following trauma, a direct injury of one of the coronary arteries must be suspected.

Rupture of the papillary muscles and interventricular valves is also seen, particularly when the blunt trauma occurs during ventricular diastole. The valvular attachments, particularly the mitral one, may be injured in this fashion and produce mitral insufficiency.

TRAUMATIC RUPTURE OF THE GREAT VESSELS

The most common great vessel to be affected by trauma is the aorta. This usually occurs secondary to a deceleration injury[13]. Although a majority of the patients will die instantly, 10 to 20% will survive the initial insult. Without proper diagnosis and surgical intervention, 50% of the survivors will perish within 24 hours[5,33]. The rupture usually occurs distal to the left subclavian artery where the aorta is the least fixed. The ascending portion of the aorta is fixed by the great vessels to the head. Beyond the left subclavian artery, the aorta is mobile and therefore can tear more easily. The tear may involve all three layers of the vessel, but may be confined to either intima, intima and media, or intima, media, and adventitia. According to the extent of the injury, the aneurysm will either have two, one or no layers. The prognosis will also vary according to the severity of the injury. The clinical symptomatology varies and a significant number of patients present no complaints[20]. Repeated radiographic examination of the chest, prompted by a high degree of suspicion from the mechanism of injury, is of invaluable assistance[7,38]. When these aneurysms become chronic they may calcify. Calcified traumatic aneurysms of the aorta may remain for years without rupturing. The opinions differ as to whether a calcified traumatic thoracic aneurysm should be repaired.

The innominate artery is the second most likely structure to be injured during trauma. Again, the severity of the injury can vary and therefore several types of lesions can be seen. A total rupture of the innominate artery is usually catastrophic and results in rapid death. False aneurysm of the innominate artery where one or two layers have been ruptured is not an uncommon lesion. This manifests by widening of the mediastinum and can be diagnosed angiographically. At times AV fistula between the innominate artery and the superior vena cava can be found. This again results in tremendous enlargement of the superior vena cava which is diagnosed on the plain film by marked widening of the mediastinum. These AV fistulae can be fairly well tolerated; however, they will eventually cause high output left ventricular failure.

Most of these lesions to the chest will result in the widening of the superior mediastinum and the aortic knob may often become indistinct[7,20,33]. As the initial examination of the chest may not be diagnostic or even suggestive, serial films are indicated. In any questionable case, arteriography is indicated and will be diagnostic.

DISSECTING ANEURYSMS

Most dissecting aneurysms are seondary to medial cystic necrosis of the aorta. This condition is seen in Marfan's disease or can be due to long standing systemic hypertension. Although the clinical signs of sudden "tearing" chest pain with radiation to the back is strongly suggestive of a dissection, its variability in occurrence and position indicates that other means and diagnostic observations be used to document the presence of the dissecting aneurysm[2,4]. Clinically, dissecting aneurysm can be mistaken for a myocardial infarction or a pulmonary embolus. This error is particularly committed in the younger patients where a dissection of the aorta is difficult to suspect. Trauma to the chest may also produce a dissection in an individual who has the predisposing factor of medial cystic necrosis of the aorta.

The radiographs of the chest in dissecting aneurysm usually show abnormalities in the contour of the aorta and serial films are important. There is usually widening of the aortic shadow and the mediastinum[2]. If the patient has intimal calcification and if this calcification is displaced away from the outer border of the aorta, a dissection of the aorta must be suspected. This sign, however, is only reliable if the displacement is seen on films obtained in several projections. Pleural effusion, displacement of the trachea, and displacement of the esophagus have also been described, but are not pathognomonic[2,5,24]. Arteriography is diagnostic and must be employed in suspected cases. Computerized axial tomography might become a very useful tool in diagnosing this condition.

EVALUATION OF THERAPY

The efficacy of the treatment given to the patient can be evaluated by observing the progression or regression of the lesions seen radiographically. With continuing scientific advancements, numerous monitoring and therapeutic devices are in common usage. Their position must be carefully studied for proper location and for potential complications caused by their use. Any intravascular monitoring device may terminate in an undesirable location. Rarely a fragment of a device may be separated and become a free intravascular foreign body[16]. Pacemakers may be placed incorrectly into the coronary sinus, right atrium, or inferior vena cava and hepatic veins. Occasionally, the pacemaker may perforate the heart. These malpositions can be easily diagnosed by plain film chest x-rays. Pacemaker wires can be broken which can also easily be seen on a chest x-ray. The condition of the pacemaker batteries can be ascertained radiographically. Thrombosis or embolus may result from the intravascular devices. The direct subclavian approach to the intravascular placement of catheters can be accompanied by the complications of local hemorrhage, pneumothorax, extravascular placement, and undesirable catheter placement.

Flow directed double lumen balloon tipped catheters (e.g. Swan-Ganz) may cause pulmonary infarction if left in place for more than 72 hours in a wedged position or with continual inflation of the balloon[27]. All of these catheters are radiopaque and their position can be monitored radiographically. If a pulmonary infarction occurs, it follows the usual roentgenographic pattern of infarction secondary to embolization.

Malposition of nasogastric or endotracheal tubes can be diagnosed in the intensive care unit by the utilization of portable x-ray equipment.

TECHNICAL FACTORS

The most critical technical factors to consider in evaluating the chest films are:

1. Is the patient supine or erect?
2. What is the degree of pulmonary inflation?

3. What is the distance from tube to film?

When the patient is supine a number of physiologic changes occur—the upper mediastinal veins, including the superior vena cava and azygos, dilate resulting in mediastinal widening; the heart may become more globular in appearance; and the usual disparity between upper lobe and lower lobe veins is abolished. Therefore, several of the signs previously described for pulmonary and systemic venous hypertension are no longer valid and detection of pathologic widening of the mediastinum becomes more difficult.

When the radiograph is taken during less than adequate pulmonary inflation (relative expiration), the pulmonary vessels appear crowded, especially in the lung bases. The upper lobe-lower lobe pulmonary venous ratio is altered and the heart may appear enlarged. Alveolar hypoventilation in the lung bases results in a relative increase in lung density and a tendency toward blurring of vascular shadows. All of these findings may mimic early changes of congestive heart failure.

The usual x-ray tube to x-ray film distance is 72" or greater. Reducing this distance results in magnification of intrathoracic structures, especially the heart, and particularly if the projection is anteroposterior (AP). This magnification is much less marked, usually no more than 10%, if the projection is AP but the tube-film distance is 72" or greater.

Although *changes* in heart size may be of great clinical significance, cardiac size must be judged with caution when technical factors differ.

CONCLUSION

It is hoped that the value of the chest radiograph in cardiac emergencies has been stressed and that the clinician dealing with cardiac emergencies will have frequent recourse to this diagnostic tool.

References

1. Baron, M.G.: Post infarction aneurysm of the left ventricle. *Circulation*, **43**: 762, 1970.
2. Baron, M.G.: Dissecting aneurysms of the aorta. *Circulation*, **43**: 933, 1971.
3. Baron, M.G.: Pericardial effusions. *Circulation*, **44**: 294, 1971.
4. Beachley, M.C.: Roentgenographic evaluation of dissecting aneurysms of the aorta. *Am. J. Roentgenol.*, **121**: 617, 1974.
5. Bennett, D.E. and Cherry, J.K.: Natural history of traumatic aneurysms of the aorta. *Surg.*, **61**: 516, 1967.
6. Black, L.F.: The pleural space and pleural fluid. *Mayo Clin. Proc.*, **47**: 493, 1972.
7. Fishbone, G. et al: Trauma to the thoracic aorta and great vessels. *Radiol. Clin. N. Am.*, **11**: 543, 1973.
8. Fishman, A.P.: Pulmonary edema. The water-exchanging function of the lung. *Circulation*, **46**: 390, 1972.
9. Fleischner, F.: The butterfly pattern of acute pulmonary edema. *Am. J. Cardiol.*, **20**: 39, 1967.
10. Fleming, P.R. and Simon, M.: The hemodynamic significance of intrapulmonary septal lymphatic lines (Lines B of Kerley). *Fact. Radiol. J.*, **9**: 33, 1958.

11. Franken, T., Thelen, M., and Thurn, P.: Roentgen examination of the thorax in acute myocardial infarction. *Fortschr. Geb. Roentg.*, **122**: 29, 1975.
12. Gaar, K.A. et al: Effect of capillary pressure and plasma protein on development of pulmonary edema. *Am. J. Physiol.*, **213**: 79, 1967.
13. Greendyke, R.M.: Traumatic rupture of the aorta with special reference to automobile accidents. *JAMA*, **195**: 527, 1966.
14. Heikkila, J., Karesoja, M., and Luomanmaki, K.: Ruptured interventricular septum complicating myocardial infarction. *Chest*, **66**: 6, 1974.
15. Heitzman, E.R.: Acute interstitial pulmonary edema. *Am. J. Roentgenol.*, **98**: 291, 1966.
16. Hipona, F. et al: Non-thoracotomy retrieval of intraluminal cardiovascular foreign bodies. *Radiol. Clin. N. Am.*, **9**: 503, 1971.
17. Hublitz, U.F. and Shapiro, J.H.: Atypical pulmonary patterns of congestive failure in chronic lung disease. *Radiol.*, **93**: 995, 1969.
18. Jacobson, G. et al: Vascular changes in pulmonary emphysema. *Am. J. Roentgenol.*, **100**: 374, 1967.
19. Keats, R. et al: Mensuration of the arch of the azygos vein and its application to the study of cardiopulmonary disease. *Radiol.*, **90**: 990, 1968.
20. Kirsch, M.M.: Roentgenographic evaluation of traumatic rupture of the aorta. *Surg. Gynec. Obstet.*, **131**: 900, 1970.
21. Lane, E.J. and Carsky, E.W.: Epicardial fat: lateral plain film analysis in normals and paricardial effusion. *Radiol.*, **91**: 1, 1968.
22. Lange, R.L. et al: Diagnostic signs in compressive cardiac disorders. *Circulation*, **33**: 763, 1966.
23. Lavender, J.P. and Doppman, J.: The hilum in pulmonary venous hypertension. *Brit. J. Radiol.*, **35**: 303, 1962.
24. Levy, S.: Acute thromboembolism associated with dissecting aneurysms of the aorta. *J. Thorac. Cardiovasc. Surg.*, **66**: 82, 1973.
25. Limsuwan, A.: VSD and ventricular aneurysm following myocardial infarction. *Chest*, **57**: 581, 1970.
26. McHugh, T.J. et al: Pulmonary vascular congestion in acute myocardial infarction: a hemodynamic and radiologic correlation. *Ann. Intern. Med.*, **76**: 29, 1972.
27. McLoud, T.C. and Putman, C.E.: Radiology of the Swan-Ganz catheter and associated pulmonary complications. *Radiol.*, **116**: 19, 1975.
28. Mellins, R.B. et al: Effect of systemic and pulmonary venous hypertension on pleural and pericardial fluid accumulation. *J. Appl. Physiol.*, **25**: 564, 1970.
29. Meyer, B.J.: Interstitial fluid pressures. *Circ. Res.*, **22**: 263, 1968.
30. Milne, E.N.C.: Correlation of physiologic findings with chest roentgenology. *Radiol. Clin. N. Am.*, **11**: 17, 1973.
31. Noble, W.H.: Lung mechanics in hypervolemic pulmonary edema. *J. Appl. Physiol.*, **28**: 681, 1975.
32. Norris, R.M. et al: Coronary prognostic index for predicting survival after recovery from acute myocardial infarction. *Lancet*, **II**: 485, 1970.
33. Parmley, L.F. et al: Nonpenetrating traumatic injury to the aorta. *Circulation*, **17**: 1086, 1958.
34. Rigler, Leo G. and Surprenant, E.L.: Pulmonary Edema. *Seminars in Roentgenol.*, **2**: 1, 1967.
35. Simon, Morris: The pulmonary vessels in incipient left ventricular decompensation. Radiologic Observations. *Circulation*, **24**: 185, 1961.
36. Staub, N.C.: The pathophysiology of pulmonary edema. *Human Path.*, **1**: 419, 1970.
37. Surette, G.D. et al: Roentgenographic study of blood flow redistribution in acute pulmonary edema in dogs. *Invest. Radiol.*, **10**: 109, 1975.
38. Sumbas, P.N.: Rupture of the aorta: a diagnostic triad. *Ann. Thorac. Surg.*, **15**: 405, 1973.

39. Waris, E.K. et al: Heart size and prognosis in myocardial infarction. *Am. Heart J.*, **71**: 187, 1966.
40. West, J.B. et al: Increased pulmonary vascular resistance in the dependent zone of the isolated dog lung caused by perivascular edema. *Circ. Res.*, **17**: 191, 1965.

CHAPTER 8

The Value of Echocardiography in Cardiac Emergencies

Alan D. Forker, M.D.; Steven Krueger, M.D.;
Robert Zucker, B.S.; Philip J. Hofschire, M.D.

One of the most recent technical advances for diagnostic evaluation of cardiac emergencies is that of echocardiography. This chapter is for non-echocardiographers seeking its appropriate use. It offers a non-invasive clinical diagnostic dimension to many recalcitrant clinical enigmas. The indications, advantages and liabilities of any new technique are fundamental to its appropriate, practical clinical implementation. The lucid summary provided should serve this current need.

Improvements in instrumentation and technique, and advances in knowledge in the past 10 years have now made echocardiography into a practical clinical tool. It now occupies a fundamental position among diagnostic techniques in cardiology. This chapter presents an overview of echocardiography as it relates to the diagnosis and management of acute cardiac emergencies. Table I lists those cardiac emergencies in which echocardiography has provided valuable information in our experience.

NORMAL ECHOCARDIOGRAM

All echocardiograms illustrated in this chapter were obtained on an Ekoline 20 echocardiograph coupled to either a Cambridge strip-chart recorder or a Honeywell 1856 Visicorder®. None of the photographs have been retouched for publication purposes. The standard technique of M-mode scan was employed[1].

The basic strategy in performing and interpreting echocardiograms is to identify a standard reference structure that is characteristic. From this standard reference structure other relationships became apparent. An example of this is found in the typical M shape and motion of the anterior leaflet of the mitral valve (Figure 1). The normal mitral valve echocardiogram has been named by the letters A-F. The A wave results from mitral opening in response to atrial contraction in late systole. Systole is present between points C and D. During this time the two mitral leaflets are in apposition and show a gradual motion towards the transducer and anterior chest wall. The E wave results from mitral valve opening in early diastole, and the E-F

TABLE I

I.   Silent mitral stenosis

II. Left atrial myxoma

III. Acute mitral insufficiency

    A. Predominant congestive cardiomyopathy

    B. Ruptured chordae tendineae

    C. Acute myocardial infarction with papillary muscle abnormality vs. ruptured interventricular septum

IV. Acute aortic valve insufficiency—bacterial endocarditis

V.   Pericardial tamponade vs. dilated left ventricle with severe congestive heart failure

VI. Unexplained syncope

    A. Left ventricular outflow tract obstruction

    B. Mitral valve prolapse

VII. Congenital heart disease

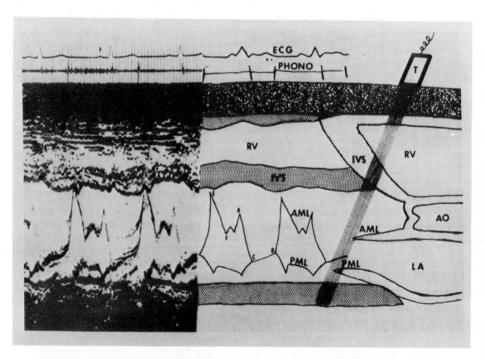

Figure 1 Normal echocardiogram with schematic representation of the anatomical structures detected by the examination. T—transducer on anterior chest wall. RV—right ventricle. IVS—interventricular septum. AML—anterior mitral leaflet. PML—posterior mitral leaflet. AO—aorta. LA—left atrium. (See text for description of normal mitral valve motion.)

slope reflects the rapidity of early diastolic left ventricular filling. The posterior mitral leaflet moves posteriorly during diastole and is a mirror image of the anterior leaflet. Due to the "tunnel vision" of the transducer on the chest wall, the transducer must be rotated along the long axis of the heart to image first the aorta and left atrium, then the mitral valve, and finally the apical region of the left ventricle[1].

Unfortunately, echocardiography is not an easy procedure to perform. Even in fully cooperative patients, complete information may not be obtained for many reasons, the most important of which is the proficiency of the echocardiographic technician. Patients with chest wall deformities create difficulty in obtaining satisfactory tracings. An acutely ill patient, who may be restless and uncooperative, and/or may have hyperinflation of the lungs due to mechanical ventilation, may make high quality echocardiography impossible.

SILENT MITRAL STENOSIS

Consider the clinical setting of a seriously ill patient with a low cardiac output and severe pulmonary hypertension. This patient could have severe mitral valve stenosis and yet have no auscultatory clues to the correct diagnosis. Due to calcification and/or severe fibrosis, the first heart sound may be soft with no audible opening snap. It may be impossible to hear a diastolic murmur due to the low flow across the mitral valve. In this setting, echocardiography can be of great diagnostic help.

The typical echocardiographic findings of mitral valve stenosis are: (1) a delayed E-F diastolic slope, (2) loss of the atrial kick of the anterior mitral valve leaflet in late diastole, and most important (3) abnormal motion of the posterior mitral valve leaflet in an anterior direction during diastole[2].

We have seen two patients with silent mitral stenosis. In both cases the echocardiogram provided the first clue to the correct diagnosis. The first was a female in her late 20's with a long history of "winter bronchitis" and recurrent bronchopulmonary infections. She had never been diagnosed as having mitral stenosis, but presented in acute pulmonary edema. Ascultation by two separate cardiologists yielded no findings of mitral valve stenosis. Echocardiography, however, was diagnostic of severe mitral valve stenosis with a flat E-F slope and anterior diastolic motion of the posterior mitral valve leaflet (Figure 2). Our second patient with silent mitral stenosis presented with a renal artery embolus.

Two recent papers have emphasized that the posterior mitral leaflet may occasionally be normal in mitral valve stenosis[3,4]. Of the 167 cases of mitral valve stenosis analyzed by Levisman et al, 16 patients had normal posterior mitral valve leaflet motion during diastole[3]. Five of these patients had severe mitral stenosis and four had significant mitral insufficiency. Despite the normal diastolic motion of the posterior mitral valve leaflet in these patients, mitral valve stenosis was still suspected because of two findings: (1) echocardiograms in all patients showed an anterior mitral valve leaflet which was

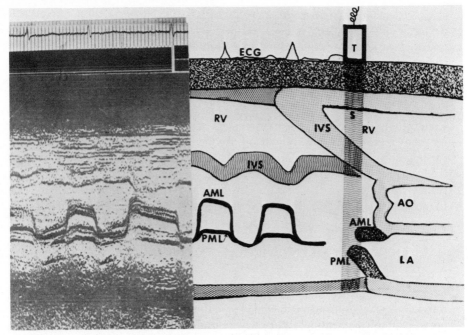

Figure 2 Echocardiogram of mitral valve stenosis. RV—right ventricle. IVS—interventricular septum. AML—anterior mitral leaflet. PML—posterior mitral leaflet. AO—aorta. LA—left atrium. Note the abnormal location during diastole of the posterior mitral leaflet, indicated by the small arrow.

thicker than normal, and (2) the late diastolic A wave height of the anterior mitral valve leaflet was reduced in all patients with normal sinus rhythm. We have seen one patient with significant mitral stenosis whose echocardiogram revealed normal posterior mitral valve leaflet motion (Figure 3).

It therefore seems reasonable that patients with unexplained symptoms of pulmonary congestion should have an echocardiogram to exclude mitral valve stenosis. Since even the echocardiogram may fail occasionally cardiac catheterization should still be considered if clinical suspicion of mitral stenosis is high.

LEFT ATRIAL MYXOMA

Patients with left atrial myxomas may present a confusing clinical picture. Classically the findings will mimic mitral valve stenosis, but occasionally a prolapsing tumor and a destroyed mitral valve may present as mitral insufficiency. The clinical picture may be further confused by systemic manifestations which falsely lead the clinician away from an intra-cardiac lesion. Echocardiography is an excellent tool for diagnosing a left atrial tumor, especially prolapsing ones. The echocardiographic diagnosis is established by demonstrating a layering of echoes behind the anterior leaflet of the mitral valve during diastole[5,6].

Sung et al recent emphasized that not all left atrial myxomas prolapse into

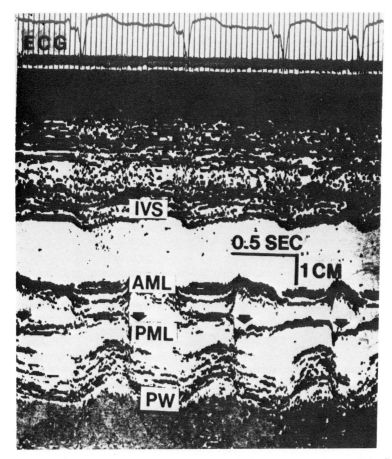

Figure 3 Echocardiogram of mitral valve stenosis with normal posterior leaflet. IVS—interventricular septum. AML—anterior mitral leaflet. PML—posterior mitral leaflet indicated by the black arrow, which shows normal posterior motion during diastole. PW—left ventricular posterior wall.

the left ventricle during diastole[7]. If the tumor does not prolapse, the clinical picture might not resemble that of mitral valve stenosis. Echocardiography may still be of diagnostic help. In this case the echocardiogram would show a layering of echoes in the left atrium immediately behind the posterior echo of the aortic root. However, the layering of echoes behind the anterior mitral leaflet during diastole, as occurs with a prolapsing atrial myxoma, may not be seen in the non-prolapsing type. It is therefore possible to overlook a left atrial myxoma if only the anterior mitral leaflet is observed, since this leaflet may move normally. A complete scan from the anterior mitral valve leaflet into the aorta and left atrium should always be performed to exclude the non-prolapsing myxoma.

Despite several attempts, we have never correctly diagnosed the presence of a left atrial thrombus. Technical problems frequently cause an artifact in the left atrium. These are usually the result of incorrect setting of the damping or gain controls. For this reason, we do not feel that echocardiography can reliably differentiate between an artifact and a thrombus.

ACUTE MITRAL INSUFFICIENCY

In the absence of coexistent mitral valve stenosis, the echocardiograph offers no clues to the diagnosis of chronic rheumatic mitral valve insufficiency. Echocardiography, however, is of value in certain acute situations, e.g. congestive cardiomyopathy with secondary mitral insufficiency and ruptured chordae tendineae. Echocardiographic findings may be present that allow the separation of acute papillary muscle dysfunction from acute ventricular septal rupture following acute myocardial infarction. These findings will be discussed individually.

Our echocardiographic experience with predominant congestive cardiomyopathy complicated by secondary mitral valve insufficiency agrees with that of Millward et al[8]. If the patient has a congestive cardiomyopathy as the most important underlying cardiac disease, there will be significant depression of left ventricular function, as measured by an increased left ventricular size and a depressed ejection fraction. The ejection fraction will be more normal in patients with predominant mitral insufficiency without myocardial dysfunction.

Two echocardiographic findings are used to diagnose ruptured chordae tendineae of the posterior mitral leaflet: pansystolic prolapse of the mitral valve, and the posterior mitral valve leaflet will appear "flail" in diastole, i.e. the posterior mitral valve leaflet will be abnormally displaced anteriorly during diastole[1,9]. In addition, mitral valve leaflets do not assume their normal mirror image configuration. Other observations, which may be of secondary help in any form of acute mitral insufficiency, are the echocardiographic findings of: (1) a smaller, more dynamic left atrium, (2) a hyperdynamic interventricular septum, (3) a hyperdynamic posterior left ventricular wall, and (4) a more normal ejection fraction. We have seen two patients with ruptured chordae tendineae of the posterior mitral valve leaflet (Figure 4). The criteria for diagnosing ruptured chordae to the anterior mitral leaflet are not as clearly established.

No echocardiographic diagnosis of papillary muscle rupture has been reported. This is not surprising since the grave clinical condition requires immediate diagnosis and surgical treatment. Since papillary muscle dysfunction is usually associated with a severely damaged left ventricle, the major indirect clues to the diagnosis are abnormal left ventricular wall motion[10] plus depressed left ventricular pump function[11]. Detection of asynergy of the ventricular septum by echocardiography is quite common with anterior infarction, but detection of posterior wall asynergy is more difficult with the single crystal technique. Left ventricular dilatation is commonly present with a poor ejection fraction. There are important limitations of measuring ejection fractions on the echocardiogram in the presence of

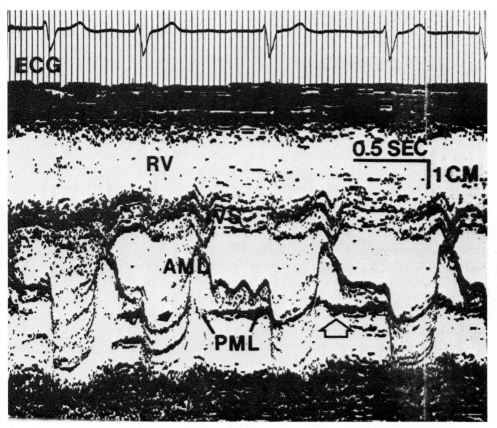

Figure 4 Echocardiogram of ruptured chordae to posterior mitral leaflet. RV—right ventricle. IVS—interventricular septum. AML—anterior mitral leaflet. PML—posterior mitral leaflet. The small black arrow indicates systole, although systolic prolapse is best identified in the last beat to the right of the picture. The large white arrow indicates the abnormal anterior position of the posterior mitral leaflet during diastole.

asynergy when one wall of the left ventricle is asynergic, i.e. the ejection fraction frequently is falsely normal.

When evaluating the etiology of a new systolic murmur after myocardial infarction, the clinical differentiation between papillary muscle dysfunction vs. ruptured interventricular septum is quite difficult. If a new murmur and thrill are localized to the left lower sternal border, it is most likely a ventricular septal defect. However, the murmur and thrill of a ruptured ventricular septum may be most prominent at the apex even in the absence of mitral valve insufficiency[12,13]. Chandraratna et al have reported their experience with echocardiography in three patients with a post myocardial infarction ventricular septal defect[14]. All three patients had dilated right ventricles ranging in size from 2.7 to 3.2 cm, with normal interventricular septal motion. Left ventricular dilatation was not found in any of the patients, and the left atrium was slightly enlarged (4.2 cm) in only one patient. For comparison, four patients with acute mitral insufficiency and pulmonary edema secondary to acute myocardial infarction were seen and evaluated by echocardiography. All four patients had normal right ventricular dimensions. Therefore, if an acute myocardial infarction patient presents with a new systolic murmur and the echocardiographic finding of a dilated right ventricle, the diagnosis of a ruptured ventricular septum should be given primary consideration[14].

DeJoseph et al recently reported one case of ventricular septal rupture studied by echocardiography[15]. First, they observed slightly paradoxic septal motion in systole with little diastolic motion; following septal rupture, large septal motion in diastole towards the anterior mitral valve leaflet developed. They reasoned that the upper portion of the septum turns flail with a basal septal infarction.

We have seen one patient with acute myocardial infarction and ruptured interventricular septum (Figure 5). This 68-year-old white male had an acute inferior wall myocardial infarction with no prior history of heart disease or murmur. Soon after hospital admission, he developed a new systolic murmur and developed severe congestive heart failure. Elevated jugular venous pressure and an enlarged pulsatile liver compatible with tricuspid valve insufficiency were present. The patient died 20 days post myocardial infarction of progressive pump failure. Autopsy revealed a ruptured interventricular septum. The initial echocardiogram, performed soon after the onset of the new murmur and congestive failure, revealed right ventricular enlargement and paradoxic ventricular septal motion (Figure 5A). This finding disagrees with the findings of Chandraratna in that all three of his patients had a normal ventricular septal motion. Our patient's paradoxic septal motion was probably due to significant tricuspid valve insufficiency creating right ventricular volume overload. The patient responded initially to vigorous diuretics and digitalis therapy. Four days following the initiation of therapy, the echocardiogram showed a smaller right ventricle and the interventricular septal motion had returned to normal (Figure 5B). A third echo was performed eight days before death. In contrast to the second echo, it again revealed an enlarged right ventricle (3.5 cm) but normal ventricular septal motion (Figure 5C). The patient had also developed a moderate posterior pericardial effusion. The left atrium did not dilate (left atrial dimension 2.8 cm, aortic root dimension 2.1 cm), and the ejection fraction by echocardiography was 66%. In this case variable right ventricular dimensions and variable types of septal motion were seen. Neither of the first two examinations would have been consistent with the previous findings of Chandraratna[14]. We postulate that an important clue to the diagnosis of ruptured interventricular septum is the preserved ejection fraction in the face of acute myocardial infarction and heart failure. As previously mentioned, patients who have papillary muscle dysfunction or rupture generally have large myocardial infarctions and greatly depressed left ventricular function.

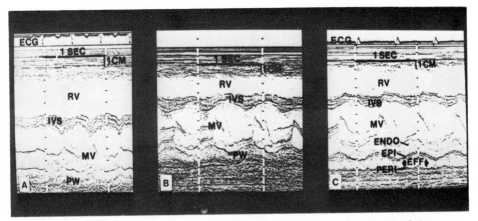

Figure 5 Serial echocardiograms in the same patient with ruptured interventricular septum post myocardial infarction. (A) Demonstrating large right (RV) and paradoxic motion of the interventricular septum (IVS). (B) Demonstrates normal right ventricular size and normal motion of interventricular septum. (C) Enlarged right ventricle with normal interventricular septal motion. Moderate size posterior pericardial effusion present. ENDO—left ventricular posterior wall endocardium. EPI—epicardium. PERI—pericardium. EFF—echo free space of the pericardial effusion.

ACUTE AORTIC VALVE INSUFFICIENCY

The first echocardiographic finding described in chronic aortic valve insufficiency was a rapid fine flutter of the anterior mitral leaflet[16]. Dillon et al first reported aortic valve vegetations secondary to bacterial endocarditis[17]. However, since neither a fluttering anterior mitral valve or vegetations are always present, the only clues to chronic aortic insufficiency may be a dilated aorta and left ventricle, plus hyperdynamic septal and posterior left ventricular wall motion. In other words, the echocardiogram may demonstrate the findings of left ventricular volume overload. However, this does not separate it from other lesions, such as mitral valve insufficiency, which could also cause left ventricular volume overload.

Two recent reports by DeMaria et al[18] and Botvinick et al[19] have summarized the current status of the echocardiographic diagnosis of acute aortic insufficiency. DeMaria emphasized that the echocardiographic findings may be diagnostic before positive blood cultures are established[18]. The diagnostic finding in acute aortic valve insufficiency is premature closure of the mitral valve in late diastole. Figure 6B demonstrates this finding in one of our patients. Normally the anterior and posterior leaflets of the mitral valve meet 40 milliseconds after the onset of the QRS complex on the electrocardiogram. In the presence of severe acute aortic insufficiency, and rapid regurgitation of blood into a normal sized left ventricular chamber, there is a rapid rise of left ventricular diastolic pressure due to decreased left ventricular compliance. The rapid rise of left ventricular diastolic pressure causes the premature closure of the mitral valve in late diastole.

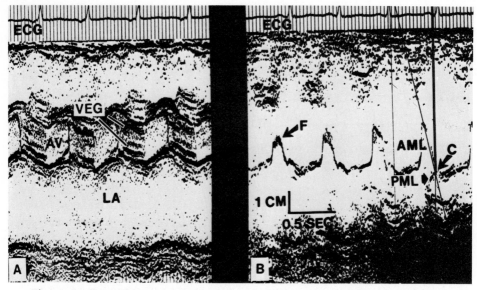

Figure 6   Echocardiogram of acute aortic insufficiency secondary to bacterial en-docarditis of aortic valve. (A) AV—aortic valve. LA—left atrium. VEG—vegetations seen during diastole on the aortic valve. (B) AML—anterior mitral leaflet. PML—posterior mitral leaflet. C—point of closure when anterior and posterior mitral leaf-lets meet. Dark vertical black line indicates closure of the mitral valve prior to onset of the QRS complex seen on the electrocardiogram. The lighter two vertical lines should be ignored. The anterior mitral leaflet has a fine fast flutter, as indicated by the black arrow (F).

Aortic valve vegetations can indeed be identified by echocardiography. The fuzzy layered echoes, seen in Figure 6A, distorting the aortic valve dur-ing diastole are caused by these vegetations. Therefore, the combination of premature diastolic closure of the mitral valve plus valvular vegetations (either aortic or mitral) is quite specific for bacterial endocarditis as the cause of aortic valvular insufficiency. Other acute causes of aortic insuf-ficiency, such as trauma or aortic root dissection, do not have vegetations.

Unfortunately, premature closure of the mitral valve is not 100% diagnostic of acute aortic valve insufficiency. Botvinick et al, reported early diastolic closure of the mitral valve in three cases without significant aortic valve insufficiency[19]. One patient had mild aortic insufficiency with a slow heart rate, and two patients had first degree AV block with a slow heart rate and no aortic insufficiency. When there is a slow ventricular rate allowing a long diastolic filling time and a higher left ventricular diastolic pressure, premature closure of the mitral valve may occur in the absence of aortic insufficiency. Finally, vasodilators such as amyl nitrite may acutely de-crease left ventricular end-diastolic pressure, either as a diagnostic test or a therapeutic trial. This has been shown to reverse the abnormal early diastolic closure of the mitral valve[19]. Therefore, if a patient presents with a murmur of aortic insufficiency and severe failure, and has already been treated with agents to decrease the afterload, such as nitroglycerin or nitroprusside, mitral valve motion may be falsely negative by echocardiography.

The echocardiographic findings of septal vibrations in the presence of aortic valve insufficiency[20] have not been diagnostically helpful in our experience.

AORTIC ROOT DISSECTION

Nanda et al first reported the echocardiographic findings in aortic root dissection[21]. Their findings were as follows: (1) a false lumen was visualized but there was maintenance of parallel echoes in all aortic wall structures; (2) all six patients studied had aortic root dilatation (range 4.2-5.3 cm); (3) four patients had widening of both anterior and posterior aortic walls (anterior wall 16-21 mm, posterior wall 10-13 mm), one patient had widening limited to the anterior aortic wall (21 mm), and one patient had widening limited to the posterior wall (10 mm); and (4) preservation of the normal aortic valve motion.

We have recently reported our experience with the false positive echocardiographic diagnosis of aortic root dissection[22]. Our findings have been confirmed by the report of Brown, Popp, and Kloster[23]. In one of our patients the false positive echo was the result of a purely technical artifact. The echocardiogram showed a normal sized aorta (2.8 cm) (Figure 7). If the echocardiographic examination in this patient had only been performed at the level of the aortic valve, two distinct echoes in the region of the posterior aortic wall would have simulated true dissection. However, by using the scanning technique and recording the scan from the aortic root to the mitral valve region, we demonstrated that the more posterior of the two parallel echoes represented the true posterior aortic wall (Figure 8). The more anterior echo represented the mitral ring or the mitral valve near the ring. The ability to record the mitral ring and the posterior aortic wall simultaneously results from the width of the ultrasound beam. Structures which are anatomically continuous, yet angulated so that echoes can be reflected from different depths, may appear to be in an anterior-posterior relationship on the same echocardiogram.

Our second patient met the criteria of Nanda et al for aortic root dissection. The aorta was dilated to 4.8 cm, and the anterior aortic wall measured 16 mm (Figure 9). At postmortem examination, however, there was no aortic root dissection, but rather a focal atherosclerotic plaque localized to the anterior wall of the ascending aorta, thus creating the false positive echocardiographic diagnosis of aortic root dissection.

We have seen a third patient who had a classic history of acute aortic root dissection, complicated by electrocardiographic and serum enzyme evidence of acute inferior wall myocardial infarction. The echocardiogram showed a dilated aorta (4.2 cm), a thickened posterior aortic wall (13 mm), and a normal anterior aortic wall thickness (5 mm) (Figure 10). She was treated for an acute aortic root dissection throughout her acute episode, but aortic root

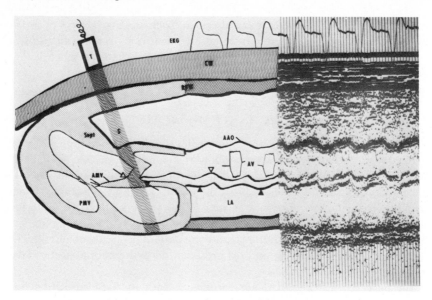

Figure 7 Echocardiogram and associated illustration of technical "false" aortic root dissection. Anatomic structures on the illustration at the left are correlated with the echocardiogram at the right. The sound beam of the transducer is broad and can be directed through the mitral valve near the annulus and the posterior aortic wall simultaneously. Mitral valve or annulus (open anterior arrow); posterior aortic wall (closed posterior arrow). Other abbreviations similar to Figure 8.

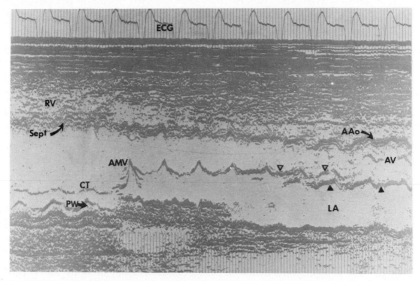

Figure 8 Echocardiogram of "false" aortic root dissection created technically. AAO—anterior aortic wall. AV—aortic valve. LA—left atrium. AMV—anterior mitral valve. CT—chordae tendineae. PW—left ventricular posterior wall. RV—right ventricle. SEPT—interventricular septum. Arrows similar to Figure 7, with the more anterior open arrow indicating the mitral valve, with the darker more posterior arrow indicating the posterior aortic wall.

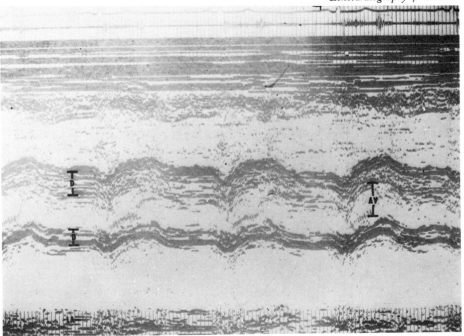

Figure 9 Echocardiogram of "false" aortic root dissection caused by directing the sound beam through atherosclerotic plaque of anterior aortic wall. AV—aortic valve. D—dimension of thickened aortic walls.

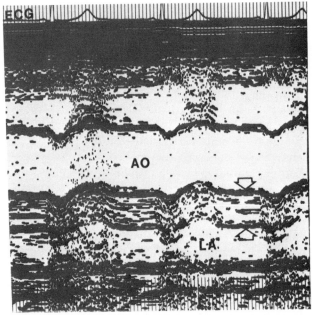

Figure 10 Echocardiogram of "false" aortic root dissection with classic dissection history. AO—aorta. LA—left atrium. Large open white arrows outline thickness of apparent posterior aortic wall.

angiography performed two months later showed no evidence of aortic root dissection. This patient is now clinically stable, asymptomatic, and no further investigation or surgery has been performed.

Brown, Popp, and Koster have emphasized that in their ten patients with a false positive aortic root dissection, none of the patients had an anterior aortic wall equal to or greater than 16 mm. This was the most reliable finding in separating true dissection from false dissection[23]. We agree with their conclusion that clinicians should be wary of the diagnosis of acute aortic root dissection made by echocardiography unless: (1) the clinical history is suggestive of dissection, (2) the anterior aortic wall is equal to or greater than 16 mm, (3) the aorta is dilated to 42 mm or greater, and (4) parallel aortic root echoes are maintained throughout systole and diastole.

Moothart et al recently described their experience with false aortic root dissection in six patients[24]. They emphasized the finding of a double aortic echo in the region of one wall as the most reliable finding along with the lack of continuity between the aorta and septum and/or mitral valve. However, some patients with just a dilated aorta may have anterior mitral leaflet-aortic discontinuity and/or septal-aortic discontinuity without dissection.

PERICARDIAL TAMPONADE

Since the first report of the echocardiographic diagnosis of pericardial effusion in 1965[25], the reliability of echocardiography has improved until it is the procedure of choice for the diagnosis of even small pericardial effusions. Generally, an echo-free space initially develops posteriorly between the pericardium and the epicardium[26]. Extremely good technique is mandatory to identify all three structures of the posterior wall (endocardium, epicardium, and pericardium) and to make sure that the fluid is between the pericardium and epicardium, and is not a pleural effusion posterior to the pericardium. In the presence of a calcified mitral annulus, incorrect identification of the posterior left ventricular wall structures is more likely to occur, resulting in a falsely positive diagnosis of pericardial effusion. Figure 11 is an example of a moderate pericardial effusion.

In a patient who presents with a severe hemodynamic problem and a big heart, echocardiography is extremely helpful to the clinician as a means of separating the patient with a large left ventricle due to left ventricular failure from the patient with a large pericardial effusion creating pericardial tamponade. With larger effusions an echo free space develops anteriorly between the anterior chest wall and the right ventricular myocardium. In the presence of pericardial tamponade, electrical alternans frequently develops on the electrocardiogram, and the swinging heart syndrome is seen on the echocardiogram[27]. This syndrome is characterized by all cardiac walls, including the septum, moving in the same direction with each heart beat. With the larger R wave of electrical alternans, the heart moves anteriorly like a pendulum hanging in a sac of fluid. With the small R wave the heart swings posteriorly. The swinging heart syndrome is an accurate predictor of a severely ill patient with a large effusion.

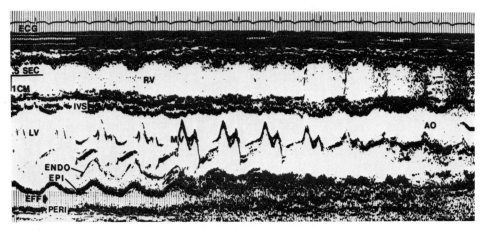

Figure 11 Echocardiogram of large posterior pericardial effusion. Also demonstrates a complete scan from the left ventricle (left) to the mitral valve (middle) to the aorta on the right of the picture. AO—aorta. RV—right ventricle. MV—mitral valve. LV—left ventricular cavity. ENDO—left ventricular posterior wall endocardium. EPI—epicardium. PERI—pericardium. EFF—echo free space of posterior pericardial effusion.

D'Cruz et al recently reported additional echocardiographic findings which accompany pericardial tamponade[28]. The three patients reported all had a paradoxical pulse, and, during inspiration their echocardiograms showed an increased right ventricular size, decreased left ventricular size, plus decreased excursion and E-F slope of the anterior mitral valve. The latter finding reflects a decreased left ventricular filling which occurs during inspiration and exaggerates the paradoxical pulse. Following pericardiocentesis the right ventricular and left ventricular size did not change dramatically between inspiration and expiration. Our experience agrees with these findings.

We have seen one patient with the unusual situation of a predominantly anterior pericardial effusion, pericardial tamponade, and electrical alternans accompanied by the swinging heart syndrome[29] (Figure 12). The anterior effusion was much greater than the posterior effusion which is exactly the opposite of the usual situation. An anterior mediastinal malignancy created the loculated anterior effusion.

UNEXPLAINED SYNCOPE

The echocardiogram may be of value in separating cardiac from noncardiac etiologies of syncope. Some cardiac causes of syncope that may be identified by echocardiography include a left atrial tumor[5], left ventricular outflow obstruction such as aortic valve stenosis[30,31] or IHSS[32,33], and the

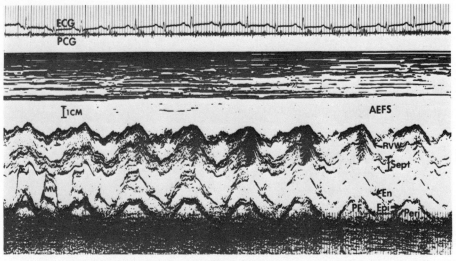

Figure 12 Echocardiogram of predominant anterior pericardial effusion with swinging heart syndrome and electrical alternans on the ECG. AEFS—anterior echo free space of the pericardial effusion. RVW—right ventricular wall. SEPT—interventricular septum. EN—left ventricular posterior wall endocardium. EPI—epicardium. PERI—pericardium. PF—posterior pericardial effusion, which is much less than the anterior effusion. MV—mitral valve.

mitral valve prolapse syndrome which frequently has associated arrhythmias[34,35]. Sometimes the echocardiogram may offer the first clue to the proper diagnosis. The following example illustrates this from our own experience. A 60-year-old negro female was initially seen at two separate times in the emergency room due to unexplained syncope and severe hypotension. On both occasions she responded to a rapid intravenous fluid challenge with return to normal of her blood pressure. The proper clinical diagnosis was not established until an echocardiogram revealed the classic findings of IHSS, including asymmetric septal hypertrophy and systolic anterior motion of the mitral valve. Only after viewing the echocardiogram did the clinicians agree that the physical findings were due to IHSS.

CONGENITAL HEART DISEASE

The differential diagnosis of cyanosis in the newborn can be confusing. A normal echocardiogram is strong evidence against the possibility of complicated cyanotic congenital heart disease[36-38]. The echocardiogram is diagnostically reliable enough in certain abnormalities that a seriously ill cyanotic infant could conceivably be taken directly for palliative surgery without an emergency heart catheterization. Later, when the patient is more stable, a complete and safer heart catheterization could then be performed. A clinical example of this might be a patient with hypoplastic right heart syndrome secondary to tricuspid or pulmonary valve atresia. The palliative procedure would be an aortico-pulmonary arterial shunt to improve pulmonary blood flow. Figure 13 is an example of one of our patients with the hypoplastic right heart syndrome.

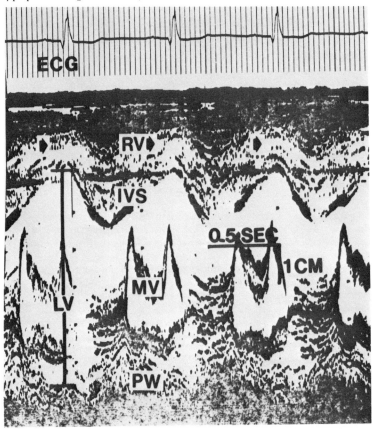

Figure 13 Echocardiogram of hypoplastic right heart syndrome. RV—right ventricle. IVS—interventricular septum. MV—anterior mitral valve. PW—left ventricular posterior wall. LV—left ventricular end-diastolic dimension or cavity size. Note the black arrow following RV, indicating the small right ventricular size in comparison to the large left ventricle.

MALFUNCTIONING PROSTHETIC VALVES

We have had no success in accurately predicting a malfunctioning prosthetic valve by echocardiography. The large amount of artifact that is seen in echocardiograms of normally functioning prosthetic valves makes it difficult to detect thrombi or abnormalities in prosthetic valves. It is, however, possible that future developments will improve the capability of echocardiography in evaluating this type of clinical problem.

SUMMARY

We have discussed in this chapter the major applications of echocardiography in the diagnosis of acute cardiac emergencies. Any patient who develops unexplained hemodynamic difficulty should have an echocardiogram to screen for unsuspected pathologic entities such as silent mitral valve stenosis, left atrial myxoma, left ventricular outflow obstruction, dissection of the ascending aorta, pericardial tamponade, and acute aortic valve insufficiency. Echocardiography may potentially separate acute mitral valve insufficiency from ruptured interventricular septum following acute myocardial infarction. For physicians dealing with pediatric patients and especially neonates, echocardiography is of value in distinguishing between dyspnea and cyanosis of pulmonary or cardiac origin.

References

1. Feigenbaum, H.: *Echocardiography.* Lea and Febiger, Philadelphia, 1972.
2. Duchak, J.M., Chang, S., and Feigenbaum, H.: The posterior mitral valve echo and the echocardiographic diagnosis of mitral stenosis. *Am. J. Cardiol.*, **29**: 628, 1972.
3. Levisman, J.A., Abbasi, A.S., and Pearce, M.L.: Posterior mitral leaflet motion in mitral stenosis. *Circulation*, **51**: 511, 1975.
4. Flaherty, J.T., Livengood, S., and Fortuin, N.J.: Atypical posterior leaflet motion in echocardiogram in mitral stenosis. *Am. J. Cardol.*, **35**: 675, 1975.
5. Schattenberg, T.T.: Echocardiographic diagnosis of left atrial myxoma. *Mayo Clin. Proc.*, **43**: 620, 1968.
6. Finegan, R.E. and Harrison, D.C.: Diagnosis of left atrial myxoma by echocardiography. *N. Engl. J. Med.*, **282**: 1022, 1970.
7. Sung, R.J., Ghahramani, A.R., Mallon, S.M., Richter, S.E., Sommer, L.S., Gottlieb, S., and Myerburg, R.J.: Hemodynamic features of prolapsing and nonprolapsing left atrial myxoma. *Circulation*, **51**: 342, 1975.
8. Millward, D.K., McLaurin, L.P., and Craige, E.: Echocardiographic studies of the mitral valve in patients with congestive cardiomyopathy and mitral regurgitation. *Am. Heart J.*, **85**: 413, 1973.
9. Sweatman, T., Selzer, A., Kamagaki, M., and Cohn, K.: Echocardiographic diagnosis of mitral regurgitation due to ruptured chordae tendineae. *Circulation*, **46**: 580, 1972.
10. Jacobs, J.J., Feigenbaum, H., Corya, B.C., and Phillips, J.F.: Detection of left ventricular asynergy by echocardiography. *Circulation*, **48**: 263, 1973.
11. Corya, B.C., Rasmussen, S., Knoebel, S.B., Feigenbaum, H., and Black, M.J.: Echocardiography in acute myocardial infarction. *Am. J. Cardiol.*, **36**: 1, 1975.
12. Seltzer, A., Gerbode, F., and Kerth, W.J.: Clinical, hemodynamic, and surgical considerations of rupture of the ventricular septum after myocardial infarction. *Am. Heart J.*, **78**: 598, 1969.
13. Forker, A.D., Tomhave, W.G., Weaver, W.F., Carveth, S.W., and Reese, H.E. Post-myocardial infarction ventricular septal defect and ventricular aneurysm. *Nebraska Med. J.*, **58**: 70, 1973.
14. Chandraratna, P.A.N., Balachandran, P.K., Shah, P.M., and Hodges, M.: Echocardiographic observations on ventricular septal rupture complicating acute myocardial infarction. *Circulation*, **51**: 506, 1975.
15. DeJoseph, R.L., Seides, S.F., Lindner, A., and Damato, A.N.: Echocardio-

graphic findings of ventricular septal rupture in acute myocardial infarction. *Am. J. Cardiol.*, **35**: 346, 1975.

16. Winsberg, F., Gabor, G.E., Hernberg, J.G., and Weiss, B.: Fluttering of the mitral valve in aortic insufficiency. *Circulation*, **41**: 225, 1970.
17. Dillon, J.C., Feigenbaum, H., Konecke, L.L., Davis, R.H., and Chang, S.: Echocardiographic manifestations of valvular vegetations. *Am. Heart J.*, **86**: 698, 1973.
18. DeMaria, A.N., King, J.F., Salel, A.F., Caudill, C.C., Miller, R.R., and Mason, D.T.: Echography and phonography of acute aortic regurgitation in bacterial endocarditis. *Ann. Intern. Med.*, **82**: 329, 1975.
19. Botvinick, E.H., Schiller, N.B., Wickramasekaran, R., Klausner, S.C., and Gertz, E.: Echocardiographic demonstration of early mitral valve closure in severe aortic insufficiency. *Circulation*, **51**: 836, 1975.
20. Cope, C.D., Kisslo, J.A., Johnson, M.L., and Meyers, S.: Diastolic vibration of the interventricular septum in aortic insufficiency. *Circulation*, **51**: 589, 1975.
21. Nanda, C., Gramiak, R., and Shah, P.M.: Diagnosis of aortic root dissection by echocardiography. *Circulation*, **48**: 506, 1973.
22. Krueger, S.K., Starke, H., Forker, A.D., and Eliot, R.S.: Echocardiographic mimic of aortic root dissection. *Chest*, **67**: 441, 1975.
23. Brown, O.R., Popp, R.L., and Kloster, F.E.: Echocardiographic criteria for aortic root dissection. *Am. J. Cardiol.*, **36**: 17, 1975.
24. Moothart, R.W., Spangler, R.D., and Blount, S.G.: Echocardiography in aortic root dissection and dilatation. *Am. J. Cardiol.*, **36**: 11, 1975.
25. Feigenbaum, H., Waldhausen, J.A., and Hyde, L.P.: Ultrasonic diagnosis of pericardial effusion. *JAMA*, **191**: 107, 1965.
26. Horowitz, M.S., Schultz, C.S., Stinson, E.B., Harrison, D.C., and Popp, R.L.: Sensitivity and specificity of echocardiographic diagnosis of pericardial effusion. *Circulation*, **50**: 239, 1974.
27. Usher, B.W. and Popp, R.L.: Electrical alternans: mechanism in pericardial effusion. *Am. Heart J.*, **83**: 459, 1972.
28. D'Cruz, I.A., Cohen, H.C., Prabhu, R., and Glick, G.: Diagnosis of cardiac tamponade by echocardiography. Changes in mitral valve motion and ventricular dimensions, with special reference to paradoxical pulse. *Circulation*, **52**: 460, 1975.
29. Krueger, S., Dzindzio, B., Zucker, B., and Forker, A.D.: Predominant anterior pericardial effusion with electrical alternans and the swinging heart syndrome. *J. Clin. Ultrasound*, in press.
30. Gramiak, R. and Shah, P.M.: Echocardiography of the normal and diseased aortic valve. *Radiology*, **96**: 1, 1970.
31. Winsberg, F. and Mercer, E.N.: Echocardiography in combined valve disease. *Radiology*, **105**: 405, 1972.
32. Shah, P.M., Gramiak, R., and Kramer, D.H.: Ultrasound localization of left ventricular outflow obstruction in hypertrophic obstructive cardiomyopathy. *Circulation*, **40**: 3, 1969.
33. Henry, W.L., Clark, C.E., and Epstein, S.E.: Assymmetric septal hypertrophy. Echocardiographic identification of the pathognomic anatomic abnormality of IHSS. *Circulation*, **47**: 225, 1973.
34. Kerber, H.E., Isaeff, D.M., and Hancock, E.W.: Echocardiographic patterns in patients with the syndrome of systolic click and late systolic murmur. *N. Engl. J. Med.*, **284**: 691, 1971.
35. Dillon, J.C., Haine, C.L., Chang, S., Feigenbaum, H.: Use of echocardiography in patients with prolapsed mitral valve. *Circulation*, **43**: 503, 1971.
36. Meyer, R.A. and Kaplan, S.: Noninvasive techniques in pediatric cardiovascular disease. *Prog. Cardiovasc. Dis.*, **15**: 341, 1973.

37. Godman, M.J., Tham, P., and Kidd, B.S.L.: Echocardiography in the evaluation of the cyanotic newborn infant. *Brit. Heart J.*, **36**: 154, 1974.
38. Goldberg, S.J., Allen, H.D., and Sahn, D.J.: *Pediatric and Adolescent Echocardiography.* Yearbook Med. Pub., Chicago, 1975.

CHAPTER 9

Prehospital Management of Acute Myocardial Infarction

A. James Lewis, M.D.; J. Michael Criley, M.D.

This Chapter describes the effect of implementation of one of the most successful American programs in pre-hospital management of acute myocardial infarction. It is designed as a comprehensive guide to others who seek to reduce the pre-hospital mortality in this fashion. A valuable portion of this Chapter is dedicated to updating cardiopulmonary resuscitation techniques and related pharmacologic treatment.

INTRODUCTION

Experience in the coronary care unit has shown that most instances of sudden death in the hospitalized patient with acute myocardial infarction (AMI) result from ventricular fibrillation (VF)[1]. When this is unassociated with cardiogenic shock or left ventricular failure (i.e., primary VF), prompt defibrillation usually results in the restoration of sinus rhythm with no adverse effect on the prognosis[1]. Suppression of ventricular ectopic beats (VEBs) with antiarrhythmic agents has successfully reduced the incidence of primary VF[1-3]. Applying these well-known principles has reduced the hospital mortality of AMI from 30% to 15%[4]. However, the impact on the overall mortality from coronary artery disease has been only 2-3%[2].

In an epidemiologic study, Kuller found that 60% of all deaths due to coronary artery disease in Baltimore occurred outside the hospital[5]. Others have reported that 40 to 75% of all deaths from AMI occur during the first symptom hour[6]. It should be clear from these data that any attempt to lower the mortality from AMI must improve treatment of the patient before he enters the hospital.

This chapter will deal with the management of the patient suspected of having AMI before he arrives in the coronary care unit (CCU), and with the prevention of sudden cardiac death, a frequent prehospital complication of acute myocardial ischemia. Emphasis will be placed both on the development of a community-level system for the early institution of definitive therapy before hospitalization, and on specific patient management.

DEVELOPMENT OF A COMMUNITY SYSTEM FOR PREHOSPITAL CORONARY CARE

Community efforts to reduce the mortality from AMI must include the

159

development of a three part integrated system. The first component is the patient, or those immediately around him. The second concerns the development of a prehospital system capable of advanced cardiac lift support (ACLS)*[7]. The third is the hospital emergency department where priority attention must be given to the potential AMI patient, and ACLS continued. Failure of any one of these parts will significantly reduce the effectiveness of the entire system.

The Patient

Symptom Recognition

In a study of 100 patients who developed an AMI, Solomon and associates[8] found that 65 experienced prodromal symtoms during a two month period prior to the AMI. Of these, 59 had chest pain. Kuller reported that 23% of persons who died suddenly of arteriosclerotic heart disease had been seen by a physician during the week before death[5].

Although the typical clinical picture of AMI is well-known, certain clinical syndromes deserve special mention since they may signal imminent AMI or sudden death[9]. In brief, these include:

1. Recent onset of angina with ordinary or less than ordinary activity.
2. Recent acceleration of a previously stable anginal pattern, so that it is precipitated by mild activity or occurs at rest (crescendo angina).
3. Anterior chest discomfort (central, diffuse, and oppressive), however mild, that is unrelieved by rest and/or nitroglycerin within five minutes.

As previously noted, these clinical syndromes herald impending danger to the life of the patient. It may become necessary to immediately institute ACLS measures. The urgency of this principle is well-documented in a study of prehospital VF by Liberthson and associates[10]. They found that, on the day of cardiac arrest, 24% of patients experienced new chest pain and/or dyspnea more than 30 minutes before the arrest (average, 3.8 hours). In 23% chest pain and/or dyspnea occurred from 1 to 30 minutes before arrest. In 53% no significant warning occurred. Several studies have documented the frequent occurrence of arrhythmias during the early hours following symptom onset in AMI. Adgey and her co-workers found that 73% (170 of 284) of AMI patients experienced arrhythmias during the first symptom hours[11]. Pantridge and Geddes found the risk of VF to be 15 times greater during the first symptom hour than during the remainder of the initial 12 hours[12]. In a study of 47 patients with AMI who were seen during the first symptom hour, Rose and associates[13] found arrhythmias in 82.9% (Figure 1). The occur-

---

*This includes the initiation of cardiopulmonary resuscitation, the use of adjunctive equipment for airway management (e.g., endotracheal intubation), monitoring for cardiac arrhythmias, defibrillation, establishment of an intravenous line and the administration of appropriate drug therapy.

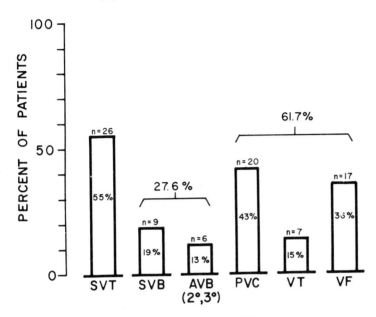

Figure 1 Arrhythmias during the first hour in 47 patients with AMI. See text for discussion.

Abbreviations: SVT = supraventricular tachycardia, SVB = supraventricular bradycardia, AVB = atrioventricular block, PVC = premature ventricular contraction, VT = ventricular tachycardia, VF = ventricular fibrillation.

rence of ventricular arrhythmias in 61.7%, and VF in 36% was particularly noteworthy.

Prompt Call for Medical Assistance

In a prospective study of 134 patients with AMI, Moss and Goldstein found that three hours was the average time between the onset of symptoms and the decision to call for medical assistance[14]. However, there is ample documentation that the highest mortality occurs during the first hour after symptoms begin[5,6]. Clearly, expert medical care is needed as soon as possible after symptom onset. Several things may prevent this: ignorance of symptom significance; the "denial syndrome", so characteristic of human nature, in which one hopes that what he suspects isn't really so; fear, either of the reality of a serious disease, or of the financial impact of illness; or, finally, inability to "get into the system". Ignorance, denial, and fear can be combated by both public and professional education. Entry into the emergency medical system may be relatively easy in some communities; in others it is quite complex. In Los Angeles County, for example, there are 54 separate telephone numbers for emergency medical service. The universal emergency telephone number (911) can greatly reduce or eliminate the confusion that the public must feel when confronted by an unexpected medical emergency.

Physicians must teach their patients the early warning symptoms of AMI and the necessity of prompt medical assistance. This is especially true for those patients with known coronary artery disease. Such patients and their families should be encouraged to form an emergency plan. This may involve calling a paramedic squad, a fire department rescue squad, a private ambulance, the family doctor, or going immediately to a nearby hospital emergency department. The appropriate emergency telephone number should be immediately available (e.g., affixed to the telephone).

The Need to Train the Public in Cardiopulmonary Resuscitation

In 1969, Pantridge and Adgey reported their experience in Belfast (Northern Ireland) with 61 patients with VF prior to hospitalization in whom resuscitation was attempted by a mobile life support unit[15]. Thirty-nine (64%) were initially resuscitated and twenty-four (39%) were long term survivors. In each of the survivors resuscitation was initiated with four minutes of cardiac arrest. Liberthson, Nagel, and associates reported 14% survival beyond hospitalization in 301 patients with prehospital VF[16]. Baum, Alvarez, and Cobb reported 17.7% long term survival during the initial three years of a program of prehospital coronary care in Seattle[17]. The long term survival rate in this program has increased to 26% after the training of a large number of citizens in cardiopulmonary resuscitation (CPR)[18]. The data from both the Belfast and Seattle groups indicate that to achieve improved survival from prehospital VF, CPR must be started within several minutes of cardiac arrest. The only way that this can occur on a large scale is by training the general public in CPR. Logical starting points for such a program would be the relatives or associates of known coronary disease patients, and elementary or high school students.

DEVELOPMENT OF A PREHOSPITAL ADVANCED CARDIAC LIFE SUPPORT SYSTEM

The primary purpose of a prehospital ACLS system is to initiate electrocardiographic (ECG) monitoring and antiarrhythmic therapy at the earliest possible time prior to hospitalization. Such systems are usually mobile, although stationary ACLS systems may be beneficial in localized areas of high population density (e.g., large office building, sports arenas, etc.).

The Mobile Advanced Cardiac Life Support System

Background

The Russians made the earliest efforts in prehospital coronary care. The impetus to develop such systems in the western world came in 1966 when Pantridge and associates demonstrated the value of antiarrhythmic therapy in AMI prior to hospitalization[12]. Initially, such mobile units consisted of specially equipped ambulances (ECG monitor, defibrillator, drugs, etc.) and were reserved exclusively for the heart attack patient[12,19,20]. This required the development of new and often expensive rescue services parallel to already existing emergency facilities. Such mobile coronary care units were often staffed by physicians and/or nurses.

One improvement was to upgrade already existing rescue resources. Such a program was developed by Nagel et al with the Miami Fire Department Rescue Service[21]. Each rescue unit was equipped with a portable radio-transceiver for transmission of voice and ECG to the hospital, and with a defibrillator.

The encouraging results of Nagel and his associates with the use of paramedical personnel to administer definitive forms of therapy outside the hospital led Criley and his co-workers to develop a pilot program in Los Angeles County in 1969[22,23]. The purpose of this program was to enhance the capabilities of already existing emergency rescue personnel and resources, permitting the institution of definitive therapy for a wide range of emergencies prior to hospitalization. This system used highly trained paramedics not only to initiate ECG monitoring and to defibrillate, but to administer essential drug therapy under the remote (i.e., radiotelemetry or telephone) supervision of a physician or specially qualified nurse. It was not restricted to heart attack patients, and hence was properly termed a mobile intensive care unit (MICU)[24]. Similar systems were developed by others[25-27].

The following discussion is based on the mobile intensive care program in Los Angeles County[22,23].

*Training of MICU Paramedics**

The training of the paramedics is the single most important element in the development and operation of a paramedic mobile intensive care program.

The curriculum for paramedic training in Los Angeles County consists of a five month program divided into three phases: a two month period in the classroom, a one month period of clinical experience in the hospital, and a two month period of field internship.

The didactic phase consists of lecture-seminar sessions with laboratory and workshops for practical demonstration. It is divided into 10 sections:

1. Basic paramedic sciences (anatomy, physiology)
2. Traumatology
3. Cardiology
4. Medical-surgical problems
5. Pharmacology and toxicology
6. Pediatrics and obstetrics

*Dr. R.D. Stewart, Director of Paramedic Training for Los Angeles County, assisted the authors in the preparation of this section.

 7. Psychiatry
 8. Assessment and reporting
 9. Advanced life support
10. Logistics

During the clinical phase students are taught technical skills (such as starting intravenous infusions) and to evaluate the patient's symptoms and signs. The student spends time in the emergency department, coronary and intensive care units, and in obstetrics.

The field internship, during which the student is expected to apply the knowledge and skills learned during the previous three months to real patients, is a vital portion of the training period. At this time, the trainee is assigned to a MICU so that he is able to work under the close supervision of experienced paramedics.

This type of curriculum can be considered only a beginning for the new paramedic. A program of required continuing education has been developed in order to maintain and improve skill levels. Recertification at two year intervals is required. This is based on satisfactory performance as a paramedic, attendance at a required number of continuing education sessions, and on the successful completion of an examination.

Legal Basis for Paramedic Operations

In California the legal basis for paramedics to perform ACLS is the Wedworth-Townsend Paramedic Act (California Health and Safety Code). It has been revised several times since its enactment in 1970. It provides for certification of paramedics after completion of a training program consisting of a minimum of 200 hours of didactic training, 100 hours of clinical experience, and 200 hours of field internship. It permits a paramedic to initiate CPR and to defibrillate. Additional features of ACLS can then be employed upon the order of a physician or a specially certified registered nurse. This is done by radio or telephone communication with the base station hospital. Under such supervision the paramedic may:

1. administer intravenous saline, glucose or volume expanding agents or solutions.
2. perform gastric suction by intubation
3. perform pulmonary ventilation by use of an esophageal airway
4. obtain blood for laboratory analysis
5. apply rotating tourniquets
6. administer parenterally, orally or topically any of the following classes of drugs or solutions:

   a. Antiarrhythmic agents
   b. Vagolytic agents
   c. Chronotropic agents
   d. Analgesic agents
   e. Alkalinizing agents
   f. Vasopressor agents
   g. Narcotic antagonists
   h. Diuretics
   i. Anticonvulsants
   j. Ophthalmic agents
   k. Oxytocic agents
   l. Antihistaminics
   m. Bronchodilators
   n. Emetics

This legislation provides that the physician or nurse shall not be liable for any civil damages resulting from instructions given to the paramedics, providing that those instructions were given "in good faith".

Mobile Intensive Care Unit Operation

Each MICU is staffed by two certified paramedics and is based at a strategic location. The type of vehicle used varies among the many agencies participating in this program. The various MICU configurations employed are[22,23]:

1. Fire department utility truck. This type of MICU is based at a fire station (Figure 2), and is staffed by two fireman-paramedics. It has no patient transport capability, hence a commercial (non-paramedic) ambulance is used. The major advantage of this type is that paramedic service may be developed without the expense of purchasing ambulances.
2. Fire department ambulance. This type of MICU is also based at a fire station, and is staffed by fire department paramedics.
3. Commercial ambulance. This type of MICU is located at the ambulance company headquarters and is staffed by civilian paramedics.
4. Helicopter. This form of MICU is used for special rescue situations, and is operated by both fire and sheriff departments.

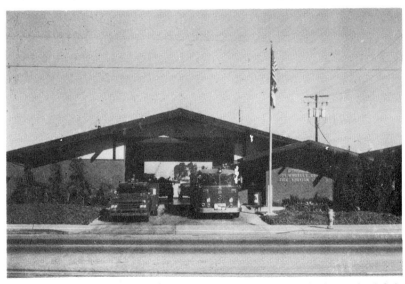

Figure 2 Typical Los Angeles County fire station. The vehicle on the left is a utility truck that has been converted into an MICU by the addition of specialized rescue equipment. It is staffed by two paramedics.

Each MICU is equipped with a radiotransceiver, defibrillator, oscilloscope, ventilation and suction apparatus, intravenous solutions, and selected drugs (Figure 3). Since this equipment is portable, the patient need not be moved before initiating therapy. A detailed list of specific drugs and equipment for an ACLS unit may be found in the standards for Cardiopulmonary Resuscitation and Emergency Cardiac Care[7]. Other types of conventional and special rescue equipment are available for the management of non-cardiac patients.

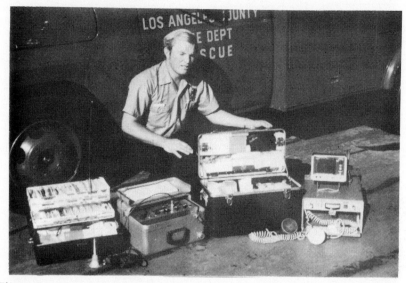

Figure 3 Paramedic equipment carried on all MICU's. From left to right: drug box containing primarily pre-filled syringes and ampules; radiotransceiver; large container for IV solutions, bandages, splints, etc.; defibrillator and oscilloscope.

Calls for emergency medical assistance are referred to the appropriate agency depending on the geographic location of the patient (e.g., fire department or civilian ambulance company) where a dispatcher receives the call, and after obtaining certain basic information (e.g., name, address, nature of emergency) deploys the nearest MICU. Upon arrival at the scene, priority is given to the initiation of necessary life saving procedures. Pertinent historical information is then obtained and the patient is briefly examined. Electrodes are connected to the patient, and the ECG is displayed on an oscilloscope. This information (voice and ECG) is then transmitted by radio or telephone to a physician (or legally certified "MICU nurse" as defined by the Wedworth-Townsend Paramedic Act) at the base station hospital (Figure 4). The base station physician or nurse directs further therapy, such as the use of various drugs. Every effort is made to stabilize the patient's condition before transport to the hospital. If these efforts are successful, a high speed ambulance ride with red light and siren is avoided.

When a private non-paramedic ambulance is used for transport by the fire department paramedics, the portable MICU equipment and a paramedic accompany the patient. Continuous radio contact is maintained with the base station during transport to the hospital. Since the base station physi-

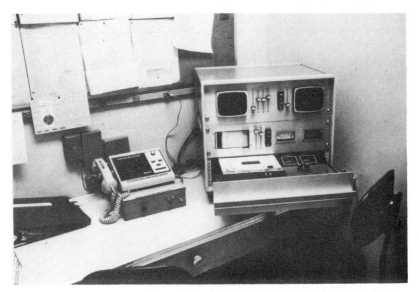

Figure 4 Hospital base station. The console at the right contains a transceiver, ECG demodulator, ECG oscilloscope, strip chart recorder and cassette tape-recorder for recording voice and ECG transmissions.

cian is in continuous communication with the MICU, he should be able to take over the direct management of the patient with minimal delay and confusion, once the patient arrives in the emergency department.

A brief written record is completed by the paramedic. At the base station, all voice and ECG communications are recorded on magnetic type. Both of these are kept as a permanent record.

Communications

A reliable communications system is an essential element in a mobile ACLS program. The development of such a system involves: (1) the initial dispatch of the rescue vehicle, (2) communication with the base station hospital for the supervision of patient therapy, and (3) the direction of the rescue vehicle to a hospital which has appropriate patient care facilities.

The initial dispatch in the Los Angeles program is accomplished over already existing communications channels (e.g., by the fire department dispatcher). A separate communications system was developed to link the paramedic in the field with the physician at the base station hospital. This system was based on the program developed by Nagel et al in Miami[21].

The essential elements of the paramedic-hospital communications network include:

1. The ability to transmit both voice and ECG.
2. The ability to transmit over radio or telephone. Since relatively few radio frequencies are available for this type of communication, it is not unusual for two or more MICUs to be communicating with a base sta-

tion hospital at the same time on the same frequency. The telephone is used whenever feasible in order to avoid this type of radio frequency overcrowding. The telephone is also useful when the radio cannot be used (e.g., due to topographic obstacles, radio interference, or equipment failure).

3. In areas where there are multiple base station hospitals using different radio frequencies, each MICU should have the capability of selecting more than one channel. Hence, if radio communication cannot be established with the primary base station (e.g., because of a topographic obstacle such as a hill or tall building), a duplexed system is used so that a second hospital can be contacted.

4. The base station hospital can interrupt ECG transmission in order to direct appropriate therapy.

The concept of "central emergency medical dispatch" is particularly pertinent to large metropolitan areas. It involves the direction of all requests for emergency response to a single center (e.g., by the use of the universal emergency telephone number, 911), and the dispatch of the rescue vehicle by that center. In addition, such a facility could maintain a current status report on all hospitals within its area (e.g., bed availability in the CCU, etc.). In this way a critically ill or injured patient would not be taken to a hospital where he cannot be treated.

The Stationary Advanced Cardiac Life Support System

The stationary ACLS unit is particularly well suited for places of high population density. It may be permanent, as in a large office building, or temporary, as in a sports arena or convention center[7,28]. Such a unit must be easily identifiable and accessible. It should possess the same capabilities to evaluate and treat the potential AMI patient, or the cardiac arrest victim, that have been discussed for mobile life support units. In addition, a mobile life support unit must be available to transport the patient to the hospital.

The Hospital Emergency Department

The final component in the emergency system is the hospital emergency department. It must be able to continue the same level of ACLS that was initiated by the MICU paramedics, or to initiate this for those patients whose initial entry into the system occurs at the hospital.

In 1970, the Los Angeles County Heart Association undertook a program designed to encourage optimal care of the potential AMI patient by hospital emergency departments[24]. The ultimate goal of this program was to have a hospital emergency department capable of delivering expert ACLS within three to five minutes to 80% of the County's population. On-site inspections of emergency room facilities were conducted by volunteer physician-nurse teams. Hospitals were asked to voluntarily subscribe to a list of standards recommended by the Heart Association. The hospitals have enthusiastically accepted this program. Many have demonstrated an eagerness to conform to the standards. The following principles are based on that program, and on the recommendations of the National Conference on Cardiopulmonary Resuscitation and Emergency Cardiac Care[7]:

1. High priority must be given to any patient suspected of having an AMI. This includes the prompt initiation of ECG monitoring and the administration of antiarrhythmic therapy.
2. There should be standing orders authorizing the emergency room nursing staff to initiate ECG monitoring, CPR and drug therapy of life threatening arrhythmias when a physician is not immediately available.
3. When the patient is transferred from the emergency room to the CCU, continuous ECG monitoring (with a portable oscilloscope) must be maintained, and a portable defibrillator must be immediately available. Trained personnel, capable of recognizing life threatening arrhythmias and of performing CPR and defibrillation must accompany the patient.
4. There should be 24 hour daily coverage of the emergency department by trained personnel. The minimal level of training for emergency department physicians and nurses should include the recognition of life threatening arrhythmias and their appropriate drug therapy, the performance of CPR and of defibrillation. Physicians should be capable of performing endotracheal intubation.
5. There should be emergency equipment and standard cardiac emergency drugs immediately available in the emergency department. This should include an ECG monitor, a defibrillator, ventilatory devices (including endotracheal tubes and laryngoscope) and suction equipment, and essential cardiac drugs (i.e., sodium bicarbonate, epinephrine, atropine, lidocaine, morphine, calcium chloride).

PRINCIPLES OF PREHOSPITAL PATIENT MANAGEMENT

The basic principles underlying patient management prior to hospitalization are: (1) Management of the suspected AMI patient, and (2) Management of the patient in cardiac arrest. In both instances, every reasonable effort should be made to stabilize the cardiac rhythm and hemodynamic state before transporting the patient to the hospital[7].

Management of the Suspected AMI Patient

Initiation of Advanced Cardiac Life Support

The first and most basic principle is that the decision to initiate ACLS is based on the patient's history, not on the ECG. During the early phase of AMI the ECG may appear normal, or show only increased amplitude of the T wave (indicative of subendocardial ischemia) in appropriate leads. In the unstable anginal syndrome, ST segment and/or T wave changes may be present during pain, but later the ECG may be normal.

Arrhythmia Monitoring

Monitoring for cardiac arrhythmias should be started early. This is best accomplished with an oscilloscope. Evidence for the high incidence of arrhythmias during the early hours of AMI has already been discussed.

Oxygen Therapy

Oxygen should be administered by mask or nasal cannula at a flow rate of 4 to 6 L/min. Although significant hypoxemia is unlikely in the uncomplicated AMI patient, there is evidence that an elevation of arterial oxygen tension may reduce infarct size[29,30].

Relief of Pain

Pain should be relieved as soon as possible not only for humane reasons, but also for the accompanying hemodynamic benefits. Sublingual nitroglycerin may be tried first if the patient is not hypotensive. If this is not successful, morphine should be administered intravenously in small (3-5 mg) doses. This may be repeated at 5 to 30 minute intervals. Morphine induces favorable hemodynamic effects by increasing venous capacitance, thereby reducing venous return. It also reduces systemic vascular resistance and hence diminishes impedance to left ventricular emptying. The result of both actions is to reduce myocardial oxygen demand[31]. These same actions may reduce left atrial pressure, and hence may have a favorable effect in pulmonary edema.

Management of Ventricular Ectopic Beats (VEB) and Rhythms

It has been axiomatic that antiarrhythmic therapy should be instituted in AMI when certain "warning arrhythmias" occur. These have included the occurrence of five or more VEBs per minute, VEBs which are closely coupled (QR'/QT less than 0.85), or which fall on the T wave of the preceding beat, or VEBs which occur in pairs, or in runs (i.e., ventricular tachycardia) or which are multiformed[32,33]. Lawrie, however, noted that when VF occurred early during the course of AMI, it was infrequently preceded by warning arrhythmias[34]. Recent studies in which continuous ECG recording was performed during the early hours of AMI indicated that VF may occur in the absence of so-called warning arrhythmias[35,36]. Ventricular ectopic beats which occur only rarely may initiate VF, as may those with long coupling intervals (QR'/QT greater than 0.85)[35]. Additional studies show that the early use of intravenous lidocaine can significantly reduce the incidence of primary VF, despite the absence of warning arrhythmias[37,38]. Hence, even in the absence of VEBs, antiarrhythmic therapy should be started at the earliest possible time. Therapy should be initiated with an intravenous bolus of lidocaine, 50 to 100 mg (approximately 1 mg/kg), followed by an infusion of 2 mg/min. An infusion rate in excess of 4 mg/min should be avoided because of possible toxicity[7,31]. Since lidocaine is metabolized in the liver, caution must be used when hepatic dysfunction is present (such as may occur in low cardiac output states, or in the presence of congestive heart failure)[31].

Management of Bradyarrhythmias

Controversy exists regarding the management of bradyarrhythmias during the course of AMI[33,39-41]. Early studies on non-ischemic hearts led to the belief that bradyarrhythmias favored the development of VF[42]. Recent investigations on ischemic myocardium indicate that slow heart rates exert a protective effect from ventricular ectopic activity[40].

The supraventricular bradyarrhythmias commonly encountered during the early phase of AMI include sinus bradycardia, junctional escape rhythm, and atrioventricular block[33]. These are often the result of increased parasympathetic tone[43]. If the ventricular rate falls between 50 to 60/min in the presence of hypotension or VEBs, atropine therapy is indicated[39]. In the absence of hypotension or VEBs, no therapy is necessary for rates above 50/min[39]. When the rate falls below 50/min, atropine should be administered to maintain an optimal cardiac output[43,44]. Atropine is administered intravenously in doses of 0.5 mg at five minute intervals until a ventricular rate of 60 to 80/min is achieved. A maximum dose is 2.0 mg[7]. Atropine can cause a supraventricular tachycardia which may lead to VF because of increased myocardial oxygen demands[45].

In the presence of a ventricular escape rhythm (ventricular rate less than 40/min), atropine is unlikely to be helpful. In the MICU this rhythm is managed with intravenous isoproterenol by constant infusion at a rate of 2 to 20 μg/min (to achieve a heart rate of approximately 60/min).

Management of Hypotension and Cardiogenic Shock

When the systolic blood pressure falls below 90 mm Hg, appropriate therapy should be instituted. If hypotension is accompanied by bradycardia, atropine is the initial agent of choice. Before vasopressor agents are used, such basic measures as oxygen administration, pain relief, and elevation of the lower extremities should be attempted. These measures may be successful in milder forms of pump failure. In more severe states, however, vasoactive agents are necessary. Dopamine is the first drug to use. At an intravenous infusion rate of between 1 to 10 μg/kg/min, it may increase cardiac contractility and renal blood flow without increasing heart rate and peripheral vascular resistance[46]. The absence of an increase in systemic vascular resistance (such as occurs with norepinephrine) and in heart rate (as with isoproterenol) may exert a favorable effect on left ventricular hemodynamics and infarct size. When dopamine is not successful, a norepinephrine infusion at a rate sufficient to attain a systolic pressure of 90 to 100 mm Hg should be started.

Management of Pulmonary Edema

The initial measures in the management of the patient with pulmonary edema before hospitalization include placing the patient in a sitting or semisitting position, and the administration of oxygen. As noted above, morphine has beneficial hemodynamic effects. With mild forms of pulmonary edema, the administration of nitroglycerin (in the absence of hypotension) may provide relief[47]. In more severe cases, rotating tourniquets should be employed. Furosemide may be administered in a dose of 40 mg intravenously over a one to two minute period (ethacrynic acid 50 mg is an alternate drug).

Management of Hypertension

Elevation of the systolic blood pressure above 140 mm Hg may be a particularly malignant feature in AMI, since it results in increased myocardial oxygen demand. The prehospital therapy includes the sublingual administration of nitroglycerin[48] and intravenous furosemide or ethacrynic acid. More effective forms of therapy, such as sodium nitroprusside or propranolol, may be considered once the patient arrives at the hospital.

Management of Prehospital Cardiac Arrest

The occurrence of sudden cardiac death outside the hospital is a common catastrophe for which immediate therapy is essential. The mechanisms responsible for cardiac arrest are VF, ventricular asystole (VA), and electromechanical dissociation (EMD)[7].

Maintenance of Circulation and Pulmonary Ventilation

The initial therapy for cardiac arrest is the institution of CPR[7]. The only exception to this rule is the occurrence of VF under observation when a defibrillator is immediately available.

An important aspect of CPR is the attainment of optimal pulmonary ventilation. The most effective way to achieve this during CPR is by endotracheal intubation and the use of 100% oxygen. Without a skilled technician endotracheal intublation may be too time consuming. An especially useful device for MICU ventilation is the esophageal obturator airway (Figure 5)[49,7]. This is a clear plastic tube approximately 15 inches long which looks like an endotracheal tube; however, the distal end is occluded. Immediately proximal to the distal end there is an inflatable cuff. There are several holes near the upper end. A face mask is fitted onto the proximal end. Grasp the lower jaw with one hand and pull it forward. Then, advance the tube through the mouth and oropharynx directly into the esophagus. The head should be flexed slightly forward during passage of the tube in order to avoid inadvertant endotracheal intubation. The distal cuffed end of the tube should lie just below the carina when the tube has been advanced so that the face mask is seated over the mouth. Now attempt ventilation, auscultating both lungs to make sure breath sounds are present. If breath sounds are absent, the airway should be withdrawn and repositioned since it probably was passed into the trachea. Once breath sounds are heard, the cuff may be inflated. Schoffermand and colleagues[50] have shown that 100% oxygen with excellent arterial oxygen tensions (mean Pa_{O_2} of 244 mm Hg) are achieved.

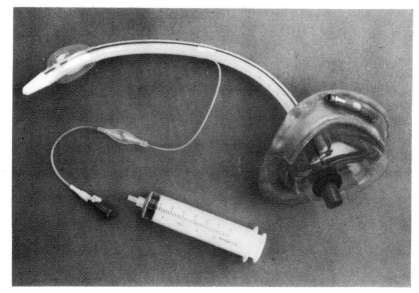

Figure 5   Esophageal obturator airway. See text for description.

Aspiration of gastric contents is prevented by the inflated cuff in the esophagus. When the patient arrives at the hospital, the esophageal airway can be replaced by an endotracheal tube. It is important to perform endotracheal intubation before the cuff of the esophageal airway is deflated in order to avoid aspiration.

Establishment of an Intravenous Line

An intravenous line must be established to allow essential drug therapy. A forearm vein or the long saphenous vein in the lower extremity is preferable. If these are not available, then cannulate the femoral vein in the groin. Use of the internal or external jugular, or the subclavian vein may necessitate the interruption of CPR, and may result in air embolism. A saphenous vein cutdown is preferable to percutaneous jugular or subclavian cannulation. A large gauge plastic catheter (14 or 16 gauge) should be used[51].

Correction of Acidosis

In the presence of cardiopulmonary arrest acidosis results from respiratory failure with carbon dioxide retention, and from anaerobic metabolism with the accumulation of lactic and pyruvic acid. The adverse effects of acidosis include suppression of diastolic depolarization in Purkinje fibers, increases susceptibility to VF, decreased ventricular contractile force, and decreased cardiac responsiveness to catecholamines[31].

The respiratory component of acidosis is managed by effective pulmonary ventilation as discussed above. The metabolic acidosis is treated by the intravenous administration of sodium bicarbonate. This drug should be administered by bolus injection rather than by continuous infusion. The initial dose is 1 mEq/kg, and this may be repeated if effective circulation is not promptly restored. Sodium bicarbonate is available in pre-filled syringes containing either 44.6 mEq or 50 mEq. As a practical measure for an average-sized adult, the initial dose is two ampules (i.e., 89.2 or 100 mEq). Thereafter, one-half the original dose is given at 10 minute intervals until effective spontaneous circulation is restored. More accurate bicarbonate administration will be possible once arterial blood gases can be obtained at the hospital. Excessive bicarbonate may result in metabolic alkalosis and hyperosmolality[52].

Management of Specific Types of Cardiac Arrest

Ventricular Fibrillation. When the patient develops VF while being monitored (witnessed VF), and when a defibrillator is immediately available, defibrillation is attempted with non-synchronized direct current countershock. If defibrillation is successful within approximately 30 seconds of VF onset, the administration of sodium bicarbonate is unnecessary. If not, one ampule should be given.

Commonly, the patient is in VF when the rescue team arrives (unwitnessed VF). The first step in resuscitation is the institution of CPR. If this has been done within two to three minutes of VF onset, defibrillation should then be attempted. In the usual case, however, cardiac arrest has been present for several or more minutes before any rescue efforts are attempted. In that case (after starting CPR) we recommend that the rescue team:

    A. establish an intravenous line,
    B. administer two ampules of sodium bicarbonate IV (repeat as indicated above) and 5 ml of 1:10,000 epinephrine IV (may repeat every 5 min),
    C. DC countershock.

Following attempted defibrillation one of four rhythms will usually result (Figure 6):

    1. Supraventricular rhythm with a normal or rapid ventricular rate (Figure 6, C-F). This may be sinus rhythm, but often is atrial fibrillation. This rhythm is the most desirable and has been associated with a more favorable prognosis[16]. It is unlikely to result unless both hypoxia and acidosis have been corrected. Once this rhythm has been established, a 100 mg bolus of lidocaine should be given, followed by a lidocaine infusion (2 mg/min).
    2. A bradyarrhythmia, commonly either junctional escape rhythm or ventricular escape rhythm (Figure 6, A-B). These two rhythms may initially be difficult to distinguish since atrial activity is often not evident and the QRS complex is wide. With proper ventilation and correction of acidosis, the QRS complex in junctional escape rhythm may become narrow. Additionally, a marked ST segment elevation may cause a supraventricular QRS to appear wide (Figure 6, F). Either rhythm may be associated with complete antrioventricular block. The appropriate therapy at this time is:

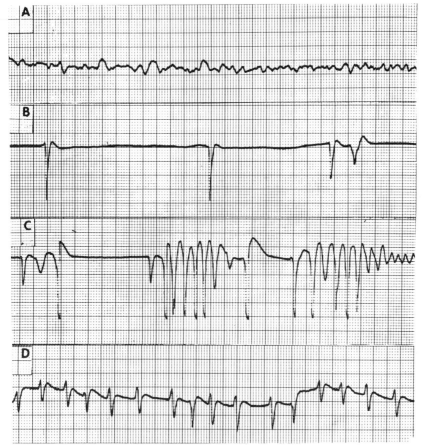

Figure 6 Electrocardiogram (lead II) received at base station hospital by radiotelemetry from MICU. The patient was a 65 year old man who sustained sudden cardiac arrest outside the hospital.

A. Ventricular fibrillation present on arrival of MICU.
B. Following defibrillation, a slow ventricular escape rhythm with a premature VEB following the third escape beat. An esophageal airway was inserted and two ampules of sodium bicarbonate were given.
C. Two brief salvos of ventricular tachycardia were initiated by closely coupled VEBs. The second salvo terminated in VF.
D. Following defibrillation atrial fibrillation with a rapid ventricular rate resulted. This was associated with a BP of 100/86.

a. Evaluate adequacy of ventilation, since hypoxia may be contributing to this arrhythmia.
b. Repeat original dose of sodium bicarbonate and epinephrine.
c. If a more rapid supraventricular rhythm does not result, administer atropine 0.5 mg IV. This dose may be repeated at 5 minute intervals. The total dose should usually not exceed 2.0 mg. Atropine is more likely to be effective if P waves are evident on the ECG

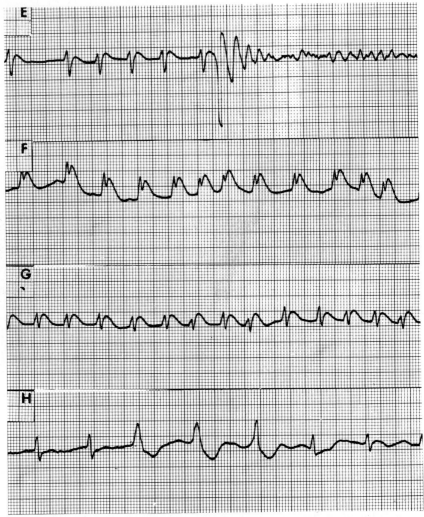

E. As a lidocaine bolus was being prepared for injection, a closely coupled VEB initiated VF.
F. Following defibrillation, atrial fibrillation with a rapid ventricular rate recurred. Note the marked ST segment elevation.
G. Atrial fibrillation, with lowering of the ST segment.
H. Supraventricular rhythm (? junctional) with transient accelerated ventricular rhythm (the third beat of which probably is a fusion beat).

monitor. Even in the absence of sinus node activity atropine may relieve sinoatrial block and restore sinus rhythm.
d. If these measures are unsuccessful, an intravenous infusion of isoproterenol 2 to 20 μg/min should be started. This may restore sinus

rhythm with normal atrioventricular conduction, or accelerate the escape pacemaker, thereby improving cardiac output. The infusion rate should be adjusted to maintain a ventricular rate of 60 to 70/min. If a stable supraventricular rhythm (e.g., sinus rhythm or atrial fibrillation) is obtained the isoproterenol can usually be discontinued.

3. Ventricular asystole. This may be an indication of uncorrected hypoxia and/or acidosis, or of extensive myocardial damage. The following measures should be taken:

   a. Evaluate adequacy of ventilation. It may be necessary, for example, to suction the patient, or to correct faulty ventilation technique (e.g., such as the lack of a proper face mask seal resulting in an oxygen leak, or improper head position during mouth-to-mouth ventilation).
   b. Repeat dose of sodium bicarbonate and epinephrine. Further details of therapy will be discussed below.

4. Ventricular fibrillation. Persistence of VF after attempted defibrillation also may be an indication of uncorrected hypoxia and/or acidosis, or of extensive myocardial damage. The following steps should be taken:

   a. Evaluate adequacy of ventilation.
   b. Repeat dose of sodium bicarbonate.
   c. Repeat dose of epinephrine if fine VF is present.
   d. Administer 5 ml of a 10% solution of calcium chloride IV. This may be repeated every 10 minutes.
   e. Repeat DC countershock.
   f. If VF persists, give lidocaine 100 mg IV and repeat countershock.

Ventricular Asystole. When cardiac arrest has resulted from ventricular asystole either a severe metabolic deficit is present and/or extensive myocardial damage has occurred. The prognosis for resuscitation is poor. In addition to beginning CPR, and inserting an endotracheal tube or esophageal airway for optimal ventilation, the following steps should be taken:

A. Administer two ampules of sodium bicarbonate and 5 ml of 1:10,000 epinephrine IV.
B. Administer 5 ml of a 10% solution of calcium chloride IV.
C. If a rhythm has not been restored, repeat the original dose of biocarbonate, and administer 5 ml of 1:10,000 epinephrine by intracardiac injection.

Electromechanical Dissociation (EMD). In EMD there is evidence of organized electrical activity on the ECG, but failure of effective myocardial contraction. Although the mechanism is not completely understood, it may result from failure in the calcium transport system[43]. This ion is essential for the coupling of the electrical event with mechanical contraction. The occurrence of EMD carries a grave prognosis. The management is similar to the therapy of ventricular asystole. In addition, an intravenous infusion of iso-proterenol 2 to 20 μg/min may be given to stimulate the resumption of effective contractions.

In any of the foregoing cardiac arrest situations, initial attempts at resuscitation and stabilization should be started where the patient is found. Therapy must be continued during transport to the hospital. In the event that cardiac arrest persists, the patient should be transported to the hospital with continuous CPR. Although it is unusual for further resuscitative efforts in the hospital to be successful, this may occur. One major advantage of the hospital setting is the ability to accurately correct metabolic deficits since arterial blood gas and electrolyte determinations can be obtained.

If resuscitation in the field has been successful and a supraventricular rhythm has been restored, a lidocaine infusion (100 mg bolus, followed by an infusion rate of 2 mg/min) should be started to prevent a recurrence of ventricular fibrillation.

References

1. Lown, B. and Ruberman, W.: The concept of precoronary care. *Mod. Concepts Cardiovasc. Dis.*, **39**: 97-102, 1970.
2. Lown, B., Klein, M.D., and Herschberg, P.I.: Coronary and precoronary care. *Am. J. Med.*, **46**: 705-724, 1969.
3. Yu, P.N.: Prehospital care of acute myocardial infarction. *Circulation*, **45**: 189-204, 1972.
4. Likoff, W.: The prognosis of myocardial infarction. In W. Likoff, B.L. Segal and W. Insull, Jr. (Eds.): *Atherosclerosis and Coronary Heart Disease*. Grune and Stratton, New York, 1972, p. 520.
5. Kuller, L.: Sudden death in arteriosclerotic heart disease. *Am. J. Cardiol.*, **24**: 617-628, 1969.
6. Fulton, M., Julian, D.G., and Oliver, M.F.: Sudden death and myocardial infarction. *Circulation*, **40** (suppl. 4): 182-191, 1969.
7. Standards for cardiopulmonary resuscitation (CPR) and emergency cardiac care (ECC). *JAMA*, **227** (suppl): 833-868, 1974.
8. Solomon, H.A., Edwards, A.L., and Killip, T.: Prodromata in acute myocardial infarction. *Circulation*, **40**: 463-471, 1969.
9. Gazes, P.C., Mobley, E.M., Jr., Faris, H.M., Jr., Duncan, R.C., and Humphries, G.B.: Pre-infarctional (unstable) angina: a prospective study—ten year follow-up. *Circulation*, **48**: 331-337, 1973.
10. Liberthson, R.R., Nagel, E.L., Hirschman, J.C., Nussenfeld, S.R., Blackbourne, B.D., and Davis, J.H.: Pathophysiologic observations in prehospital ventricular fibrillation and sudden cardiac death. *Circulation*, **49**: 790-798, 1974.
11. Adgey, A.A.J., Geddes, J.S., Webb, S.W., Allen, J.D., James, R.G.G., Zaidi, S.A., and Pantridge, J.F.: Acute phase of myocardial infarction. *Lancet*, **2**: 501-504, 1971.
12. Pantridge, J.F. and Geddes, J.S.: A mobile intensive care unit in the management of myocardial infarction. *Lancet*, **2**: 271-273, 1967.
13. Rose, R.M., Lewis, A.J., Fewkes, J., Clifton, J.F., and Criley, J.M.: Occurrence of arrhythmias during the first symptom hour in acute myocardial infarction (abstract). *Circulation*, **50** (suppl. III): 121, 1974.
14. Moss, A.J. and Goldstein, S.: The pre-hospital phase of acute myocardial infarction. *Circulation*, **41**: 737-742, 1970.

15. Pantridge, J.F. and Adgey, A.A.J.: Prehospital coronary care. *Am. J. Cardiol.*, **24**: 666-673, 1969.
16. Liberthson, R.R., Nagel, E.L., Hirschman, J.C., and Nussenfeld, S.R.: Prehospital ventricular defibrillation. *N. Engl. J. Med.*, **291**: 317-321, 1974.
17. Baum, R.S., Alvarez, H. III, and Cobb, L.A.: Survival after resuscitation from out-of-hospital ventricular fibrillation. *Circulation*, **50**: 1231-1235, 1975.
18. Shaffer, W.A. and Cobb, L.A.: Recurrent ventricular fibrillation and modes of death in survivors of out-of-hospital ventricular fibrillation. *N. Engl. J. Med.*, **293**: 259-262, 1975.
19. Grace, W.J. and Chadbourn, J.A.: The mobile coronary care unit. *Dis. Chest*, **55**: 452-455, 1969.
20. Lewis, R.P., Frazier, J.T., and Warren, J.V.: An approach to the early mortality of myocardial infarction. *Am. J. Cardiol.*, **26**: 644, 1970.
21. Nagel, E.L., Hirschman, J.C., Nussenfeld, S.R., Rankin, D., and Lundblad, E.: Telemetry—medical command in coronary and other mobile emergency care systems. *JAMA*, **214**: 332-338, 1970.
22. Lewis, A.J., Ailshie, G., and Criley, J.M.: Prehospital cardiac care in a paramedical mobile intensive care unit. *Calif. Med.*, **117**: 1-8, 1972.
23. Criley, J.M., Lewis, A.J., and Ailshie, G.E.: Mobile emergency care units, implementation and justification. *Adv. Cardiol.*, **15**: 9-24, 1975.
24. Lewis, A.J. and Criley, J.M.: An integrated approach to acute coronary care. *Circulation*, **50**: 203-205, 1974.
25. Cobb, L.A., Conn, R.D., Samson, W.E., and Philbin, J.E.: Early experience in the management of sudden death with a mobile intensive/coronary care unit. *Circulation*, **42** (Suppl III): 144, 1970.
26. Rose, L.B. and Press, E.: Cardiac defibrillation by ambulance attendants. *JAMA*, **219**: 63-68, 1972.
27. Lambrew, C.T., Schuchman, W.L., and Cannon, T.H.: Emergency medical transport systems: Use of ECG telemetry. *Chest*, **63**: 477-482, 1973.
28. Carveth, S.: Cardiac resuscitation program at the Nebraska football stadium. *Dis. Chest*, **53**: 8-11, 1968.
29. Maroko, P.R., Radvany, P., Braunwald, E., and Hale, S.L.: Reduction of infarct size by oxygen inhalation following acute coronary occlusion. *Circulation*, **52**: 360-368, 1975.
30. Saltzman, H.A.: Efficacy of oxygen enriched gas mixtures in the treatment of acute myocardial infarction. *Circulation*, **52**: 357-359, 1975.
31. White, R.D.: Essential drugs in emergency cardiac care. In: *Advanced Cardiac Life Support*. American Heart Association, 1975, Ch. 7.
32. DeSanctis, R.W., Block, P., and Hutter, A.M.: Tachyarrhythmias in myocardial infarction. *Circulation*, **45**: 681-702, 1972.
33. Kimball, J.T. and Killip, T.: Aggressive treatment of arrhythmias in acute myocardial infarction. Procedures and results. *Prog. in Cardiovasc. Dis.*, **10**: 483-504, 1968.
34. Lawrie, D.M.: Ventricular fibrillation in acute myocardial infarction. *Am. Heart J.*, **78**: 424-426, 1969.
35. Lie, K.I., Willens, H.J.J., Downar, E., and Durrer, D.: Observations on patients with primary ventricular fibrillation complicating acute myocardial infarction. *Circulation*, **52**: 755-759, 1975.
36. Dhurandhar, R.W., MacMillan, R.L., and Brown, K.W.G.: Primary ventricular fibrillation complicating myocardial infarction. *Am. J. Cardiol.*, **27**: 347-351, 1971.
37. Lie, K.I., Wellens, H.J., van Capelle, F.J., and Durrer, D.: Lidocaine in the prevention of primary ventricular fibrillation. *N. Engl. J. Med.*, **291**: 1324-1326, 1974.

38. Wyman, M.G. and Hammersmith, L.: Comprehensive treatment plan for the prevention of primary ventricular fibrillation in acute myocardial infarction. *Am. J. Cardiol.*, **33**: 661-667, 1974.
39. Rotman, M., Wagner, G.S., and Wallace, A.G.: Bradyarrhythmias in acute myocardial infarction. *Circulation*, **45**: 703-722, 1972.
40. Epstein, S.E., Goldstein, R.E., Redwood, K.R., et al: The early phase of acute myocardial infarction: Pharmacological aspects of therapy. *Ann. Int. Med.*, **78**: 918-936, 1973.
41. Grauer, L.E., Gershen, B.J., Orlando, M.M., and Epstein, S.E.: Bradycardia and its complications in the prehospital phase of acute myocardial infarction. *Am. J. Cardiol.*, **32**: 607-611, 1973.
42. Han, J., Millet, D., Chizzonnitti, B., and Moe, G.K.: Temporal dispersion of recovery of excitability in atrium and ventricle as a function of heart rate. *Am. Heart J.*, **71**: 481, 1966.
43. James, T.N.: The coronary circulation and conduction system in acute myocardial infarction. *Prog. in Cardiovasc. Dis.*, **10**: 410-449, 1968.
44. Gregory, J.J. and Grace, W.J.: The management of sinus bradycardia, nodal rhythm and heart block for the prevention of cardiac arrest in acute myocardial infarction. *Prog. in Cardiovasc. Dis.*, **10**: 505-517, 1968.
45. Massumi, R.A., Mason, D.T., Amsterdam, E.A., DeMaria, A., Miller, R.R., Scheinman, M.M., and Zelis, R.: Ventricular fibrillation and tachycardia after intravenous atropine for treatment of bradycardias. *N. Engl. J. Med.*, **287**: 336-338, 1972.
46. Goldberg, L.I.: Dopamine—clinical uses of an endogenous catecholamine. *N. Engl. J. Med.*, **291**: 707-710, 1974.
47. Gold, H.K., Leinbach, R.C., and Sanders, C.A.: Use of sublingual nitroglycerine in congestive failure following acute myocardial infarction. *Circulation*, **46**: 839-845, 1972.
48. Epstein, S.E., Kent, K.M., Goldstein, R.E., Borer, J.S., and Redwood, D.R.: Reduction of ischemic injury by nitroglycerine during acute myocardial infarction. *N. Engl. J. med.*, **292**: 29-35, 1975.
49. Don Michael, T.A., Lambert, E.H., and Mehran, A.: "Mouth-to-lung airway" for cardiac resuscitation. *Lancet*, **2**: 1329, 1968.
50. Schofferman, J., Oill, P., and Lewis, A.J.: The esophageal obturator airway: a clinical evaluation. *Chest*, in press.
51. Kaye, W.E.: Intravenous techniques. In: *Advanced Cardiac Life Support*, American Heart Association, 1975, Ch. 6.
52. Mattar, J.A., Weil, M.H., Shubin, H., and Stein, L.: Cardiac arrest in the critically ill. II. Hyperosmolal states following cardiac arrest. *Am. J. Med.*, **56**: 162-168, 1974.

CHAPTER 10

Current Concepts in the Management of Acute Uncomplicated Myocardial Infarction

Mark Schnee, B.Sc., M.R.C.P. (U.K.); Alan D. Forker, M.D.;
Barry Dzindzio, M.D.; Helen Starke, M.D.;
James Buell, M.D.; Robert S. Eliot, M.D.

This Chapter summarizes the management of uncomplicated myocardial infarction and forms the basis for subsequent discussions. It comprehensively reviews the technical, therapeutic and rehabilitative aspects of this condition. Complicated forms of infarction are handled in subsequent chapters.

It is the aim of this chapter to review some of the current concepts of therapy with acute uncomplicated myocardial infarction. Uncomplicated infarctions are characterized by a lack of serious arrhythmias, conduction abnormalities, or overt pump failure. We will consider the patient from the time he is admitted to the coronary care unit until he is discharged from the hospital. The therapeutic conclusions will be largely based on a review of the literature and on our own observations and experiences.

RELIEF OF PAIN

Acute myocardial infarction may have several different manifestations, but chest pain is the commonest presenting symptom. Prompt relief of pain is essential. Intravenous analgesic administration is the most effective route to achieve rapid pain relief and it avoids confusion from elevated serum enzymes that may result from intramuscular injections. Unfortunately, no analgesic agent is ideal in all respects. The choice of a drug depends upon its analgesic and sedative effectiveness, weighed against its potential side effects. Furthermore, the hemodynamic consequences of treatment are important if therapy is to be rational. Although there are many analgesics to choose from, including methadone, diamorphine, pentazocine and meperidine, long-standing experience and predictable clinical effectiveness continue to favor morphine as the drug of choice. In addition to its analgesic effect, morphine is an excellent sedative.

Experimental animal work indicates that morphine sulfate reduces peripheral vascular resistance while venous capacitance increases, contributing to a reduction in venous return to the heart[1]. In normal volunteers, intravenous morphine sulfate increases forearm blood flow with a decline in the forearm vascular resistance, but with no change in arterial blood pressure[2]. This is thought to represent a vasodilator action on the peripheral circulation, but the mechanism is probably indirect, due to central nervous system inhibition of sympathetic nervous discharge.

A recent study compared the hemodynamic effects of intravenous morphine and pentazocine during cardiac catheterization in patients with coronary artery disease[3]. The effect of 8 mg of intravenous morphine was compared to the effect of 48 mg of intravenous pentazocine. Morphine significantly decreased cardiac index, left ventricular end-diastolic pressure, pulmonary artery wedge pressure, left ventricular work index, and oxygen consumption. There was no significant effect on aortic pressure. In contrast, pentazocine significantly elevated mean aortic pressure, left ventricular end-diastolic pressure, pulmonary artery wedge pressure, and left ventricular work index. Cardiac work was decreased 8.2% by morphine and increased 22.1% by pentazocine. In the setting of acute myocardial infarction, the hemodynamic effects of pentazocine could be deleterious because of elevation of myocardial oxygen demands. On the other hand, morphine would be more advantageous because of a lowering of left ventricular end-diastolic pressure, cardiac output and left ventricular work, thus lowering myocardial oxygen demand. These hemodynamic data favor the use of morphine in acute myocardial infarction.

Possible adverse side effects of morphine are respiratory depression due to a direct effect on the brain stem, nausea and vomiting due to direct stimulation of chemoreceptors in the medulla, and exaggerated vagal tone with resultant sinus bradycardia. Secondary hypotension may sometimes result, especially in patients already hypovolemic or vasoconstricted, but can be corrected by elevating the legs. The respiratory depression from morphine is dose related and rarely occurs with the usual clinical doses in patients with normal lung function; but morphine must be used with great caution in patients with diminished respiratory reserve. In summary, the favorable hemodynamic response, potent analgesic and sedative effect, and long-standing experience favor intravenous morphine as the drug of choice in acute myocardial infarction.

SEDATION

Because anxiety and emotional stress are common during an acute myocardial infarction, sedation is an important part of therapy. Those patients given frequent doses of morphine during the first 24 to 48 hours of the event will probably be receiving adequate sedation from their analgesic. But as the patient begins to recover and feel well, an oral tranquilizer is frequently indicated. A most important facet of the patient's care is a good patient-physician relationship, where an understanding sympathetic physician can alay many anxieties. However, we believe that oral diazepam (Valium®) is a suitable tranquilizer; it is clinically effective, well tolerated without serious side effects, and it does not appear to have any significant interaction with Coumadin® anticoagulation.

Diazepam also appears to have desirable hemodynamic effects. The acute hemodynamic effects of intravenous diazepam at cardiac catheterization were recently reported[4]. Aortic pressure, left ventricular end-diastolic pressure, tension-time index, and myocardial oxygen consumption were all significantly decreased. Heart rate was unchanged. This combination of effects has been described at nitroglycerin-like, since it can potentially reduce myocardial wall tension and left ventricular oxygen demand. While the acute hemodynamic effects of intravenous diazepam have been studied, no clinical studies are available on the acute and chronic effects of oral diazepam. Our practice is to use Valium® 2-5 mg t.i.d. It is an effective tranquilizer which is relatively safe and free of adverse hemodynamic effects.

OXYGEN

Traditionally, we have routinely administered humidified oxygen at 4-6 liters/minute by a rebreathing face mask to all patients with acute myocardial infarction. The major clinical rationale is the frequent, unsuspected, associated hypoxia arising from ventilation perfusion abnormalities, diffusion abnormalities, reduced cardiac output, atelectasis, or respiratory depression following morphine administration.

The question of routine oxygen administration to a patient who is comfortable and not clinically or chemically hypoxic is more difficult to answer. One could raise some theoretical objections about the use of oxygen in this situation, since oxygen causes an increased systemic vascular resistance and a small rise of 5-10 mm Hg in systolic pressure[5,6]. Oxygen also decreases cardiac output by up to 15%. This combination of changes could conceivably increase myocardial oxygen demands and jeopardize muscle adjacent to the area of acute myocardial infarction. On the other hand, an elevation of peripheral resistance and arterial pressure might sufficiently augment coronary artery perfusion pressure to offset the increased demand. No controlled clinical trials have been performed to study the effect of oxygen therapy on either mortality or morbidity in acute myocardial infarction.

Of interest, however, is a recent report by Moroko et al[7], concerning the effects of oxygen therapy on the extent of myocardial necrosis in dogs following acute coronary occlusion. Their data demonstrated that 40% oxygen inhalation decreased the amount of ST elevation and CPK rise in comparison to 20% oxygen. One hundred percent oxygen did not decrease myocardial injury further. However, they postulated that an increased availability of oxygen to ischemic areas was the mechanism by which 40% oxygen reduced the extent of myocardial damage. These recent experimental animal observations provide further justification for our traditional practice of giving oxygen to patients with acute myocardial infarction, but we must admit that similar data is not yet available for humans.

ANTICOAGULANT THERAPY IN ACUTE MYOCARDIAL INFARCTION

The anticoagulant dilemma persists, and questions regarding their long-term and short-term value in acute myocardial infarction remain unanswered after thirty years of experience.

There are several considerations arguing against anticoagulant treatment in acute myocardial infarction: (1) Blood coagulation plays a relatively minor role in the formation of the arterial or white thrombus, since the initial step is the formation of platelet aggregates with subsequent fibrin deposition[8]. (2) Some evidence suggests that acute myocardial infarction can occur without coronary thrombosis, and coronary thrombosis may even be a secondary rather than primary event in acute myocardial infarction[9-12]. While coronary thrombi are frequently found at postmortem examination in the setting of transmural infarction and late death, they are found in only 10% of cases manifesting acute subendocardial infarction or sudden death[10]. An additional practical consideration is that many drugs interact with oral anticoagulants and complicate anticoagulant control[8]. Finally, unpredictable long-term patient compliance frequently results in either subtherapeutic levels or hemorrhagic complications.

Two recent retrospective analyses favor the concept of routine anticoagulant use. Modan et al[13] reported a reduction in 21-day hospital mortality from 27.3 to 8.3% with the use of anticoagulants. Tonascia et al[14] supported these findings in a retrospective analysis demonstrating a 2½ fold greater mortality in non-anticoagulated patients. In contrast, prospective clinical trials[15,16] do not show improved mortality with routine anticoagulant therapy. The Working Party on Anticoagulant Therapy in Coronary Thrombosis to the Medical Research Council found no significant reduction in mortality in a concurrently randomized clinical trial, although the incidence of thromboembolic complications was markedly less in the anticoagulated group[15].

Given these considerations, it is our practice to employ oral anticoagulants as a prophylactic measure to prevent deep venous thrombosis and subsequent pulmonary thromboembolism. They also may limit the development of mural thrombi and prevent systemic emboli. We do not routinely anticoagulate myocardial infarction patients, but select high risk cases hoping to prevent pulmonary or systemic emboli. The important indications are the following: (1) complicated myocardial infarction requiring prolonged bedrest and usually characterized by increasing cardiac size and/ or congestive heart failure, (2) clinical, ECG and/or x-ray evidence of ventricular aneurysm, (3) prominent varicose veins, (4) history of prior pulmonary or systemic emboli. If anticoagulation is employed, we seriously attempt to discontinue it when the patient is fully ambulatory. We do not use long-term anticoagulation unless there is evidence of recurrent pulmonary emboli.

Fibrinolytic agents such as streptokinase and urokinase promote the dissolution of arterial thrombi by activating plasmin. It was originally hoped that such treatment might reduce mortality in acute myocardial infarction. However, the composite results of ten studies[17], although suggestive of a beneficial effect, are inconclusive and indications for thrombolytic therapy in coronary care units will require further investigations.

Data on the prophylactic effects of antiplatelet agents in myocardial infarction remain sparse. Indirect evidence that aspirin may exert protective effects was suggested by the finding at autopsy that myocardial infarction was significantly less common in arthritics than among the general population[18]. Although statistically inconclusive, a randomized controlled trial with prophylactic aspirin, given in a single daily dose to men with recent myocardial infarction, noted a reduction of 12% in total mortality at six months and 25% at twelve months[19]. The Boston Collaborative Drug Surveillance Program studied two independent patient groups, one with a discharge diagnosis of myocardial infarction, and the other with a different discharge diagnosis[20]. They showed a negative association between regular aspirin intake and nonfatal myocardial infarction. Such data suggest that further controlled clinical trials of aspirin on a prophylactic basis are warranted and cooperative trials have been started under supervision of the National Heart and Lung Institute. Nevertheless, neither aspirin nor fibrinolytic therapy have an established role in the management of myocardial infarction in our institution at the present time.

PROPHYLACTIC ANTIARRHYTHMIC DRUGS

Halkin has recently summarized the reported information on prophylactic antiarrhythmic drugs in acute myocardial infarction up to 1974[21]. Bloomfield et al[22] and Koch-Weser et al[23] analyzed the results of group I drugs (quinidine and procainamide) and found no improvement in mortality between treated and untreated patients. Analyzing the effects of lidocaine (a group II drug) in four separate studies[24-27], no consistent improvement could be demonstrated using either intravenous or intramuscular lidocaine in hospitalized patients with acute myocardial infarction. No controlled prospective studies have been reported using prophylactic diphenylhydantoin, propranolol, or bretylium.

Since Halkin's analysis, two papers have been published regarding prophylactic lidocaine. Lie et al[28] reported a double-blind randomized study involving 212 consecutive patients. Intravenous lidocaine was given as a 100 mg IV bolus followed by an infusion at 3 mg per minute for the next 24 hours. Ventricular fibrillation occurred less often in the treated group, but mortality rates were equal in the treated and controlled groups. A high incidence of side effects occurred in the treated group, especially in older age patients. Valentine et al[29] reported their experience with a double-blind prospective study in pre-hospital patients treated with 300 mg of intra-muscular lidocaine by 233 different physicians. During the first two hours after injection, three out of 156 lidocaine-treated and 8 out of 113 placebo-treated patients died (P<.03). It was disappointing, however, that no significant difference was found between treated and untreated groups in either late death or total mortality (16% in the placebo group and 13% in the lidocaine group).

A major criticism of all reported studies of this type is the exclusion of high risk patients. These excluded patients represent a large proportion of the acute myocardial infarction patients who would be expected to have a higher rate of lethal arrhythmias and sudden death.

In institutions with an adequate coronary care facility, we still recommend the compulsive monitoring of acute myocardial infarction patients. We still treat arrhythmias according to exact diagnosis and specific warning signs, such as frequent PVC's, multifocal PVC's, consecutive PVC's or the R on T phenomenon. We do not advise the routine prophylactic use of anti-arrhythmic agents, because the risk of routine prophylaxis with current available drugs probably outweighs the benefits. Nevertheless a certain percentage of patients with primary ventricular fibrillation will not exhibit warning signs before the onset of their fibrillation[30].

Prophylactic agents may diminish the frequency of ventricular ar-rhythmias when adequate blood levels are achieved, but most smaller community hospitals are not prepared to measure and monitor routine pro-cainamide, quinidine, or lidocaine blood levels. Inadvertent high levels of such drugs are easily produced and readily result in drug toxicity.

The pre-hospital administration of prophylactic antiarrhythmic agents requires further investigation. Routine administration of myocardial suppressant drugs can have unpredictable effects on a damaged heart already manifesting a decreased cardiac output, especially when renal and hepatic excretory functions are additional unknown factors. Also mitigating against the routine use of prophylactic antiarrhythmics in the pre-hospital setting are significant sinus bradycardia, hypotension, congestive heart failure, and distal conduction abnormalities, such as high grade AV block and bundle branch blocks.

Another issue worthy of comment concerns the practice of routinely administering atropine to patients with sinus bradycardia. Initial coronary care experience suggested that sinus bradycardia was an important trigger event leading to electrical instability and ventricular fibrillation; and, therefore, prophylactic atropine was frequently used in the past to treat sinus bradycardia. Recent experimental evidence questions this rationale[31]. Acute coronary occlusion in dog models has demonstrated that increasing heart rate enhances vulnerability to ventricular fibrillation, and that slow heart rates are not associated with an increased incidence of ventricular ar-rhythmia. In addition, pooled patient data relating to short-term survival in acute myocardial infarction suggest a better prognosis in those with un-treated sinus bradycardia[31].

Therefore, it does not seem reasonable to administer atropine prophylactically to all patients just because the sinus rate is less than 60 per minute. If a patient has sinus bradycardia with no hemodynamic side effects, further observation is warranted. However, if the bradycardia is accompanied by signs of inadequate organ perfusion, hypotension, or escape arrhythmias, atropine is administered in a dose of 0.6 to 1.0 mg intravenously.

THE ROLE OF DIGITALIS IN ACUTE MYCARDIAL INFARCTION

Let us assume that a patient is in the coronary care unit 24 hours following an acute myocardial infarction. He now displays mild dyspnea, moist audible rales at both lung bases, and an audible third sound gallop at the apex. Is digitalis and/or diuretic therapy advisable?

The use of digitalis in acute myocardial infarction remains quite controversial, as summarized in the recent article by Rahimtoola and Gunnar[32]. One of the frequently stated concerns about the use of digitalis is the possibility of increased myocardial sensitivity and vulnerability to ventricular arrhythmias. Nevertheless, Constant[33] reviewed the literature and reported in 1970 that no clinical study had demonstrated an increased incidence of arrhythmias. Considerable debate has arisen over the hemodynamic effects of digitalis in acute myocardial infarction and several authors including Hodges et al[34], Lipp et al[35], and Forrester et al[36] were unable to show any improvement in left ventricular function in the acute stage of infarction. In contrast, Rahimtoola et al[37] administered ouabain to 16 patients within 48 hours of acute myocardial infarction. Although cardiac output did not improve, there was a decrease in left ventricular end-diastolic pressure and pre-ejection period, with an increase in left ventricular stroke work, dP/dt and Vmax. This improvement occurred in patients both with and without clinical heart failure.

Newer concerns about the use of digitalis have arisen since the experimental studies of Maroko et al demonstrated that digitalis may extend the area of myocardial infarction in experimental animals[38]. Cardiac glycosides increase myocardial oxygen demands in the nonfailing heart by enhancing contractility, increasing systemic resistance, and elevating mean arterial blood pressure. All of these would increase left ventricular work and myocardial oxygen consumption, thus extending the limit of myocardial infarction. However, applying the same precordial mapping techniques to experimental animals in heart failure, ouabain tends to limit the area of ischemic injury[38]. It must be kept in mind that the dose of digitalis used in these animal studies was two to three times the maximum digitalizing dose employed in humans. It is difficult to extrapolate from animal models to the clinical setting, and more clinical investigation will be needed before this controversy can be settled.

The efficacy of diuretic therapy in the management of heart failure due to myocardial infarction is clearer. Recent data with hemodynamic intracardiac monitoring indicates that intravenous furosemide[39] actually lowers pulmonary artery wedge pressure prior to the diuretic response. Therefore, furosemide is effective not only as a diuretic, but probably also acts to increase venous capacitance. We have not observed serious intravascular depletion or secondary hypotension with the use of intravenous furosemide.

In summary, when a patient exhibits signs of heart failure in the absence of supraventricular tachyarrhythmias following a myocardial infarction, we usually begin with a diuretic. If the patient manifests supraventricular tachyarrhythmias, digitalis is readily employed to control the ventricular rate. Finally, if cardiomegaly is present and persists despite diuretic therapy, we believe oral digoxin is definitely indicated as in other patients with congestive heart failure. We basically follow the clinical rule: the larger the heart, the more useful digoxin therapy will be.

NITROGLYCERIN AND PROTECTION OF THE MYOCARDIUM

It was previously taught that nitroglycerin was contraindicated in acute myocardial infarction because it caused hypotension and reflex tachycardia. Both of these effects could extend the limits of the acute infarction. Nevertheless, recent clinical and hemodynamic experiences tend to disprove this thesis[31,40]. Not only has nitroglycerin therapy been recently vindicated of therapeutic guilt, but experimental[31] and clinical observations[40] approve its use. Epicardial mapping studies in dogs show that nitroglycerin results in less ST segment elevation and CPK depletion in acute myocardial infarction[31]. This appears to be especially true if hypotension and reflex tachycardia are minimized by the simultaneous use of an alpha receptor stimulant, such as methoxamine or phenylephrine[40]. However, another clinical study suggested that adding phenylephrine was not beneficial[41].

In patients with congestive heart failure following acute myocardial infarction, invasive monitoring has shown that sublingual nitroglycerin decreases left ventricular stroke work, pulmonary artery wedge pressure, and improves cardiac output[42]. Finally, two more recent documented effects argue in favor of the use of nitroglycerin: (1) sublingual nitroglycerin enhances ventricular electrical stability by raising the ventricular fibrillation threshold[31]; and (2) nitroglycerin reduces the extent of left ventricular asynergy secondary to myocardial ischemia, as observed in humans during left ventricular angiography[43]. The angiographic left ventricular response to nitroglycerin is being proposed as a method of separating infarcted from ischemic myocardium.

Given these considerations, we do not believe that nitroglycerin is contraindicated in the immediate postmyocardial infarction patient unless severe hypotension or shock is present. Hemodynamic intracardiac monitoring has shown minimal hypotensive effects in the majority of patients, and we use sublingual nitroglycerin freely in the postmyocardial infarction patient. The sublingual method provides the best absorption, and it is usually administered at 1½-2 hour intervals. The drug is ineffective in the oral form, but appears to be well absorbed through the skin as a 2% nitroglycerin ointment. While we have had limited clinical experience with nitroglycerin ointment, studies by Reicheck et al[44] suggest that nitroglycerin ointment is an effective means of maintaining a sustained effect. Since we have observed no serious hypotensive effects with sublingual nitroglycerin, we support its use by physicians in community hospitals where complex instrumentation for invasive monitoring is absent. However, if stronger agents, such as nitroprusside, are used to relieve afterload, we definitely recommend the routine use of invasive hemodynamic monitoring, i.e., Swan-Ganz catheter placement, because of potential serious hypotension. We also recommend that all patients with evidence of pump failure have invasive monitoring.

We do not recommend the routine prophylactic use of "long acting" nitrates in convalescent patients following acute myocardial infarction because none have been shown to prolong life, prevent infarction, or improve collateral vessel development. Oral nitrates are less freely recommended for relief of angina because of questionable gastrointestinal absorption and possible biotransformation in the liver.

CORTICOSTEROIDS

The possibility that corticosteriods might limit infarct size has been suggested, but clinical trials have yielded conflicting results. As Semple and Dall have emphasized, this may be partly due to a lack of distinction between the physiologic versus the pharmacologic effects of steroids[45]. A multicenter, double-blind trial by the Scottish Society of Physicians, using decreasing doses of oral hydrocortisone following an initial parenteral 400 mg bolus, found no difference in mortality between treated and control groups[46]. Subsequently, a large trial involving 446 acute infarction patients given the larger dose, 500 mg intravenous bolus of hydrocortisone followed by a continuous infusion of 500 mg over 8-10 hours, showed a significant reduction in mortality from 23.2% to 14.5%[47]. The study's validity, however, was somewhat in question since the patients were not graded for severity of infarction and the comparison group was not well controlled. Much larger doses of steroids (2 gm methylprednisolone) have demonstrated a reduction in infarct size when comparison is made between predicted and completed infarct estimates as measured by early and total CPK data[48].

On the other hand, some evidence suggests that steroids delay healing following acute myocardial infarction and could conceivably promote the development of ventricular aneurysm[49]. Therefore, while some observations suggest that a fresh look at steroid therapy in acute myocardial infarction might be appropriate, we do not recommend the routine use of oral or intravenous corticosteroids at this time for patients with acute myocardial infarction.

MOBILIZATION

Levine was possibly the first to challenge the rigid rule of prolonged immobilization for postmyocardial infarction patients[50]. Several papers have appeared over the last eight years challenging the concept of prolonged immobilization. Groden et al published the first control trial in the United Kingdom, demonstrating that mobilization on the 15th day after a myocardial infarction did not increase the incidence of complications[51]. Since that time, several other studies[52-55] have shown no increased risk from early as opposed to late mobilization following acute uncomplicated myocardial infarctions.

These observations suggest that a patient may safely begin mild activity once he is free of failure, shock, pain, and arrhythmias. Indeed, considering the documented adverse effects of prolonged bedrest[56], we believe judicious early mobilization is both reasonable and preferable to a routine program of extended immobilization. Consequently, if a patient is stable and has had an uncomplicated myocardial infarction, we allow the patient to feed himself and use a bedside commode by the second day. On the third day, he may sit in a chair, and by the fourth day, ambulate near the bed. On day five, if stable, he is moved from the coronary care unit to a progressive care area and is usually walking in the hall within seven days. Patients having uncomplicated myocardial infarctions are usually discharged within 12-14 days.

References

1. Henney, R.P., Vasko, J.S., Brawley, R.K., et al: The effects of morphine on the resistance and capacitance vessels of the peripheral circulation. *Am. Heart J.*, **72**: 242-250, 1966.
2. Capone, R., Mansour, E., Mason, D.T., Amsterdam, E.A., and Zelis, R.: "Central Sympatholysis—The mechanism of morphine induced peripheral arteriolar dilation. *Clin. Res.*, **19**: 111, 1971.
3. Alderman, E.L., Barry, W.H., Graham, A.F., and Harrison, D.C.: Hemodynamic effects of morphine and pentazocine in cardiac patients. *N. Engl. J. Med.*, **287**: 623-627, 1972.
4. Cote, P., Gueret, P., and Bourassa, M.G.: Systemic and coronary hemodynamic effects of diazepam in patients with normal and diseased coronary arteries. *Circulation*, **50**: 1210-1216, 1974.
5. McNicol, M.W. and Kirby, B.J.: Oxygen Therapy in Myocardial Infarction. In L.E. Meltzer and A.J. Dunning (Eds.): *Textbook of Coronary Care*, The Charles Press, Philadelphia, 1972, pp. 521-530.
6. Davidson, R.M., Ramo, B.W., Wallace, A.G., Whalen, R.E., and Starmer, C.F.: Blood-gas and hemodynamic responses to oxygen in acute myocardial infarction. *Circulation*, **47**: 703-710, 1973.
7. Maroko, P.R., Radvany, P., Braunwald, E., and Hale, S.L.: Reduction of infarct size by oxygen inhalation following acute coronary occlusion. *Circulation*, **52**: 360-368, 1975.
8. Robinson, D.S.: Anticoagulants Updated—Application in Coronary Artery Disease. In K. Melmon (Ed.): *Cardiovascular Drug Therapy*, F.A. Davis Co., Philadelphia, 1974, pp. 9-22.
9. Chandler, A.B., Chapman, I., Leif, E.R., Roberts, W.C., Schwartz, C.J., Sinapius, D., Spain, D.M., Sherry, S., Ness, P.M., and Simon, T.L.: Coronary thrombosis in myocardial infarction: report of a workshop on the role of coronary thrombosis in the pathogenesis of acute myocardial infarction. *Am. J. Cardiol.*, **34**: 823-833, 1974.

10. Roberts, W.C. and Buja, L.M.: The frequency and significance of coronary arterial thrombosis and other observations in fatal acute myocardial infarction: a study of 107 necropsy patients. *Am. J. Med.*, **52**: 425-443, 1972.

11. Baroldi, G.: Coronary heart disease: significance of the morphologic lesions. *Am. Heart J.*, **85**: 1-5, 1973.

12. Eliot, R.S., Baroldi, G., and Leone, A.: Necropsy studies in myocardial infarction with minimal or no coronary luminal reduction due to atherosclerosis. *Circulation*, **49**: 1127, 1974.

13. Modan, B., Shani, M., Schor, S., and Modan, M.: Reduction of hospital mortality from acute myocardial infarction by anticoagulant therapy. *N. Engl. J. Med.*, **292**: 1359-1362, 1975.

14. Tonascia, J., Cordis, L., Schmerler, P.H., and And, B.A.: Retrospective evidence favoring use of anticoagulants for myocardial infarction. *N. Engl. J. Med.*, **292**: 1362-1366, 1975.

15. Report of the Working Party on Anticoagulant Therapy in Coronary Thrombosis to the Medical Research Council: Assessment of short term anticoagulant administration after cardiac infarction. *Brit. Med. J.*, **1**: 335, 1969.

16. Results of a Cooperative Clinical Trial: Anticoagulants in acute myocardial infarction. *JAMA*, **225**: 724-729, 1975.

17. Simon, T.L., Ware, J.H., and Stengle, J.M.: Clinical trials of thrombolytic therapy in myocardial infarction. *Ann. Intern. Med.*, **79**: 712-719, 1973.

18. Isomaki, H.A.: Aspirin and myocardial infarction in patients with rheumatoid arthritis. *Lancet*, **2**: 831, 1972.

19. Elwood, P.C., Cochrane, A.L., Burr, M.L., and Sweetnam, P.M.: A randomized controlled trial of acetyl salicylic acid in the secondary prevention of mortality from myocardial infarction. *Brit. Med. J.*, **1**: 436-440, 1974.

20. Boston Collaborative Drug Surveillance Group: Regular aspirin intake and myocardial infarction. *Brit. Med. J.*, **1**: 440-442, 1974.

21. Halkin, H.: Considerations for prophylactic use of antiarrhythmic drugs in acute myocardial infarction. In K.L. Melmon (Ed.): *Cardiovascular Drug Therapy*, F.A. Davis Co., Philadelphia, 1974, pp. 119-129.

22. Bloomfield, S.S., Romhilt, D.W., Chou, T., and Fowler, N.O.: Quinidine for prophylaxis of arrhythmias in acute myocardial infarction. *N. Engl. J. Med.*, **285**: 979-986, 1971.

23. Koch-Weser, J., Klein, S.W., Foo-Canto, L.L., Kastor, J.A., and Desanctis, R.W.: Antiarrhythmic prophylaxis with procainamide in acute myocardial infarction. *N. Engl. J. Med.*, **281**: 1253-1260, 1969.

24. Chopra, M.P., Thadani, V., Portal, R.W., and Aber, C.P.: Lignocaine therapy for ventricular ectopic activity after acute myocardial infarction: a double blind trial. *Brit. Med. J.* **3**: 668-670, 1971.

25. Darby, S., Bennet, M.A., Cruickshank, J.C. et al: Trial of combined intramuscular and intravenous lignocaine in prophylaxis of ventricular tachyarrhythmias. *Lancet*, **1**: 817, 1972.

26. Pitt, A., Lipp, H., and Anderson, S.T.: Lignocaine given prophylactically to patients with acute myocardial infarction. *Lancet*, **1**: 612, 1971.

27. Mogensen, L.: A controlled trial of lignocaine prophylaxis in the prevention of ventricular tachyarrhythmias in acute myocardial infarction. *Acta Med. Scan*, **513**: 39, 1971.

28. Lie, K.I., Wellens, H.J., Van Capelle, F.J., and Durrer, D.: Lidocaine in the prevention of primary ventricular fibrillation. A double blind randomized study of 212 consecutive patients. *N. Engl. J. Med.*, **291**: 1324-1326, 1974.

29. Valentine, P.A., Frew, J.L., Mashford, M.L., and Sloman, J.G.: Lidocaine in the prevention of sudden death in the prehospital phase of acute infarction. *N. Engl. J. Med.*, **291**: 1327-1331, 1974.

30. Lie, K.I., Wellens, H.J.J., Downar, E., and Durrer, D.: Observations on patients with primary ventricular fibrillation complicating acute myocardial infarction. *Circulation,* **52**: 755, 1975.

31. Epstein, S.E., Goldstein, R.E., Redwood, D.R., Kent, K.M., and Smith, E.R.: The early phase of acute myocardial infarction; Pharmacologic aspects of therapy. *Ann. Intern. Med.,* **78**: 918-936, 1973.

32. Rahimtoola, S.H. and Gunnar, R.M.: Digitalis in acute myocardial infarction: help or hazard. *Ann. Intern. Med.,* **82**: 234-240, 1975.

33. Constant, J.: Digitalis in myocardial infarction: therapy concepts. *N.Y. State J. Med.,* **70**: 650-658, 1970.

34. Hodges, M., Friesinger, G.C., Riggins, R.C.K., and Dagenais, G.R.: Effects of intravenously administered digoxin on mild left ventricular failure in acute myocardial infarction in man. *Am. J. Cardiol.,* **29**: 749-755, 1972.

35. Lipp, H., Denes, P., Gambetta, M., et al: Hemodynamic response to acute intravenous digoxin in patients with recent myocardial infarction and coronary insufficiency with and without heart failure. *Chest,* **63**: 862-867, 1972.

36. Forrester, J.S., Bezdek, W., Chatterjee, K., et al: Hemodynamic effects of digitalis in acute myocardial infarction. *Ann. Intern. Med.,* **76**: 863-864, 1972.

37. Rahimtoola, S.H., Sinno, M.Z., Chuquimia, R., Loeb, H.S., Rosen, K.M., and Gunnar, R.M.: Effects of ouabain on impaired left ventricular function in acute myocardial infarction. *N. Engl. J. Med.,* **287**: 527-531, 1972.

38. Maroko, P.K., Wattanabe, T., Covell, J.W., Braunwald, E., Bernstein, E.F., and Ross, J., Jr.: The effect of positive inotropic agents and counterpulsation on myocardial ischemic injury following experimental coronary occlusion. *Circulation,* **42 (Suppl III)**: III-81, 1970.

39. Dikshit, K., Vyden, J.K., Forrester, J.S., Chatterjee, K., Prakash, R., and Swan, H.J.C.: Renal and extrarenal hemodynamic effects of furosemide in congestive heart failure after acute myocardial infarction. *N. Engl. J. Med.,* **288**: 1087-1090, 1973.

40. Borer, J.S., Redwood, D.R., Levitt, R., Cagin, N., Bianchi, C., Vallin, H., and Epstein, S.E.: Myocardial ischemia treated with nitroglycerin plus phenylephrine. *N. Engl. J. Med.,* **293**: 1008-1012, 1975.

41. Come, P.C., Flaherty, J.T., Baird, M.G., et al: Reversal by phenylephrine of beneficial effects of intravenous nitroglycerin in acute myocardial infarction. *N. Engl. J. Med.,* **293**: 1003-1007, 1975.

42. Gold, H.K., Leinbach, R.C., and Sanders, C.A.: Use of sublingual nitroglycerin in congestive failure following acute myocardial infarction. *Circulation,* **46**: 839-845, 1972.

43. Dumesnil, J.G., Ritman, E.L., Davis, G.D., Gau, G.T., Rutherford, B.D., and Frye, R.L.: Regional left ventricular wall dynamics before and after sublingual administration of nitroglycerin. *Am. J. Cardiol.,* **36**: 419-425, 1975.

44. Reichek, N., Goldstein, R.E., Nager, M., et al: Sustained effects of nitroglycerin ointment in patients with angina pectoris. *Circulation,* **46 (Suppl. II)**: 209, 1972.

45. Semple, T. and Dall, J.L.C.: Steroids in myocardial infarction. *Am. Heart J.,* **70**: 716-717, 1965.

46. Scottish Society of Physicians Trial. Hydrocortisone in severe myocardial infarction. *Lancet,* **2**: 785, 1964.

47. Barzilai, D., Plavnick, J., Hazani, A., Einath, R., Kleinhaus, N., and Kantery: Use of hydrocortisone in the treatment of acute myocardial infarction. *Chest,* **61**: 488-491, 1972.

48. Maley, T., Gulotta, S., and Morrison, J.: Effect of methylprednisone on predicted infarct size in man. *Clin. Res.,* **14**: 193, 1966.

49. Bulkley, B.H. and Roberts, W.C.: Steroid therapy during acute myocardial infarction: a cause of delayed healing and of ventricular aneurysm. *Am. J. Med.*, **56**: 244-250, 1974.

50. Levine, S.A.: Some harmful effects of recumbency in the treatment of heart disease. *JAMA*, **126**: 80-84, 1944.

51. Groden, B.M., Allison, A., and Shaw, G.B.: Management of myocardial infarction: the effects of early mobilization. *Scot. Med. J.*, **12**: 435-440, 1967.

52. Harpur, J.E., Kellet, R.J., Conner, W.T., et al: Controlled trial of early mobilization and discharge from hospital in uncomplicated myocardial infarction. *Lancet*, **2**: 1331-1334, 1971.

53. Hutter, A.M., Jr., Sidel, V.W., Shine, K.I., and Desanctis, R.W.: Early hospital discharge after myocardial infarction. *N. Engl. J. Med.*, **288**: 1141-1144, 1973.

54. Hayes, M.J., Morris, G.K., and Hampton, J.R.: Comparison of mobilization after two and nine days in myocardial infarction. *Brit. Med. J.*, **3**: 10-13, 1974.

55. Abraham, A.S., Sever, Y., Weinstein, M., Dollberg, M., and Menczel, J.: Early ambulation after myocardial infarction. *N. Engl. J. Med.*, **292**: 719-722, 1975.

56. Fareeduddin, K. and Abelman, W.H.: Impaired orthostatic tolerance after bed rest in patients with myocardial infarction. *N. Engl. J. Med.*, **280**: 345-350, 1969.

CHAPTER 11

The Treatment of Congestive Failure and Acute Pulmonary Edema

James S. Forrester, M.D.; Protasio L. DaLuz, M.D.;
David D. Waters, M.D.; H.J.C. Swan, M.D., Ph.D.

This Chapter briefly redefines the various pathophysiologic forms (sub-sets) of congestive failure seen in cardiac emergencies. The therapeutic agents are then discussed and highlighted for quick reference in tabular form. Finally, the proper therapeutic agents are matched with each subset of cardiac failure.

An important consequence of hemodynamic monitoring in coronary care units during the last decade has been the identification of subsets of patients with various degrees and types of circulatory impairment. Identification of subset is not at all an academic exercise, since the hemodynamic and metabolic effects of therapeutic agents vary substantially within each sub-set. The fact that the effects of therapeutic agents can be reasonably predicted within a given subset provides a rational basis for the therapy of cardiac failure.

SUBSETS OF PATIENTS WITH HEART FAILURE

The concept of subsets is in no way unique to the problem of acute heart failure. In most therapeutic decision making, we seek to establish recognizable sub-groups of patients about whom we can make relevant statements concerning prognosis or therapy which do not necessarily apply to the entire patient population. In an earlier chapter, we discussed heart failure in terms of pulmonary congestion and peripheral hypoperfusion, each of which has a specific and independently variable hemodynamic cause. Elevating pulmonary capillary pressure results in pulmonary congestion and reducing cardiac index causes peripheral hypoperfusion. Since pulmonary congestion and peripheral hypoperfusion can occur either independently or together, four subsets of patients can be recognized:

1. No pulmonary congestion or peripheral hypoperfusion.
2. Pulmonary congestion without hypoperfusion.
3. Peripheral hypoperfusion without congestion.
4. Combined pulmonary congestion and peripheral hypoperfusion.

The major justification for establishing subjects is its relevance to clinical care. This subset classification is particularly relevant for three reasons. First, the hemodynamic determinants of pulmonary congestion and peripheral hypoperfusion, pulmonary capillary pressure and cardiac index, represent the two axes of the Starling relationship ("performance" vs. "preload"). Thus, the four subsets represent different levels of cardiac function. Second, because survival in acute heart failure is directly related to the level of cardiac function, the subsets are of major prognostic value (Table I). Third, both the primary goals of therapy and the response to drugs are different in each subset of cardiac function.

TABLE I
MORTALITY RATES IN CLINICAL AND HEMODYNAMIC SUBSETS

Subset	Pulmonary Congestion (PCP > 18 mm Hg)	Peripheral Hypoperfusion (CI < 2.2 L/ Min/M²)	% Mortality Clinical	% Mortality Hemodynamic
I	-	-	1	3
II	+	-	11	9
III	-	+	18	23
IV	+	+	60	51

The two basic principles of therapy for heart failure are to: (1) reduce pulmonary congestion by decreasing pulmonary capillary pressure when it is elevated, and (2) reduce hypoperfusion by increasing cardiac output when it is depressed. When heart failure is secondary to acute myocardial infarction, there is an additional goal. Since therapy directed at improving cardiac performance by altering cardiac output and pulmonary capillary pressure may substantially affect both myocardial oxygen supply and demand, attention also must be given to the effects of therapeutic agents upon the degree of myocardial ischemia (Figure 1). Therapy which increases contractility, afterload (arterial systolic pressure), preload (pulmonary capillary pressure), or heart rate, increases myocardial oxygen demand. Because it is unlikely that medical therapy will increase flow to ischemic areas in the presence of fixed proximal coronary artery stenoses, an increase in oxygen demand carries a substantial risk for increasing infarct size. In acute myocardial ischemia, therefore, an agent which improves cardiac performance may also increase infarct size[1] if changes in the four major determinants of oxygen demand are not carefully controlled.

THE RESPONSE TO THERAPY

Because of the advances in hemodynamic monitoring made in the past several years, it is now possible to reasonably predict the response to a given therapy in an individual with heart failure. To accomplish this, it is necessary to understand the two major determinants of this response: (1) the resting

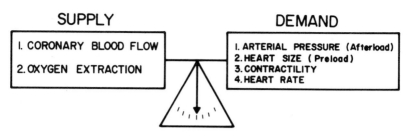

Figure 1 The determinants of myocardial oxygen supply and demand. Increases in arterial pressure, heart size, contractility, and heart rate augment oxygen demand. An appropriate balance is maintained whenever changes in oxygen demand are followed by directionally and quantitatively similar changes in supply. Since myocardial oxygen extraction is normally high (approximately 70-80%), an increase in coronary blood flow is the major mechanism by which an increased oxygen demand is met.

level of cardiac function and (2) the drug's mechanism of action which varies with the level of cardiac function and the state of compensatory response mechanisms.

Therapeutic agents employed to improve cardiac function are usefully considered in three classes: diuretics, vasodilators, and inotropic agents. There is also a fourth miscellaneous group of agents which do not fit these categories. This classification is particularly suitable in clinical practice, for although there are substantial variations in the magnitude of effects, the direction of the hemodynamic response to various drugs within each subset is similar.

Diuretic Agents

Diuretic agents reduce pulmonary capillary pressure with little change in cardiac output or heart rate in patients with heart failure[2,3]. There are two mechanisms by which these agents reduce elevated pulmonary capillary pressure. The most immediate effect is extrarenal and has been described for both furosemide and ethacrynic acid. These agents produce a rapid and substantial increase in venous capacitance, resulting in a redistribution of venous blood toward the periphery and a consequent reduction in pulmonary capillary pressure. An important characteristic of this effect is that it occurs within approximately 5 minutes of the drug administration, thus preceding the diuretic effect and making these drugs useful in acutely ill patients.

The second mechanism increases sodium and water excretion by the kidney. The resulting diuresis produces a decrease in intravascular volume, and a consequent decrease in left ventricular volume and pressure. This leads to a reduction in pulmonary capillary pressure and relief of pulmonary congestion. When pulmonary capillary pressure is reduced from high levels to 15 to 18 mm little change in cardiac output occurs. As pulmonary capillary pressure is reduced from this range to lower levels, however, a substantial decrease in cardiac output may be observed, as the left ventricle descends on its Starling function curve (Figure 2). Therefore, patients with isolated pulmonary congestion (Subset II) improve clinically, when pulmonary capillary pressure decreases with no change in cardiac index; whereas in those patients without pulmonary congestion (Subsets I and III), clinical deterioration may occur secondary to diminished cardiac index. In subset IV (both pulmonary congestion and peripheral hypoperfusion) diuretics will relieve pulmonary congestion but have no effect on the signs and symptoms of peripheral hypoperfusion, since cardiac index does not increase.

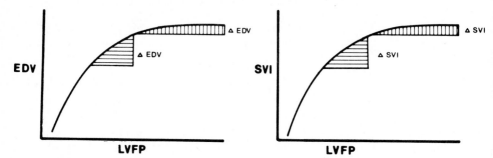

Figure 2 The effect of initial left ventricular volume upon the hemodynamic response to therapeutic reduction in preload. In the left panel, the relationship between end-diastolic volume (EDV) and left ventricular filling pressure (LVFP) is shown. When the left ventricular volume is high (i.e., the flat part of the pressure-volume curve) a substantial reduction in LVFP can occur with only a small reduction in LVEDV. In contrast, the magnitude reduction in LVFP beginning from a normal volume (i.e., on the ascending part of the pressure-volume curve) is associated with a large decrease in LVEDV. This phenomenon is related to cardiac output in the right panel, which illustrates the relationship between stroke volume index (SVI) and LVFP (the Frank-Starling mechanism). In the flat portion of the function curve (i.e., at high left ventricular volume, as in heart failure) a decrease in LVFP is associated with a relatively small change in LVEDV. Therefore, little change in SVI occurs because preload is little altered. On the ascending portion of the function curve (normal LVFP), however, since a similar change in LVFP is associated with a substantial change in LVEDV, a substantial fall in SVI can occur secondary to decreased preload. Thus when diuretics or vasodilators are allowed to produce a marked decrease in LVFP, a substantial reduction in cardiac output may occur.

The advantages and disadvantages, mechanisms of action and doses of the most commonly used diuretics are shown in Table II. Thiazide diuretics act at the ascending limb of the loop of Henle and distal tubule to prevent reabsorption of sodium. Furosemide and ethacrynic acid, the most potent diuretics, exert their effect through the entire loop of Henle as well as the distal tubule. Spironolactone, the aldosterone antagonist, acts only on the distal renal tubule to prevent sodium potassium exchange. Therefore, it is less potent than the other agents, but conserves potassium, which other agents cause to be excreted in large amounts. Furosemide and ethacrynic acid are best used when rapid and profound diuresis is required, as in the treatment of acute pulmonary edema. Since these drugs cause a potent kaluresis, serum potassium levels should be monitored during such therapy.

TABLE II
DIURETICS

	Mechanism of Action	Advantages	Disadvantages	Initial Dose
1. Furosemide	Block Na^+ reabsorption in loop of Henle and distal tubules	Potency 4+ Fast acting Safe	May cause sudden hypotension. Tendency to refractoriness. Rebound phenomenon after withdrawal Kaluresis	40 mg IV or oral
2. Ethacrynic acid	Same as above	Potency 4+ Fast acting Safe	Same as above	50 mg IV or oral
3. Thiazides	Na^+ reabsorption in distal tubules Inhibits free water formation	Potency 3+ Fast acting	Kaluresis Tendency to refractoriness	25-50 mg oral
4. Aldosterone antagonists	Prevent Na^+-K^+ exchange at distal renal tubule by competing with aldosterone	No K^+ loss	Immediate effectiveness is less than with furosemide, ethacrynic acid or thiazides	25-100 mg oral

Peripheral Vasodilators

These agents are dramatically effective in improving cardiac hemodynamics in patients with heart failure. Cardiac output increases substantially, pulmonary capillary pressure falls, and there is little change in heart rate. The mechanism for this response is shown in Figure 3. Reduction in resistance to ejection results in an increase in ejection fraction, which is translated into an increase in stroke volume and cardiac output. The increase in systolic emptying leads to a decreased left ventricular diastolic volume, and decreased pulmonary capillary pressure.

Like diuretic agents, the effect of peripheral vasodilators differs between patients in the heart failure subsets and those classified as normal. Peripheral vasodilators *increase* stroke volume in patients with elevated pulmonary capillary pressure (Subsets II and IV), but *decrease* stroke volume and increase heart rate in patients with normal levels of pulmonary capillary pressure (Subsets I and III). The mechanisms responsible for these differences are illustrated in Table III. Individuals with normal cardiac function (Subset I) have a normal ejection fraction. Therefore, they have little

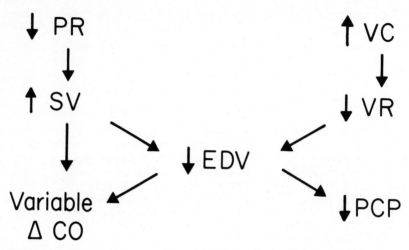

Figure 3 Mechanism of action of peripheral vasodilators. PR = peripheral vascular resistance, SV = stroke volume, EDV = end-diastolic volume, CO = cardiac output, VC = venous capacitance, VR = venous return, PCP = pulmonary capillary pressure.

There are two major effects of peripheral vasodilators. The first is to reduce resistance to ejection, thus increasing stroke volume and decreasing EDV or PCP. The second is to dilate veins, thus increasing VC and decreasing VR: these effects also reduce EDV and PCP. The final effect on CO is variable, depending upon the relative effect of the agent upon the arteriolar and venular beds, and the level of PCP at the time of drug administration.

TABLE III
VASODILATORS

	Mechanism of action	Advantages	Disadvantages	Dose range
1. Nitroprusside	Relaxation of smooth muscle of arteries and veins	Potency 4+ Immediate effect Half-life extremely short	Requires hemo-dynamic monitoring	15-400 μg/min IV
2. Phentolamine	Relaxation of smooth muscle primarily in arterial walls	Potency 4+ Fast acting	Requires hemo-dynamic monitoring	0.25-1.0 mg/min IV
3. Isosorbide Dinitrate	Relaxation of smooth muscle of arteries and veins	Sublingual administration	Less potent than nitroprusside or phentolamine Effect for only 1½ hours	2.5-5 mg
4. Nitroglycerin Ointment	Relaxation of smooth muscle of arteries and veins	Prolonged duration of action—up to 6 hours Removable	Topical use not well accepted by all patients	1.5-4.0 inches

capability to increase ejection fraction above the normal range by reducing peripheral vascular resistance. Since peripheral vasodilators also dilate peripheral veins, resulting in peripheral venous pooling, reduction in stroke volume occurs due to the Starling effect. In contrast, individuals with increased pulmonary capillary pressure due to heart failure, exhibit an increase in ejection fraction with reduction in peripheral vascular resistance which in turn leads to an increase in stroke volume and a decrease in pulmonary capillary pressure[4].

The specific peripheral vasodilators, their advantages and disadvantages, and doses are shown in Table III. Nitroglycerin[5] exerts its effect primarily on the venous system, phentolamine[6,7] primarily on the arterial system, and nitroprusside[8,9] acts somewhere between the two. The most potent agents are nitroprusside and phentolamine. Phentolamine is seldom used because it is considerably more expensive than nitroprusside. The use of nitroprusside to improve cardiac performance has several major advantages. Its effect on hemodynamics is immediate, and its half life is extremely short (about 30 seconds in the systemic circulation). Its major disadvantage is that intravascular hemodynamic monitoring is required to control drug administration. Of the nitrates which have so far been studied, isosorbide dinitrate[10] and nitroglycerin ointment[11] have received the most attention. These two agents are approximately equally potent. Sublingual Isordil's® major disadvantage is that it lasts a relatively short time, about 1½ hours, and therefore requires frequent administration. Nitroglycerin ointment is an exceptionally effective drug for the treatment of both acute and chronic heart failure and has a medium range duration (4-6 hours). Its disadvantage is that cutaneous application may be unpleasant to some individuals.

The use of vasodilating agents is limited by their propensity to aggravate hypotension in patients with severe heart failure. The response to infusion of a peripheral vasodilator, however, generally follows a three step progression determined by dose level (Table IV). At low doses, cardiac output increases and pulmonary capillary pressure decreases with little change in arterial pressure. If the infusion rate is then increased, a further increase in cardiac output and fall in pulmonary capillary pressure occurs, but arterial pressure also begins to decrease. If the infusion rate is again increased, profound vasodilatation occurs, and cardiac output, pulmonary capillary pressure, and arterial pressure all fall. At this infusion rate peripheral vasodilating agents are potentially lethal. For this reason to avoid overdosage, two guidelines are employed in vasodilator therapy: (1) pulmonary capillary pressure should not fall below 15 to 18 mm Hg (if the patient is being evaluated clinically, these drugs should not be administered in the absence of rales) and (2) arterial pressure should be kept within the physiologic range (generally, greater than 100 mm Hg peak systolic pressure).

Inotropic Agents

Inotropic agents increase cardiac output and decrease pulmonary capil-

TABLE IV

DOSE DEPENDENT RESPONSE TO PERIPHERAL VASODILATORS

	AP	LVP	CO
Low dose	↔	↓	↑
Medium dose	↓	↓↓	↑↑
High dose	↓	↓↓	↓

AP = arterial pressure
LVFP = left ventricular filling pressure
CO = cardiac output

lary pressure by improving myocardial contractility. These agents, therefore, are quite effective in the treatment of Subsets II (isolated pulmonary congestion) and IV (both pulmonary congestion and peripheral hypoperfusion). Because increased myocardial contractility also increases myocardial oxygen demand, these agents are of limited value when acute myocardial ischemia accompanies acute heart failure. Table V illustrates the advantages and disadvantages, mechanisms of action, and dose levels of the commonly used inotropic agents.

Digitalis compounds[12,13] have three important cardiovascular effects: they increase myocardial contractility, slow atrioventricular conduction and heart rate, and constrict both peripheral arterioles and venules. They are effective agents for increasing cardiac output and decreasing pulmonary capillary pressure in patients with heart failure, but have little effect on cardiac output in normal individuals.

Digoxin is currently the most commonly used digitalis preparation in patients with heart failure. It is approximately 80% absorbed in the gastrointestinal tract, and its serum half-life is approximately 1.5 days. Most digoxin is excreted by the kidneys at a rate proportional to the glomerular filtration rate, but a small percentage is metabolized by the liver. When given intravenously, the effect of digoxin can be detected at 10 minutes, and at approximately 30 minutes to an hour its peak effect is attained. Little therapeutic advantage can be gained by using a more rapidly acting digitalis preparation.

Few drugs have a more narrow therapeutic-to-toxic dose ratio than digitalis: the prevalence of digitalis toxicity in hospitalized patients has been reported to be as high as 20 to 30%. Therefore, the dosage employed and the rate of administration should be governed by the clinical circumstances. For instance, in a situation of moderate urgency, such as rapid atrial fibrillation associated with moderate pulmonary congestion, it would be appropriate to administer 1 mg of digoxin intravenously followed by 0.25 mg intravenously every four hours until the ventricular rate decreases to less than 100 beats/min. The loading dose of digitalis should be related to body size and the maintenance dose related to renal function. 0.25 mg of digoxin per day is

TABLE V
INOTROPIC AGENTS

Drug	Dosage	Action	Adverse Effects
Digoxin	loading: 1 to 1 ½ mg Maint.: variable	Na-K ATPase blocker	↑MVO$_2$, freq. toxicity, electrophysiol. effects
Norepinephrine	titrate to AP	α & β stimulation	↑MVO$_2$, arrhythmias, renal vasoconstriction
Dopamine	5-10μgm/kg/min	β1 stimulation	↑MVO$_2$, arrhythmias
Isoproterenol	1-5μgm/kg/min	β stimulation	↑MVO$_2$, arrhythmias

AP = arterial pressure
MVO$_2$ = myocardial oxygen consumption
Maint. = maintenance

an average maintenance dose for an averaged sized individual with normal renal function.

Catecholamines, including epinephrine, norepinephrine[14,15], isoproterenol[16], glucagon[17] and dopamine[18,19] all reduce pulmonary capillary pressure and increase cardiac output in patients with heart failure. The differences in mechanisms of action relate predominantly to the magnitude of effects of these agents upon the so-called α- and β-adrenergic receptors. The α-receptors are responsible for adrenergic medicated peripheral vasoconstriction and the β-receptors are responsible for cardiac stimulation (β1 receptors) and sympathetic vasodilatation (β2 receptors). Isoproterenol and glucagon are peripheral vasodilators, and can increase cardiac output by this mechanism, whereas both dopamine and norepinephrine are dominantly β-adrenergic at low doses and α-adrenergic at high doses. Inotropic agents therefore differ predominantly in their effect upon arterial pressure: in the clinical dosage usually employed, dopamine and norepinephrine increase and isoproterenol and glucagon cause no change or decrease arterial pressure. Because it is the most potent inotropic agent, isoproterenol is probably the most effective in increasing cardiac output and decreasing pulmonary capillary pressure, but is also most prone to aggravate myocardial ischemia if it is present. Dopamine may be used for the Subset IV patient with concomitant hypotension, and norepinephrine should be utilized when immediate restoration of arterial systolic pressure takes precedence over all other considerations.

Other Agents

Morphine is perhaps the most important agent used in the treatment of acute pulmonary edema. It has three important actions: it is a potent peripheral vasodilator, has minor inotropic effects, and it is a central nervous system sedative. Given intravenously to a patient with acute pulmonary edema, its peripheral venous and arterial vasodilating effects cause a substantial reduction in pulmonary capillary pressure, and may increase cardiac output if it is depressed. As with other peripheral vasodilating agents, excessive drug administration can cause a fall in cardiac output and arterial pressure. Although the drug is a respiratory depressant, when cautiously administered it does not produce respiratory failure nor aggravate CO_2 retention associated with acute pulmonary edema.

Oxygen increases peripheral vascular resistance, and can lead to a reduction in cardiac output. This disadvantage, however, is outweighed by its beneficial effects. Acute pulmonary edema is associated with hypoxemia due to veno-arterial intrapulmonary shunting. Administration of oxygen therefore serves partially to reduce hypoxemia, and thereby increse oxygen delivery to ischemic tissues. Recent experimental evidence also suggests that oxygen administration during acute myocardial infarction may reduce the severity of ischemic injury to the myocardium.

AN APPROACH TO THE TREATMENT OF ACUTE HEART FAILURE

In this section we will outline a practical physiologically based approach to the management of patients with acute heart failure. In the most acutely ill patients, two series of treatment decisions are required. The first concerns selection of an appropriate treatment within the first several minutes, and of necessity must follow the most cursory of evaluations. The second set of treatment decisions involves those made within the first several hours, in which both a more careful evaluation is required and a greater range of therapeutic alternatives is presented.

When a patient is first seen with severe acute heart failure the predominant symptoms are either those associated with marked elevation in pulmonary capillary pressure—signs of severe pulmonary congestion, or the symptoms of acute reduction in cardiac output—the signs of peripheral hypoperfusion. This initial distinction provides the basis for treatment within the first several minutes.

Acute Pulmonary Edema: The First Few Minutes

Prior to therapy one critical question must be answered: is there clear evidence that the patient has pulmonary congestion and not acute respiratory failure secondary to other causes? The administration of morphine to a patient with primary respiratory failure, for instance, can substantially aggravate this disorder, whereas it may be lifesaving in acute pulmonary congestion of cardiac origin. If the diagnosis of acute pulmonary congestion secondary to heart failure is established within the first minutes of seeing the patient, three emergency procedures are indicated: (1) administer oxygen by face mask, nasal cannula, or endotracheal tube, (2) place a large bore intravenous line, (3) administer five to 10 mg morphine sulfate IV slowly over several minutes. If for any reason morphine cannot be immediately given, a sublingual peripheral vasodilator such as nitroglycerin

may be an extremely effective alternative. If these therapies are not immediately effective, phlebotomy (range 100 to 500 cc) may be performed, or rotating tourniquets may be employed.
quets may be employed.

Peripheral Hypoperfusion: The First Few Minutes

As with pulmonary congestion, one critical question must be answered prior to therapy: is the acute hypoperfusion due to a cardiac or non-cardiac cause; specifically, is there cardiogenic shock or hypovolemia? A rapid evaluation for evidence of pulmonary congestion, most importantly the presence of rales on auscultation, is critical to this distinction. Although the distinction may seem to be relatively straightforward, it can be deceptively difficult in a patient with severe peripheral hypoperfusion who has shallow breathing, or when only a few rales are audible. If hypovolemia is present, fluid replacement takes immediate priority. In all other cases with associated hypotension, three procedures must be initiated immediately:

1. Place both an intravenous cannula and intraarterial line.
2. Continuously infuse a pressor agent through the intravenous line (norepinephrine, 5 µg/min or dopamine, 5-10 µg/min are both suitable). Systolic arterial pressure should be titrated to a level of 90 to 120 mm Hg.
3. Administer oxygen by face mask, nasal cannula, or endotracheal intubation.

The above therapies are administered as emergency measures without regard to the etiology of the presenting symptomatology, and are dominantly directed toward immediate reduction of pulmonary capillary pressure in acute pulmonary congestion and increase in cardiac output or arterial pressure in acute peripheral hypoperfusion. As soon as these emergency procedures have been completed, the second phase of emergency treatment for acute heart failure should begin.

The First Few Hours

The process of therapeutic decision making during this time depends upon subset identification and upon the immediate cause of acute heart failure. *Subset I* (normal function) is not germane to this discussion.

Subset II is characterized by isolated pulmonary congestion, i.e., an isolated increase in pulmonary capillary pressure. Although an increase in pulmonary capillary pressure is most commonly due to depressed function, cardiac index is not necessarily decreased. Most compensatory mechanisms are geared to preserve cardiac output, even at the expense of pulmonary capillary pressure. For instance, dilatation, hypertrophy, and renal mechanisms can all increase cardiac index but also increase pulmonary capillary pressure. Thus, the clinical manifestations of increased pulmonary capillary pressure generally precede those of decreased cardiac index in heart failure, and isolated pulmonary congestion is probably the most common of the subsets of heart failure.

Treatment in this subset is directed primarily at reducing pulmonary capillary pressure. The most effective agents for this purpose are the diuretics, because they can be readily administered with few side effects. When diuretics are ineffective in relieving pulmonary congestion in the absence of acute myocardial ischemia, digitalis is also effective, but carries a greater risk of toxicity than the diuretics. Other inotropic agents are of limited value in this subset. If diuretics are ineffective and acute ischemia is present, a trial of sublingual or topical nitrates is appropriate.

Patients in *Subset III* have circulatory failure, often without a cardiac abnormality. There are three major causes. The majority of patients in this subset demonstrate reduction in stroke volume with a compensatory tachycardia. Such patients often exhibit substantial improvement with volume loading. The amount of volume administration is controlled by the hemodynamic response. In general, cardiac output will increase with volume infusion until the level of pulmonary capillary pressure reaches approximately 15-18 mm Hg after which further increase in cardiac output is minimal. Depending upon the etiology of the signs of peripheral hypoperfusion, patients may or may not return to normal cardiac function. For instance, the patient is Subset III who presents with bleeding as the etiology for peripheral hypoperfusion will respond quite well to volume replacement; on the other hand a patient with acute myocardial infarction may still exhibit substantial reduction in cardiac output after pulmonary capillary pressure is brought to the high normal range. Such patients may then be identified as part of Subset IV (combined peripheral hypoperfusion and pulmonary congestion) and treated with additional agents such as peripheral vasodilators, but only after adequate volume replacement.

A small group of patients in this subset have a normal stroke volume and a reduced heart rate. This group of patients may respond quite favorably to a therapeutic increase in heart rate, the most substantial increases in cardiac output being observed in patients with heart rates in the range of 5-70 beats/min, with little response in cardiac index beyond 90-100 beats/min. In units equipped with temporary transvenous pacemaking capability, this is the therapy of choice because the response can be titrated directly to heart rate. In the absence of pacemaking capability, intravenous atropine may increase heart rate and cardiac output in this group of patients.

The third group of patients presenting as clinical Subset III are those with marked reduction in peripheral vascular resistance, frequently secondary to arterial-venous shunting. In this group, cardiac output may be within the normal range, although peripheral perfusion is markedly reduced. Appropriate therapy for this group has not been clearly defined. The most effective therapy for these patients is that directed at the underlying disease itself (e.g., specific antibiotic therapy for septicemic shock, epinephrine and steroids for anaphylaxis).

After a patient has been identified in *Subset IV*, attention should center upon the level of arterial pressure. If arterial pressure is in the physiologic range, the choice of therapies lies between inotropic agents and peripheral vasodilators, which are of comparable effectiveness in improving cardiac function. Both groups are limited by the side effects which they produce. In the presence of acute myocardial infarction, the use of peripheral vasodilators is much to be preferred, since these agents reduce myocardial oxygen requirement, whereas inotropic agents increase myocardial oxygen requirement and by so doing may increase infarct size. Vasodilator administration, on the other hand, may be limited by development of hypotension. In the absence of both myocardial ischemia and hypotension, isoproterenol is the most potent inotropic agent, but should be used with caution in patients with known disease of any type. Digitalis is most commonly the inotropic agent of choice in the absence of myocardial ischemia, although its potency is not as great as other inotropic agents or intravenous peripheral vasodilators. The potency of peripheral vasodilators varies widely between the intravenous agents (nitroprusside and phentolamine) which increase cardiac output by 25-75%[8] and the sublingual, oral, or topical agents (nitroglycerin, isosorbide) which increase cardiac output by about 25% when optimally administered.

When arterial pressure is less than 100 mm Hg, the inotropic agents with a pressor action are generally the drugs of choice. Dopamine offers a considerable advantage in this situation. It has a mild pressor action which is readily titrated and also increases cardiac index. In addition, its selective action on important vascular beds promotes distribution of blood flow to desired areas: specifically, it increases renal and mesenteric perfusion. In contrast, norepinephrine offers more potency for increasing arterial pressure, but is more difficult to titrate. The increased arterial pressure generally is a reflection of a more substantial increase in peripheral vascular resistance than in cardiac output and the agent may be less effective than dopamine in increasing flow to vital organs. For this reason, administration of agents such as norepinephrine is seldom of lasting benefit and should be viewed primarily as a temporizing measure to obtain control of arterial pressure until a more effective therapy can be administered. As with patients with normal arterial pressure, digitalis may also be effectively employed to increase cardiac index in the hypotensive patients in Subset IV, although a substantial increase in arterial pressure should not be expected.

In summary, the therapy of acute heart failure is predicated upon an understanding of the hemodynamic basis of the presenting symptoms. Based upon this understanding, subsets of patients can be identified. The response to a therapeutic agent in each subset is different, because drugs have multiple effects on the myocardium, the peripheral vasculature, and the determinants of myocardial oxygen supply and demand. Through an understanding of these complex interactions, it is possible to select an appropriate therapy and predict its effect in a substantial majority of patients with heart failure.

References

1. Maroko, P.R., Kjekshus, J.K., Sobel, B.E., et al: Factors influencing infarct size

208 / Cardiac Emergencies

following experimental coronary artery occlusion. *Circulation*, **43**: 67-82, 1971.

2. Dikshit, K., Vyden, J.K., Forrester, J.S., et al: Renal and extrarenal hemo-dynamic effects of furosemide in congestive heart failure after acute myocardial infarction. *N. Engl. J. Med.*, **288**: 1087-1090, 1973.

3. Mond, H., Hunt, D., and Sloman, G.: Haemodynamic effects of furosemide in patients suspected of having acute myocardial infarction. *Brit. Heart. J.*, **36**: 44-53, 1974.

4. da Luz, P.L. and Forrester, J.S.: Influence of vasodilators upon function and metabolism of ischemic myocardium. *Am. J. Cardiol.*, In press.

5. Gold, H.K., Leinbach, R.C., and Sanders, C.A.: Use of sublingual nitro-glycerin in congestive failure following acute myocardial infarction. *Circulation*, **46**: 839-845, 972.

6. Walinsky, P., Chatterjee, K., Forrester, J., et al: Enhanced left ventricular per-formance with phentolamine in acute myocardial infarction. *Am. J. Cardiol.*, **33**: 37-41, 1974.

7. da Luz, P.L., Subin, H., and Weil, M.H.: Effectiveness of phentolamine for reversal of circulatory failure (shock). *Critical Care Medicine*, **1**: 135, 1973.

8. Chatterjee, K., Parmley, W.W., Ganz, W., et al: Hemodynamic and metabolic responses to vasodilator therapy in acute myocardial infarction. *Circulation*, **48**: 1183-1193, 1973.

9. Franciosa, J.A., Guiha, N.H., Limas, C.J., et al: Improved left ventricular func-tion during nitroprusside infusion in acute myocardial infarction. *Lancet*, **1**: 650-654, 1972.

10. Gray, R., Chatterjee, J., Vyden, J.K., et al: Hemodynamic and metabolic effects of isosorbide dinitrate in chronic congestive heart failure. *Am. Heart J.*, **90**: 346-352, 1975.

11. Taylor, W.R., Forrester, J.S., Magnusson, P., et al: The hemodynamic effects of nitroglycerin ointment in congestive heart failure. Submitted to *Am. J. Cardiol.* for publication.

12. Rahimtoola, S.H., and Gunnar, R.M.: Digitalis in acute myocardial infarction: help or hazard? *Ann. Intern. Med.*, **82**: 234-240, 1975.

13. Rahimtoola, S.H., Sinno, M.Z., Chuquimia, R., et al: Effects of ouabain on im-paired left ventricular function in acute myocardial infarction. *N. Engl. J. Med.*, **287**: 527-531, 1972.

14. Abrams, E., Forrester, J.S., Chatterjee, K., et al: Variability in response to norepinephrine in acute myocardial infarciton. *Am. J. Cardiol.*, **32**: 919-923, 1973.

15. Mueller, H., Ayres, S.M., Giannelli, S. Jr., et al: Cardial performance and metabolism in shock due to acute myocardial infarction in man: response to catecholamines and mechanical cardiac assist. *Trans. N.Y. Acad. Science*, **34**: 309-333, 1972.

16. Misra, S.N. and Kezdi, P.: Hemodynamic effects of adrenergic stimulating and blocking agents in cardiogenic shock and low output state after myocardial in-farction. *Am. J. Cardiol.*, **31**: 724-735, 1973.

17. Diamond, G.A., Forrester, J.S., Danzig, R., et al: Haemodynamic effects of glucagon during acute myocardial infarction with left ventricular failure in man. *Brit. Heart. J.*, **33**: 290-295, 1971.

18. Talley, R.C., Goldberg, L.I., Johnson, C.E., et al: A hemodynamic comparison of dopamine and isoproterenol in patients in shock. *Circulation*, **39**: 361-378, 1969.

19. MacCannell, K.L., McNay, J.L., Meyer, M.B., et al: Dopamine in the treat-ment of hypotension and shock. *N. Engl. J. Med.*, **275**: 1389-1398, 1966.

CHAPTER 12

Treatment of Myocardial Infarction Shock *

Dean T. Mason, M.D.; Ezra A. Amsterdam, M.D.;
Richard R. Miller, M.D.; Anthony N. DeMaria, M.D.;
Louis A. Vismara, M.D.; Garrett Lee, M.D.;
Melvin Tonkon, M.D.; James Price, M.D.

Since the relative success in controlling fatal cardiac arrhythmias, pump failure has emerged as the dominant cause of death in acute myocardial infarction. Shock is the most extreme and clinically complicated form of such pump failure. This Chapter clearly encompasses the pathophysiologic basis for management of myocardial infarction shock. The use of new therapeutic techniques and agents is presented with either sophisticated invasive monitoring or with bedside clinical judgment. The indications for and value of surgical interventions are also discussed.

The rapidly expanding scope of therapy for myocardial infarction complicated by severe cardiac pump failure, including diverse pharmacologic agents, mechanical circulatory assist, and direct cardiac surgery, has substantially enhanced therapeutic potential in this syndrome. However, rational, effective, and safe use of these potent treatment alternatives is based on appropriate patient selection. Because the indications for differing types of therapy may be quite specific in relation to pattern of altered physiology, proper application of treatment is essential both for maximum efficacy and avoidance of deleterious effects. Thus, selection of therapy involves, in each case, a systematic approach to patient assessment, including evaluation of clinical status, quantitative definition of hemodynamic function, and estimation of prognostic class.

PATHOPHYSIOLOGIC BASIS OF THERAPY

Consideration of the structural and pathophysiologic aspects of myocardial infarction provides an understanding of the mechanisms of the effects produced in this setting by current therapeutic modalities. Myocardial infarction results in a zone of central necrosis surrounded by an area of

*Supported in part by Research Program Project Grant HL 14780 from the National Heart and Lung Institute, NIH, Bethesda, Maryland; and Research Grants from California Chapters of the American Heart Association, Dallas, Texas.

ischemia outside of which is relatively normal or uninvolved tissue[1]. The central zone is irreversibly damaged and in some instances this is so extensive as to preclude survival with any form of therapy. However, in the absence of this extreme, the region of greatest potential for influencing survival and thereby of principal therapeutic interest, is the acutely ischemic area which, although depressed, remains viable. The anatomical outcome in the ischemic area is a primary determinant of the clinical course in patients with cardiac function compatible with survival after acute myocardial infarction. Thus, to the extent that the nonlethally injured zone can be influenced toward recovery of structural and functional integrity, left ventricular performance and prognosis may be favorably altered. By contrast, factors promoting ischemia will result in increased myocardial injury, further cell death, and continued deterioration of ventricular function.

LIMITATIONS OF CARDIOTONIC AGENTS

A wide spectrum of drugs is currently available for support of the failing myocardium in myocardial infarction shock. However, until recently, pharmacologic therapy was principally limited to the conventional positive inotropic drugs, usually sympathomimetic agents[2-4]. This approach is capable, in most instances, of at least transiently elevating the blood pressure in myocardial infarction shock and it has been suggested that it has produced some improvement in survival[5]. However, most studies have indicated that mortality is not significantly affected by such treatment, remaining at 90%[6-8]. Indeed, the current multiplicity of these agents and continuing pursuit of more effective forms of pharmacotherapy to some extent reflects their lack of success.

Recent investigations have suggested several bases for the observed failure of traditional drug therapy in myocardial infarction shock. Experimental studies have indicated that the basis for the enhancement of hemodynamic function by positive inotropic drugs is their action upon normal areas of myocardium, since their action on injured myocardium is markedly attenuated[9-11]. The massive degree of myocardial loss which characterizes myocardial infarction shock[12,13], severely reduces the extent of uninvolved and thereby normally responsive cardiac muscle upon which a positive inotropic agent can exert its effect. As a result, these agents have a limited potential for significantly improving cardiac function in the large majority of patients with myocardial infarction shock. In addition, acutely infarcted myocardium is characterized by passive, systolic expansion resulting from the distending force produced by contraction of the uninvolved areas of the ventricle[14,15]. In experimental myocardial infarction, this paradoxical expansion is augmented by positive inotropic agents because of their enhancement of contractile function of normal myocardium with little effect on injured areas. There may thus be diversion of a significant portion of the stroke volume into the expansile area of the ventricle during systole. These factors result in counterproductive dissipation of contractile energy and exacerbation of the already deranged ventricular function. Finally, recent experimental studies have demonstrated that positive inotropic interventions may augment the intensity and extent of myocardial ischemia in myocardial infarction[16]. This results from their elevation of myocardial oxygen requirements in a setting in which a concomitant rise in coronary blood flow is precluded by structural restrictions in the coronary arteries. Thus the zone of ischemia and necrosis may be enlarged.

REGULATION OF MYOCARDIAL OXYGEN CONSUMPTION

Since development of cardiac pump failure is more closely related to cumulative quantity of myocardium destroyed by both previous and new infarction, it is relevant to consider the therapeutic implications of recent investigations concerned with modification of infarct size. These studies have demonstrated the potential for reduction of ischemia and thereby infarct size by favorable alteration of the cardiac oxygen supply-demand relationship. They are based on the concept that myocardial ischemia and necrosis in coronary heart disease result from an imbalance between myocardial oxygen needs and availability and that myocardial injury can be limited by favorable alteration of this balance[17,18]. Understanding of the regulation of myocardial oxygen consumption and supply is fundamental to this approach[19]. The major determinants of myocardial oxygen consumption and cardiac energetics are (1) left ventricular wall tension (product of systolic pressure and volume of the ventricle); (2) left ventricular contractility; and (3) heart rate (Figure 1).

DETERMINANTS OF MYOCARDIAL OXYGEN CONSUMPTION

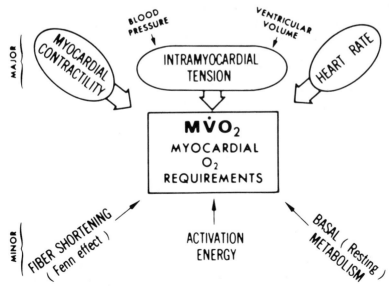

Figure 1   Hemodynamic-related determinants of myocardial oxygen consumption (MVO_2).

REGULATION OF MYOCARDIAL OXYGEN SUPPLY

Myocardial oxygen supply is principally related to coronary blood flow which is governed by mechanical, neural, humoral, and metabolic factors normally integrated by autoregulatory mechanisms which modulate coronary vascular resistance and thereby coronary blood flow[20]. In coronary artery disease these autoregulatory mechanisms are limited in maintenance of adequate coronary flow because of the unresponsiveness of obstructive narrowing in the vessels; mechanical factors assume preeminence. Thus, coronary perfusion pressure, as produced by aortic diastolic pressure, is normally a primary determinant of coronary blood flow and becomes even more critical. It must be maintained within a relatively narrow range because of the diminished capacity of the coronary circulation to compensate for alteration in this factor[20]. Therefore, the crucial importance of maintaining normal blood pressure in cardiogenic shock due to mycardial infarction should be recognized.

In myocardial infarction shock with low coronary arterial perfusion pressure, autoregulation of myocardial blood flow is impaired in the diseased coronary bed and the coronary vessels become dependent on adequate levels of systemic arterial diastolic pressure to maintain coronary blood flow. With very low levels of arterial blood pressure, the critical closing pressure of the coronary vasculature may be reached. Therefore, prolonged hypotension produces death of ischemic but potentially viable myocardium surrounding the infarcted area and results in greater depression of left ventricular function. Thus, there is further decline of cardiac output and more profound lowering of arterial pressure, which leads to additional reduction of coronary blood flow, continued deterioration ôf cardiac function, and ultimately a fatal outcome. Consequently, in myocardial infarction shock, primary therapeutic consideration should be given to maintenance of coronary perfusion pressure to supply adequate flow through the stenotic atherosclerotic vessels, thus improving the contractile state of the ischemic myocardium.

MODIFICATION OF INFARCT SIZE

Improved understanding of the factors governing myocardial oxygen supply and demand has recently led to experimental evaluation, with some extension to clinical trials, of a number of treatment modalities designed to reduce the extent of acute myocardial infarction[16-18]. Minimizing the area of infarction and ischemia improves left ventricular function and diminishes the incidence of tachyarrhythmias. Therapeutic approaches to the limitation of infarct size include: (1) reduction of myocardial oxygen needs by propranolol[21-23], nitroglycerin[24-28], long-acting nitrates[29-31], nitroprusside[32-35], phentolamine[35,36], and Arfonad [37]; (2) improvement of myocardial oxygen delivery by phenylephrine[25,26,28], norepinephrine[39], external counterpulsation[40], internal balloon counterpulsations[41-44], inspiration of oxygen-enriched air[45], thrombolytic agents[46], and coronary artery bypass reperfusion[47,48]; (3) decrease in myocardial edema and inflammation by hydro-cortisone[49], hyaluronidase[50], hypertonic mannitol[51-54], and cobra venom[55]; and (4) augmentation of myocardial anaerobic metabolism by glucose-insulin-potassium[56-58], and hypertonic glucose[59].

The clinical value of many of these manipulations in acute myocardial infarction remains to be firmly established. In addition, their use in patients must be individualized and application depends upon the hemodynamic setting associated with the acute coronary event. Thus, propranolol is effective in protecting the ischemic myocardium in preinfarction angina[60], but should not be employed in heart failure due to acute infarction because of the agent's action of depressing pump function[21]. Nitroprusside is useful in reducing myocardial oxygen requirements in preinfarction angina and in also improving pump performance in heart failure with acute infarction[32-34], whereas the drug may not be applicable in hypotension associated with myocardial infarction shock. In the latter situation, norepinephrine may be necessary to maintain coronary perfusion pressure[39]; however, this agent should not be employed in the absence of refractory hypotension. Nitrates are beneficial in decreasing cardiac oxygen needs in the intermediate coronary syndrome, and in also reducing pulmonary congestion in myocardial infarction with normal cardiac output[28], but are hazardous because of their cardiac output lowering effect in low output heart failure and cardiogenic shock due to myocardial infarction[28].

In myocardial infarction with congestive heart failure, certain combinations of therapy, such as nitroprusside and dopamine with counter-pulsation, may be employed to optimize pump function by achieving the most favorable alterations of contractility and peripheral vascular resistance, while attempting to protect the ischemic myocardium. Further, in therapeutic trials designed to limit acute infarct size, phenylephrine has been added to nitroglycerin to counteract the hypotensive and reflex tachycardia effects of the nitrate[26]. Concerning the effects of inotropic stimuli on the function of the ischemic heart, a difference in response has been observed in experimental animals with global ischemia produced by partial obstruction of the left main coronary artery compared to segmental ventricular ischemia caused by occlusion of the left circumflex coronary artery[61]. Thus isoproterenol depressed left ventricular function in global ischemia because of inotropic-induced increased myocardial oxygen demand without a concomitant increase in coronary blood flow[61], while the catecholamine improved cardiac performance in segmental ischemia[61]. In contrast, propranolol or nitroglycerin enhanced cardiac function in global ischemia due to a reduction of myocardial oxygen requirements[61]. Finally, it should be pointed out that the positive inotropic action of cardiotonic agents may be attenuated in the ischemic ventricle[62,65] (Figure 2), and that myocardial depression by negative inotropic agents may be enhanced in coronary heart disease[66].

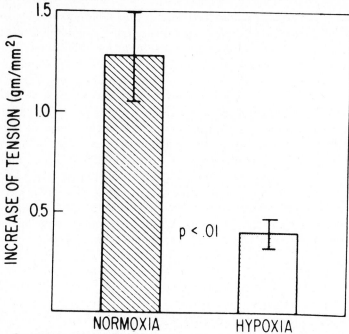

Figure 2   Attenuation of the positive inotropic action of digitalis in the hypoxic cat papillary muscle. The positive cardiotonic action of isoproterenol was not diminished at this level of hypoxia. (From Mason, D.T., Amsterdam, E.A., Miller, R.R., et al: Recent advances in pathophysiology and therapy of myocardial infarction shock. In H. Russek (Ed.): *Cardiovascular Disease: New Concepts in Diagnosis and Therapy*. University Park Press, Baltimore, 1974, pp. 143, with permission.)

In the context of the therapy of myocardial infarction shock, these studies have several significant implications. The theoretical importance of maintenance of coronary perfusion pressure in association with positive inotropic therapy is supported as is simultaneous increase in myocardial oxygen supply and reduction of demand by counterpulsation. In addition and perhaps of most relevance in relation to shock, attenuation of myocardial injury suggests the therapeutic potential for aversion of the continuing evolution of ischemic damage responsible for shock in many patients in whom the syndrome is not an early complication of infarction. In these patients, in whom cardiac pump function is commonly adequate initially, interventions which reduce myocardial oxygen demand, such as beta blocking drugs and nitrates, may frequently be given with beneficial effect and without deleterious results[67,68]. However, because such agents do not support and may seriously impair ventricular performance, they have no place in the therapy of established shock. Similarly, a drug such as nitroprusside, which by its unloading effects improves pump performance and reduces ischemic injury in myocardial infarction with congestive failure, is contraindicated in shock with significant hypotension because of its hypotensive action. On the other hand, intra-aortic balloon counterpulsation has most advantageous potential in shock in that it supports coronary perfusion pressure by diastolic augmentation (Figure 3) and reduces myocardial oxygen demand by systolic pressure unloading. Thus potential for modification of infarct size must be viewed in terms of the clinical setting. Whereas in uncomplicated infarction with adequate ventricular function, modest negative contractile action or reduction of blood pressure may be associated with a net favorable effect on the balance between myocardial oxygen supply and demand and thereby reduction of injury, these alterations contribute to further deterioration in the patient with little or no functional cardiac pump reserve.

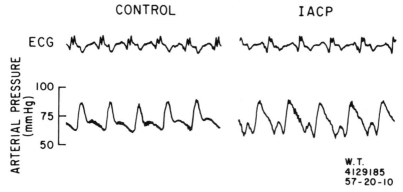

Figure 3 Electrocardiogram (ECG) and intraarterial pressure tracings in a patient with acute myocardial infarction shock before (control) and during intra-aortic balloon counterpulsation (IACP). Note reduction in systolic pressure and augmentation of diastolic pressure above peak systolic pressure during counterpulsation. (From Amsterdam, E.A., DeMaria, A.N., Hughes, J.L., et al: Myocardial infarction shock: mechanisms and therapy. In D.T. Mason (Ed.): *Congestive Heart Failure*. Yorke Medical Books, New York City, 1976, with permission.)

PATIENT EVALUATION

Early, accurate diagnosis of shock and prompt institution of appropriate treatment are essential in order to maximize therapeutic potential in this syndrome in which delay exacts an inordinate toll in terms of progressive myocardial damage and functional deterioration. The diagnosis of shock in myocardial infarction is usually, but not always, readily apparent. It is based on evidence of severely reduced tissue perfusion and the clinical manifestations of the underlying, marked derangement of cardiac pump function (Table I in Chapter 2). Systolic blood pressure is generally reduced to less than 80 mm Hg, or 40 mm Hg or more below the usual systolic level if there was prior hypertension. Because of the inaccuracy of sphygomanometric determination of blood pressure in states of severe vasoconstriction[69], reliable evaluation is facilitated by measurement of intra-arterial pressure. Significant arterial hypoxemia is usually present. When direct hemodynamic analysis of ventricular function is not available, indirect estimation of circulatory status can be achieved by clinical evaluation. Thus adequacy of systemic blood flow can be inferred from clinical assessment of renal, cerebral, and integumentary status. Inadequate renal blood flow is indicated by oliguria; cerebral hypoperfusion is manifested by altered sensorium; and cold, diaphoretic, or cyanotic skin reflects reduced peripheral blood flow and heightened sympathetic activity.

HEMODYNAMIC ASSESSMENT

Therapeutic efficacy in cardiogenic shock is predicated on accurate evaluation of cardiac function which may now be obtained by direct hemodynamic analysis. This involves cardiac catheterization for determination of left ventricular filling pressure and cardiac output, and insertion of a small polyethylene catheter into a systemic artery for accurate measurement of blood pressure. Peripheral vascular resistance may then be calculated. These procedures are facilitated by current techniques which allow right or left ventricular catheterization at bedside with or without fluoroscopic guidance[70,71]. However, left ventricular filling pressure can be accurately determined from pulmonary artery and pulmonary capillary wedge pressures which are readily obtained by right heart catheterization with a flow-directed catheter[71]. This catheter also allows withdrawal of blood from the central circulation for determination of arterial blood gases and pH, and provides a secure route for the administration of drugs.

Central venous pressure, although widely accessible, has distinct disadvantages in the hemodynamic evaluation of patients with myocardial infarction. It provides a measure of right, rather than left, ventricular filling pressure and thus may be normal in the presence of considerable elevation of filling pressure of the injured left ventricle[72]. It is also affected by the degree of venoconstriction present. However, central venous pressure has been found useful as a guide to volume expansion[73], as its alteration during such therapy in myocardial infarction may reflect directional, although not quantitative, changes in left ventricular filling pressure[74]. However, even for this purpose there is controversy based on findings which indicate central venous pressure monitoring may be misleading[72]. Thus caution must be exercised in utilizing changes in central venous pressure in the evaluation of response to volume therapy.

ASSESSMENT OF PROGNOSIS

To obviate delay in identifying patients at high risk of death from cardiac pump failure, a precise, objective means of evaluation is essential. Clinical estimation, while generally useful for classification of the patient with acute myocardial infarction, is not sufficiently sensitive to predict outcome in the individual[74] and may vary widely from hemodynamic status[75]. Hemodynamic analysis provides a more direct means of assessing prognosis. Studies of quantitative assessment of hemodynamic function in acute myocardial infarction have yielded a high degree of accuracy in predicting survival and mortality related to cardiac pump dysfunction. Certain critical variables are closely related to prognosis in these studies which achieve an accuracy of 80-100 percent in predicting outcome[76-79]. The variables chiefly utilized are left ventricular stroke work[76], stroke work index[77,78], cardiac index[77,80], cardiac work[81], and cardiac work index[78] alone or in combination with left ventricular filling pressure. Recent innovations that are promising in this regard are noninvasive techniques for estimating extent of myocardial damage and thereby prognosis in acute myocardial infarction. These include serum myocardial enzyme disappearance curves[82] and isotopic myocardial scanning[83].

In our experience utilizing right and/or left heart catheterization for assessment of prognosis related to cardiac pump dysfunction in over 200 patients with acute myocardial infarction, cardiac work index > 0.7 kg · M/min/M², stroke work index of 11.0 gm · M/M², and the ratio of stroke work index to left ventricular filling pressure of 0.5 are associated with survival in greater than 90 percent of patients[80]. In patients in whom these values were lower, mortality rate from cardiac pump dysfunction was greater than 85 percent. This information on clinical outlook afforded by hemodynamic assessment allows selection of appropriate treatment in patients with myocardial infarction and provides a rational basis for early institution of recently available aggressive forms of therapy when prognosis is grave.

SPECIFIC THERAPEUTIC MODALITIES

The goal of therapy in this syndrome is to achieve a cardiac output and perfusion pressure sufficient to meet systemic requirements, support cardiac function, and prevent extension of infarction. Advances in diagnostic techniques and therapeutic methods have afforded more specific and systematic treatment of myocardial infarction shock and thereby enhanced potential for reduction of the nearly always fatal outcome in this condition.

Volume Expansion

When cardiogenic shock persists after elimination of all reversible factors as previously delineated (Table I in Chapter 2), a trial of volume expansion is employed if appropriate[84-88]. This may in itself improve cardiac output and blood pressure or, if severe hemodynamic dysfunction persists, it will provide optimum plasma volume and left ventricular filling pressure prior to initiation of specific drugs or other means of therapy.

Volume expansion may increase cardiac output by augmenting venous return to the heart, thereby elevating left ventricular filling pressure and end-diastolic fiber length. This enhancement of cardiac pump function is provided by the Starling principle which, within limits, affords augmented performance of the ventricle with increased end-diastolic fiber length. Despite injury to the left ventricle from myocardial infarction with the result that the beneficial effect on ventricular performance following elevation of filling pressure is diminished in comparison with the normal heart, the increment of improvement may be of critical importance in the patient in cardiac pump failure. Increase in filling pressure in itself is not without hazard, however, and excessive elevation may result in pulmonary congestion or pulmonary edema. Clinical experience has demonstrated that while increases in cardiac output may result from volume expansion, little or no improvement is associated with elevation of left ventricular filling pressure above 20 mm Hg[85],[88]. Further, improvement in cardiac output is not a necessary concomitant of increase in left ventricular filling pressure, as has been previously noted in large infarctions resulting in severely diminished cardiac reserve. Volume expansion in this setting results only in increased filling pressure and the potential hazard of pulmonary congestion. It therefore follows that this form of therapy should be undertaken with caution, especially in the presence of a large infarction, and that therapeutic response in the individual patient, rather than a predetermined level of filling pressure, be utilized as the most prudent guide to volume expansion. Therapeutic efficacy will be evident from improved hemodynamic function on the readily observable variables of blood pressure and urine flow which will increase if cardiac output improves.

On the basis of the preceding discussion, volume expansion is most rationally administered in conjunction with accurate assessment of left ventricular filling pressure. This is accomplished by the methods previously described to measure left ventricular pressure directly[70] or indirectly[71]. A trial of volume expansion is indicated if left ventricular filling pressure is low or even normal. This is accomplished by rapid infusion of one of a number of substances: 10% Dextran 40 (Rheomacrodex®), 6% Dextran 75 (Macrodex®), or normal saline solution. When the hazard of pulmonary congestion is high or the filling pressure is normal initially, 5% dextrose in water can be employed, although it is not as useful a plasma expander as are the other materials. Initial administration consists of infusion of 100 to 200 ml of fluid relatively rapidly over five to ten minutes. If a salutary effect occurs (increase in cardiac output, blood pressure, or urine flow) without evidence of pulmonary congestion, this can be continued to a total of 500 to 1,000 ml over 30 to 60 minutes with care not to exceed left ventricular filling pressure of 18 to 20 mm Hg. Observation of the patient for dyspnea and pulmonary rales also guides continuation of fluid administration. If volume expansion produces an increase in filling pressure and no enhancement of function, it is probable that the ventricle cannot respond to an increased volume load. The danger of pulmonary congestion is therefore imminent and fluid therapy should not be pursued. If volume expansion results in correction of the deranged hemodynamic status, further therapy may not be required. However, if adequate function is not restored by fluid administration or elevated filling pressure precludes this approach, further treatment is necessary and consists of utilization of specific pharmacologic agents and/or surgical intervention to enhance depressed ventricular performance.

The necessity of eliminating hypovolemia and attaining optimum left ventricular filling pressure before instituting treatment with cardiac and vasoactive drugs is reemphasized. Administration of pharmacologic agents after maximizing left ventricular function by fluid administration will increase their efficacy, reduce required dose, and decrease the hazard of untoward effects. As previously indicated, because of excessive left ventricular filling pressure not uncommonly associated with myocardial infarction shock, volume expansion will often be contraindicated.

Pharmacologic Therapy

Despite its limitations, drug therapy retains an important role in the treatment of shock. An enlarged spectrum of differing drugs and increased understanding of pathophysiologic mechanisms have provided a more rational approach to their use. Further, newer techniques utilizing mechanical cardiac assist and direct cardiac surgery are limited in their availability and applicability.

Augmentation of depressed cardiac output in shock can be effected by several means pharmacologically: (1) as aforementioned, increase in venous return by volume expansion may raise cardiac output; (2) positive inotropic agents may increase cardiac output by enhancing myocardial contractility as well as possess a combination of effects on the myocardium and peripheral vasculature; and (3) reduction of impedance to left ventricular outflow, or cardiac unloading, may increase cardiac output as accomplished by certain vasodilator agents which diminish left ventricular impedance. As has been previously noted, maintenance of adequate coronary perfusion pressure is critically important in myocardial infarction shock. In addition to enhancing myocardial function and thereby improving systemic circulation, support of coronary perfusion is essential for preservation of the ischemic zone surrounding the infarct and prevention of extension of the area of necrosis. Since the vasodilating agents usually reduce blood pressure, their applicability in shock is limited. However, in those instances of shock characterized by markedly elevated peripheral vascular resistance and adequate blood pressure, they may be useful.

On the basis of these considerations, the hemodynamic pattern, which is not a consistent one in cardiogenic shock, is a major determinant in the proper selection of a therapeutic agent. If systolic blood pressure is markedly reduced a drug with vasoconstrictive as well as positive inotropic effects (norepinephrine or metaraminol) is indicated in order to support coronary blood flow. On the other hand, if peripheral resistance is excessive and blood pressure adequate or mildly lowered, a vasodilating agent with positive inotropic effects (dopamine) or without inotropic action (nitroprusside) is appropriate.

Catecholamines

The most commonly utilized drugs for cardiogenic shock and thus those about which most information is available are the sympathomimetic agents which include the catecholamines and certain noncatecholamine drugs with similar structural and pharmacologic properties. The catecholamines are characterized by a benzene ring with two adjacent hydroxyl groups (comprising the catechol nucleus) to which is attached a short carbon chain with an amine group. The noncatecholamine sympathomimetic drugs are structurally similar but lack the distinct catechol nucleus. The catecholamines include both endogenously synthesized compounds and synthetic forms. The endogenously produced catecholamines are dopamine, norepinephrine, and epinephrine. Of the large number of synthetically produced catecholamines (Table I), those of pertinence to this discussion are norepinephrine (Levophed®), dopamine (Intropin®), isoproterenol (Isupres®), epinephrine (Adrenalin®), metaraminol (Aramine®), and mephentermine (Wyamine®).

TABLE I

MYOCARDIAL INFARCTION SHOCK – PHARMACOLOGIC THERAPY

AGENT	Positive inotropic effect of stimulation of myocardial beta-adrenergic receptors		Increase in PVR by stimulation of arteriolar alpha-adrenergic receptors		Decrease in PVR by direct stimulation of arteriolar beta-adrenergic receptors	Decrease in PVR by nonadrenergic, direct dilating effects	ADMINISTRATION
	Direct	Indirect	Direct	Indirect			
I. Positive inotropic effect; increase in PVR:							
1. Norepinephrine (Levophed®)	+		+				9 to 32 mg (4 to 16 ml) of the bitartrate in 1,000 ml of 5 percent dextrose in H_2O; initial rate 1 to 2 μg per minute intravenously; may also be given intramuscularly, 2 to 10 mg.
2. Metaraminol bitartrate (Aramine®)	+	+	+	+			50 to 200 mg (5 to 20 ml) in 1,000 ml of 5 percent dextrose in H_2O; initial intravenous rate 1 to 2 μg per minute intravenously; may also be given intramuscularly, 2 to 10 mg.
II. Positive inotropic effect; decrease in PVR:							
1. Isoproterenol hydrochloride (Isuprel®)	+				+		1 to 5 mg (10 to 50 cc) in 500 ml of 5 percent dextrose in H_2O; initial rate 0.5 to 1.0 μg per minute intravenously.
III. Positive inotropic effect; mixed effect on PVR:							
1. Epinephrine (Adrenalin®)	+		+		+		1 to 5 mg (1 to 5 ml) in 500 ml of 5 percent dextrose in H_2O; initial rate 1 to 2 μg per minute intravenously.
2. Dopamine (Intropin®)	+		+			+	200 mg (5 ml) in 1,000 ml of 5 percent dextrose in H_2O; initial rate 0.2 to 0.4 μg per minute intravenously.
3. Mephentermine sulfate (Wyamine®)		+	+			+	500 to 1,000 mg (16.7 to 33.3 ml) in dextrose in H_2O; initial rate 0.24 to 0.50 mg per minute intravenously; may also be given intravenously 30 to 45 mg in single injection.

Abbreviations: PVR = peripheral vascular resistance.

The effects of adrenergic stimuli are mediated by receptors, the nature of which has not fully been elucidated, in the effector organs. These receptors are termed alpha and beta and their presence has been postulated in most organs subserved by the adrenergic nervous system. Endogenous catecholamines, synthetic catecholamines, and other sympathomimetic agents can activate these receptors and are therefore adrenergic stimulating agents, but other types of chemical agents lacking structural similarity to the catecholamines are without effect at these sites. In the cardiovascular system both alpha and beta receptors are present in the smooth muscle of blood vessels and beta receptors are present in the myocardium; there is no evidence of alpha receptors in the myocardium itself. Contraction of blood vessel smooth muscle by adrenergic agents causing vasoconstriction is mediated by alpha receptors in the smooth muscle; relaxation of this tissue resulting in vasodilation is mediated by beta receptors. In the heart, beta receptor stimulation is excitatory causing increases in contractility, heart rate, and metabolic activity. Drugs which stimulate the respective adrenergic receptors are termed alpha-adrenergic or beta-adrenergic stimulating agents. The actions of an adrenergic drug may stimulate alpha receptors of one organ and beta receptors of another. Thus, norepinephrine activates myocardial beta receptors (cardiac stimulation) and produces predominant alpha receptor excitation in blood vessel smooth muscle (vasoconstriction).

The effects of the catecholamines on adrenergic receptors can be direct or indirect. The latter refers to the mechanism of action of the indirect-acting catecholamines which themselves have little or no intrinsic effect on adrenergic receptors and produce their effects by stimulation of release of the stored neurotransmitter, norepinephrine, from sympathetic nerve terminals. Norepinephrine, epinephrine, dopamine, and isoproterenol directly stimulate adrenergic receptor sites. Mephentermine possesses only indirect adrenergic effects and metaraminol acts via both modes (Table I). Whereas the activity of the direct-acting catecholamines is independent of endogenous norepinephrine stores, indirect-acting agents are totally dependent on adequate endogenous norepinephrine stores for their effects. Thus, long-term administration of norepinephrine-depleting drugs (reserpine or guanethidine) or prolonged use of an indirect-acting catecholamine (metaraminol or mephentermine) can markedly limit responsiveness to the latter class of agents because of depletion of norepinephrine from sympathetic nerve terminals.

Norepinephrine and Metaraminol

Norepinephrine and metaraminol, the hemodynamic effects of which are quite similar, have been the two most widely employed drugs in the treatment of cardiogenic shock. Norepinephrine acts directly and metaraminol, as previously noted, acts in part directly and partially by causing norepinephrine release from endogenous stores. These drugs stimulate both alpha and beta-adrenergic receptors and thus possess vasoconstrictor and positive inotropic properties. Consequently, they have the potential in cardiogenic shock to simultaneously raise cardiac output and arterial blood pressure. However, their actual effects vary with the condition of the individual patient and the dosage employed. With small doses, cardiac output and blood pressure are increased, mainly as a result of predominant beta adrenergic stimulating action on the heart[89]. With large doses, vascular resistance is markedly increased and cardiac output may actually fall despite the positive inotropic effects of these drugs. Such an adverse effect can also occur with administration of norepinephrine or metaraminol to patients in whom the peripheral resistance is already excessive and in whom the need may actually be for reduction in vascular resistance. This inordinate elevation of peripheral resistance may have the deleterious effect of decreasing cardiac output and increasing the metabolic needs of the heart without a proportionate rise in coronary blood flow and myocardial perfusion, resulting in further ischemia and deterioration of an already injured myocardium[90]. In the treatment of cardiogenic shock with norepinephrine or metaraminol, cardiac output is usually increased with maintenance of systolic blood pressure at 90 to 100 mm Hg[89],[90]. Such an approach will maximize positive cardiac inotropic effects while obviating excessive systemic vasoconstriction, thereby enhancing cardiac output without undue increases in cardiac workload. Therefore, these drugs should be administered in the smallest effective dosage with frequent attempts at withdrawal.

Several undesirable pharmacologic effects may be associated with the use of norepinephrine and metaraminol. Aggravation of oliguria may result from renal artery constriction produced by these drugs. Prolonged therapy may produce a decrease in plasma volume when fluid transudates at the capillary level because of post-capillary venoconstriction[91]. The resultant hypovolemia may aggravate the shock state with production of apparent intractability. Indeed, in some instances cardiogenic shock requiring constant therapy with these drugs has been abolished by administration of fluids. The necessity is again stressed for use of minimal effective dosage as well as careful attention to fluid requirements during sustained administration of these vasoconstrictor agents.

Although the hemodynamic actions of norepinephrine and metaraminol are similar, certain differences merit emphasis. As previously noted, metaraminol should be avoided in patients previously treated with catecholamine-depleting drugs. Norepinephrine, if extravasated, produces local tissue necrosis, an effect not shared by metaraminol which can be administered intramuscularly as well as intravenously. As with other indirect-acting catecholamines the effects of metaraminol are somewhat prolonged, lasting for up to 20 minutes after its discontinuance, in comparison to those of norepinephrine, the onset and offset of which are more abrupt.

Mortality in cardiogenic shock remains distressingly high after all forms of medical therapy, and substantiation of suggested beneficial effects on survival by these vasopressor-positive inotropic agents is difficult because of the grave and multifactorial nature of the problem. However, their use in patients with myocardial infarction cardiogenic shock is often successful in improving coronary blood flow, systemic blood pressure, and cardiac output, the therapeutic goals upon which reduction in mortality is based.

Dopamine

Because of its unique properties, dopamine possesses several advantages for use in the shock state (Table I)[92],[93]. In addition to its beta-adrenergic stimulating effect on the myocardium, it produces direct non-adrenergic dilation of the renal, mesenteric, coronary, and intracerebral vascular beds, and also causes skeletal muscle vasoconstriction by alpha adrenergic stimulation. Thus, its effect on total peripheral vascular resistance is the net result of the agent's separate actions on the regional circulations. In general, total peripheral vascular resistance is unaltered or mildly reduced, heart rate is not changed or rises mildly, and cardiac output rises. Blood pressure is thus increased as a result of the enhanced cardiac output[92]. At high doses, the predominant effect of dopamine is alpha adrenergic stimulation in all vascular beds and thus vasoconstriction.

In patients with coronary artery disease, peripheral resistance is reduced and cardiac output and blood pressure elevated by dopamine without impairment of overall myocardial energy metabolism[93,94]. In comparative studies of patients in shock dopamine has produced greater increments in cardiac output and urine flow than norepinephrine[93] and its potential value in this syndrome is further supported by additional experimental and clinical studies[92-94]. The salutary effects of dopamine on renal blood flow have been of particular importance in oliguric patients with shock[92]. It should be emphasized, however, that because of its peripheral vascular effects, dopamine may not be capable of supporting adequate blood pressure in patients in whom it does not increase cardiac output. Norepinephrine has been required in such patients. The most serious adverse effect of dopamine is ventricular arrhythmias. Hypotension has also occurred particularly at lower doses. Other side effects include angina, nausea, and vomiting.

Isoproterenol

This drug is a relatively pure beta-adrenergic agonist with potent stimulatory effects on the heart, thus augmenting contractility and cardiac rate, and causing peripheral vasodilation (Table I). Cardiac output may therefore be significantly increased by its actions. In patients with chronic coronary artery disease, isoproterenol has not only produced increases in cardiac output but also raised overall coronary blood flow more than myocardial oxygen demands[95,96]. Thus, no metabolic evidence of ischemia was present in association with increased myocardial contractility and mechanical effort. The effect of isoproterenol on blood pressure is the net result of its combined actions on cardiac output and systemic vascular resistance. When cardiac output increases in excess of fall in peripheral resistance, blood pressure rises. Volume expansion may be necessary with the use of isoproterenol because of the increased vascular capacitance associated with its vasodilatory effects.

Isoproterenol has been beneficial, in some studies, in the treatment of patients with myocardial infarction shock. Elevations in both cardiac output and blood pressure have been obtained with isoproterenol in patients with cardiogenic shock[96]. The combination of isoproterenol and volume expansion has also been useful in this syndrome. However, further evaluation has demonstrated that its usefulness is largely limited to shock of mild degree. In patients with shock and severe hypotension, the drug has not been beneficial and in some instances it has had deleterious effects on clinical course[4]. This is largely due to the substantial increase in myocardial oxygen requirements produced by the drug without concomitant rise in coronary blood flow. This latter has resulted from the inability of isoproterenol to augment the reduced blood pressure in patients with profound hypotension[3,5]. Indeed, in such situations, isoproterenol may actually further reduce the blood pressure. Increased myocardial ischemia and further depression of cardiac pump function as well as ventricular irritability result. Intensified myocardial ischemia after the administration of isoproterenol has been demonstrated experimentally[17,18]. Its role in cardiogenic shock is therefore limited.

Epinephrine

Epinephrine acts directly on cardiac beta-adrenergic receptors as a potent cardiac stimulant increasing myocardial contractility and frequency of contraction (Table I). Its effect on the peripheral vasculature, however, is mixed since it has predominantly alpha-stimulating effects in some vascular beds (skin, mucosa, and kidney) and beta-stimulating actions in others (skeletal muscle)[92]. These effects are also dose-dependent, intensity of alpha stimulation increasing with increasing dosage of epinephrine. Thus the net effect of epinephrine on total peripheral vascular resistance is the result of its effects on the various regional circulations and, importantly, a function of the dosage utilized. At therapeutic doses, beta-adrenergic effects predominate on the peripheral vessels and total peripheral vascular resistance is mildly reduced. However, constriction is maintained in the renal and cutaneous circulations due to predominant alpha-adrenergic effects in these areas. Thus because of the redistribution of the circulating blood volume, the rise in cardiac output after epinephrine results in increased regional blood flow primarily to skeletal muscle with no enhancement or actual reduction of flow to vital organs such as the kidney. Cardiac arrhythmias, resulting from increased automaticity, are a potential hazard with epinephrine. There has been limited use and little systematic investigation of epinephrine in the treatment of cardiogenic shock.

Mephentermine

Mephentermine produces release of norepinephrine from sympathetic nerves and thus its primary actions are similar to those of metaraminol (Table I)[92]. Its effects on vascular resistance are, however, somewhat complex in that in current studies, they have varied with dosage and patient population. In normal subjects mephentermine increased cardiac output, heart rate, and peripheral vascular resistance. In patients with shock, however, large doses of mephentermine have resulted in decreases in peripheral resistance, apparently by a direct non-adrenergic effect on peripheral blood vessels[91,92].

Pure Alpha-Adrenergic Stimulating Agents

It is to be noted that those sympathomimetic amines with alpha-adrenergic stimulating properties and absence of positive inotropic effect have little or no place in the treatment of cardiogenic shock. Such agents include methoxamine (Vasoxyl®) and phenylephrine (Neosynephrine®). Although blood pressure is usually increased by their action, cardiac output is often diminished because of their lack of supportive action on the myocardium at the same time that they impose a greater work load (increased peripheral vascular resistance) on the heart. Further cardiac deterioration is the consequence of such a combination of actions. Those very uncommon cases of hypotension in which the primary defect is reduced peripheral vascular resistance in the presence of minimal myocardial damage and normal cardiac output are the only situations in which use of the pure alpha-adrenergic agonists is rational.

Other Drugs

The lack of notable success in the treatment of cardiogenic shock with traditional medical therapy has spurred development of differing pharmacologic agents and new application of old ones to this syndrome. Initial therapeutic trials have been carried out with the positive inotropic agents, digitalis and glucagon, and the vasodilator drugs, nitroprusside, phentolamine, phenoxybenzamine, chlorpromazine, and corticosteroids.

Digitalis

Because of its demonstrated efficacy in enhancing performance of the failing myocardium and the view that cardiogenic shock is an extreme form of heart failure, the potential role of digitalis in this syndrome has received attention. In addition to its direct, positive inotropic effect, which is unrelated to adrenergic mechanisms, digitalis directly constricts peripheral arteries[97]. However, when increased cardiac output is associated with digitalis therapy in congestive heart failure, reduction in peripheral vascular resistance occurs. This is the result of sympathetic withdrawal associated with improved cardiac pump function which overrides the relatively weak constricting action of the glycoside[98].

In experimental cardiogenic shock, digitalis has produced beneficial effects on cardiac function[98]. However, similar results have not been forthcoming from clinical studies in myocardial infarction shock. Although inconsistent hemodynamic benefit has occurred with digitalis in congestive heart failure without shock associated with myocardial infarction (Figure 4)[98-104], the glycoside has been of no benefit in myocardial infarction shock[104] and has proved potentially deleterious because of its acute vasoconstricting effects[105]. Attenuation of the hemodynamic effects of digitalis in this setting appears to be related to diminished contractile action of the drug on ischemic myocardium as demonstrated experimentally (Figure 2)[11].

Glucagon

Extensive investigations of glucagon have established that it possesses a

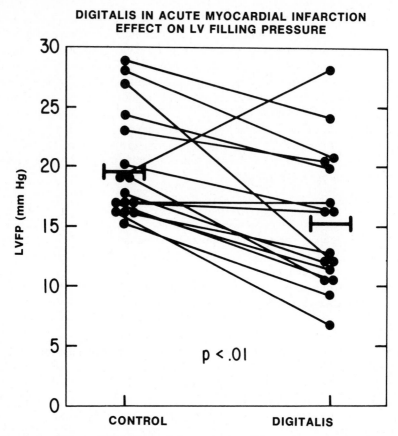

Figure 4 Effects of digitalis on left ventricular filling pressure (LVFP) in acute myocardial infarction patients in whom this variable was elevated (>12 mm Hg) prior to the glycoside. (From Mason, D.T.: Digitalis pharmacology and therapeutics: recent advances. *Ann. Intern. Med.*, **80**: 520, 1974, with permission.)

positive inotropic effect independent of beta-adrenergic receptor stimulation and mildly dilates peripheral arteries. Clinical evaluation of its use in patients with severe cardiac pump failure has been disappointing, however, in that significant beneficial effects have not been consistent (Figure 5)[106]. This may stem from the inability of glucagon to augment contractility in the chronically failing heart. On the other hand, its positive inotropic action may provide adjunctive therapy for other positive inotropic agents in patients with recent onset of cardiac pump dysfunction. Its role in cardiogenic shock is, however, a limited one.

Systemic Vasodilator Drugs

These agents have been demonstrated to improve hemodynamic function in cardiac failure by reduction of left ventricular afterload and preload[107].

GLUCAGON AND SYMPATHOMIMETIC AMINES IN CARDIAC PUMP FAILURE

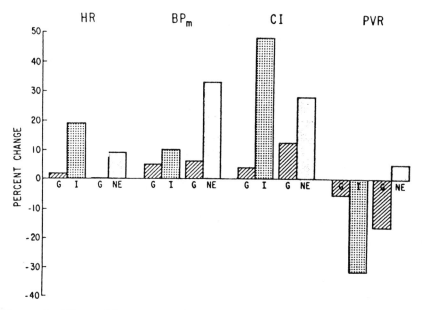

Figure 5 Effects of intravenous glucagon (G), compared to catecholamines, on hemodynamic variables in patients with chronic coronary artery disease. I = isoproterenol; NE = norephinephrine; HR = heart rate; BP_m = mean systemic arterial blood pressure; CI = cardiac index; PVR = peripheral vascular resistance. (From Amsterdam, E.A., Mansour, E.J., Hughes, J.L., et al: Present status of glucagon and bretylium tosylate. In H. Russek and B. Zohman (Eds.): *Changing Concepts in Cardiovascular Disease*. Williams & Williams Co., Baltimore, 1972, p. 215, with permission.)

They produce no direct inotropic effects and thus alteration of ventricular function is achieved entirely by their extra-myocardial actions. The relative effects on afterload and preload vary with the individual agents[108].

The vasodilator agents which have received principal attention and application are intravenous nitroprusside and intravenous phentolamine. They are capable of substantially improving depressed ventricular performance in cardiac failure, as manifested by increase in cardiac output and diminution in left ventricular filling pressure. These salutary effects are achieved while myocardial oxygen consumption is simultaneously reduced (Figure 6), suggesting potential for limitation of infarct size and also enhancement of intrinsic contractile state by decrease in ischemia.

Reduction in myocardial oxygen demand is the result of conversion of contractile effort to flow work rather than the metabolically more costly pressure work[19] by lowering of left ventricular afterload. However, because of this vasodilating and consequently hypotensive effect, these agents have limited use in cardiogenic shock in which, as previously noted, elevation of reduced coronary perfusion pressure is a prime therapeutic requisite. In

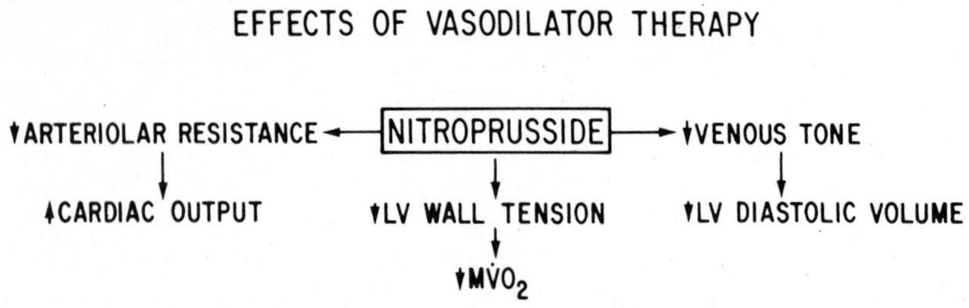

EFFECTS OF VASODILATOR THERAPY

↑ARTERIOLAR RESISTANCE ←⟨NITROPRUSSIDE⟩**→ ↑VENOUS TONE**

↓CARDIAC OUTPUT **↑LV WALL TENSION** **↑LV DIASTOLIC VOLUME**

↑MV̇O₂

Figure 6 Effects of intravenous nitroprusside on variables of pump performance, left ventricular (LV) filling, and myocardial energetics in ischemic heart disease.

those cases of shock characterized by extreme vasoconstriction and reduced cardiac output, however, impedance and afterload reduction would be rational treatment with potential to raise cardiac output, maintain adequate blood pressure, and favorably influence the metabolic status of the mechanically overburdened myocardium.

Other agents with vasodilating action which have received experimental attention and clinical consideration in the treatment of cardiogenic shock are dibenzyline, chlorpromazine, and corticosteroids[2]. The potential hazards of these agents in this syndrome and the impropriety of their use in the presence of hypotension, where they could produce catastrophic consequences, are reemphasized.

MECHANICAL CARDIAC ASSIST

The limitations of conventional medical therapy in cardiogenic shock have resulted in innovative therapeutic methods, among the most significant of which is mechanical cardiac assist. This approach is based on the principle of increasing coronary blood flow and reducing myocardial oxygen demands while providing support of the systemic circulation. This unique capability has the potential to alleviate myocardial ischemia and injury, and thereby reverse hemodynamic deterioration.

In the development of mechanical devices for temporary support of the failing heart, two general approaches have been utilized: (1) modifications of total cardiopulmonary bypass techniques used in open-heart surgery and (2) counterpulsation by phasic alterations of aortic pressure applied synchronously with the cardiac cycle. The bypass approach has included various forms of partial venoarterial pumping which can be carried out for several hours with or without a membrane oxygenator. Although left-heart bypass can be accomplished clinically by a transseptal technique not requiring thoracotomy[109], these shunt methods have not usually been feasible or effective in shock following myocardial infarction but have been useful as postoperative adjuncts in cardiac surgery.

Intra-Aortic Balloon Counterpulsation

The second approach of synchronous pressure assistance or arterioarterial pumping utilizes the concept of counterpulsation in which, as originally designed, blood is withdrawn from the aorta during systole and returned during diastole by a reciprocating pump[110,111]. An important advance in the practical application of this approach has been the introduction of intra-aortic balloon counterpulsation which is the most frequently applied of these methods in the treatment of cardiogenic shock. In this system, a balloon attached to a catheter is inserted into the descending thoracic aorta through the femoral artery[112]. Diastolic augmentation of coronary blood flow is achieved by raising ascending aortic diastolic pressure by rapid inflation of the balloon during ventricular relaxation (Figure 3). During subsequent deflation of the balloon in systole, resistance to left ventricular ejection is reduced, ventricular outflow is enhanced, and myocardial oxygen requirements are diminished. Balloon counterpulsation can be carried out safely for several days with little discomfort to the patient.

Results with intra-aortic balloon counterpulsation in myocardial infarction shock indicate improvement in cardiac output, increase in mean aortic pressure, augmentation of coronary blood flow, and resultant beneficial effects on myocardial metabolism, as reflected in evidence of increased myocardial oxygenation[111,113]. Abnormally elevated myocardial oxygen extraction fell toward normal and lactate production by the myocardium, indicating cellular hypoxia, decreased or shifted to extraction. Although in some patients in cardiogenic shock, prognosis is enhanced in association with these salutary hemodynamic effects[111], deterioration of pump function often follows discontinuance of circulatory assistance and a minority of patients with myocardial infarction shock unresponsive to pharmacologic management have recovered as a result of counterpulsation[113,114]. Prolonged counterpulsation beyond 48 hours in patients who do not improve sufficiently within this period to allow withdrawal of mechanical assist does not provide additional benefit on clinical outcome. A major application of counterpulsation in this setting is support of patients during left-heart catheterization and selective coronary arteriography in preparation for a definitive surgical procedure[115]. Complications of intra-aortic counterpulsation have been relatively infrequent and include thromboembolism from the balloon surface, which is avoidable by anticoagulation, trauma to the aorta, arterial insufficiency related to the site of balloon insertion, and destruction of blood elements, which has not been a serious problem[111].

The response of the patient to counterpulsation in the first 24 hours is indicative of subsequent course and provides the basis for systematic application of this form of therapy[116,117]. After 24 hours of counterpulsation, assistance is discontinued and the patient assessed. If improvement and stability are evident, counterpulsation may be reinstituted to attempt further benefits. Reevaluation is performed within 24 hours and if no additional gains have occurred in functional status, gradual discontinuation of counterpulsation is achieved over 24 hours. If, however, further improvement results, continued periods of counterpulsation are undertaken until a stable level of function is achieved. If hemodynamic deterioration ensues after the first 24 hours of assist, counterpulsation is reinstituted for another 24 hours with reassessment after its cessation. Deterioration at this time indicates balloon dependence and consideration is directed toward evaluation of potential for definitive therapy by cardiac surgery.

External Counterpulsation

Noninvasive counterpulsation devices have been developed which utilize intermittent external body compression synchronized with the cardiac cycle[110]. These atraumatic external synchronous methods are currently undergoing clinical evaluation. Present evidence indicates that both morbidity and mortality are reduced in patients with acute myocardial infarction complicated by mild left ventricular failure[118]. One such device consists of a system of arm and leg cuffs for sequenced pulsation of the extremities. Another technique (Cardioassist) utilizes the lower extremity body boot or wet suit which hydraulically provides phasic positive and negative ambient pressures in diastole and systole, respectively (Figure 7). External assistance may also be achieved by the technique of body acceleration applied synchronously with the heartbeat (BASH procedure); the patient is abruptly moved in a caudal direction on a shake-bed during cardiac ejection, thereby enhancing the delivery of stroke volume from the left ventricle into the ascending aorta. There are no data which demonstrate that external pressure circulatory assist modalities improve survival in the extreme condition of left heart failure of cardiogenic shock.

CARDIAC SURGERY

The excessive mortality associated with the major complications of acute myocardial infarction has stimulated the development of innovative approaches to the management of these problems. Among these has been the application of emergency cardiac surgery[119], until recently not considered feasible in the hazardous setting of acute myocardial infarction (AMI). This section deals with our experience at the School of Medicine of the University of California at Davis (UCD) in the surgical treatment of cardiogenic shock, extending infarction, and ventricular tachycardia-fibrillation in AMI unresponsive to pharmacological and related noninvasive treatment alone[120]. It is principally concerned with the approach to evaluation and results of operative intervention by our medical-surgical team in the management of these intractable complications of the acute phase of myocardial infarction.

Angiographic Evaluation

During a recent four-year period, 35 patients underwent emergency left heart catheterization with angiography for assessment of possible surgical treatment because of complicated AMI. This group constituted 28 AMI patients with refractory cardiogenic shock (primary pump failure); two with

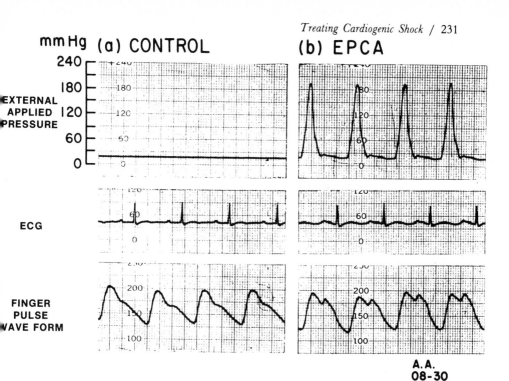

Figure 7 Simultaneously recorded external applied pressure and finger pulse wave form in a patient with acute myocardial infarction before: (a) control and (b) during external counterpulsation (external pressure circulatory assist = EPCA). Note augmentation of diastolic pressure during counterpulsation. (From Amsterdam, E., Banas, J., Criley, M., et al: Clinical evaluation of external pressure circulatory assist in acute myocardial infarction. Submitted, *N. Engl. J. Med.*, 1976, with permission.)

threatened extension of transmural infarction; and five with intractable, recurrent primary ventricular tachycardia-fibrillation (secondary pump failure). Indications for complete cardiac catheterization included unresponsiveness to conventional medical therapy[119] and absence of other serious concomitant disease. Further, AMI patients with intractable cardiac failure were, in general, selected for examination by left heart catheterization for surgically approachable lesions on the basis of relative youth (less than 60 years of age), absence of ECG evidence of old myocardial infarction, lack of symptoms of pump dysfunction prior to the AMI, and/or presence of cardiac murmurs at the time of the present AMI.

Since 100 to 125 patients with transmural AMI are admitted to our Coronary Care Unit each year, these 35 patients who underwent complete heart catheterization for possible operative intervention were selected from 70 AMI patients with complicated AMI admitted to the UCD-Sacramento Medical Center over the four-year period. This somewhat increased frequency of complicated AMI reflects a selected patient population resulting from our position as a cardiac referral center.

The complete procedure of emergency cardiac catheterization to identify surgically approachable complications carried out in each of these 35 AMI patients consisted of, in addition to initial hemodynamic measurements by Swan-Ganz right heart catheterization[71], complete retrograde left heart catheterization including determination of intraventricular pressures, cardiogreen indicator-dilution cardiac output, biplane left ventricular cineangiography, and selective coronary arteriography[121]. Left heart catheterization and angiography were performed without the aid of mechanical circulatory assistance in all patients. The studies were performed within 6 hours to 14 days after AMI occurrence and within a few hours of the occurrence of the complication which was refractory to vigorous management by medical means. The clinical and hemodynamic criteria by which we judge cardiogenic shock to be refractory to medical therapy with prognosis approaching 100% fatality rate have been described in detail previously[78,80].

Left heart and coronary angiography in the refractory state of AMI complications was accomplished with remarkable patient safety in this critical condition with only one death related to the catheterization procedure itself. In this, the second patient in our series, intractable cardiogenic shock terminated in fatal outcome during coronary arteriography which precipitated acute electromechanical dissociation unresponsive to cardiopulmonary resuscitation[122]. Further, this death represents our single instance of mortality attributable to emergency coronary arteriography carried out for identification of surgically approachable abnormalities in 77 patients in the difficult setting of acute coronary insufficiency related to intermediate coronary syndrome (42 patients)[123] and refractory AMI complications reported herein (28 with pump failure, two with extending infarction, and five with recurrent ventricular tachycardia-fibrillation). There has been no mortality associated with cardiac catheterization and angiography in acute coronary disease in our series in the past three years.

Patient Selection for Emergency Surgical Therapy

Of the patients who underwent left heart catheterization and angiography for complicated AMI, 23 out of 35 (66%) were considered candidates for surgical intervention. These 23 patients included 16 with cardiac pump failure, two with extending AMI, and five patients with recurrent ventricular tachycardia and fibrillation. The group comprised 18 males and 5 females who ranged in age from 30 to 75 years (mean 58 years). The 16 patients with cardiac pump failure had extensive infarctions with: (1) major left ventricular segmental dysfunction alone in five; (2) acute ventricular septal rupture in six; and (3) acute mitral regurgitation in five. The two patients with threatened extension of infarction had established transmural AMI. Of the five patients with intractable ventricular tachycardia, two had transmural myocardial infarction while the infarction was nontransmural in the other three.

Results of Surgical Therapy

All 12 catheterized patients who were not considered suitable candidates for operative intervention had cardiac pump failure related to massive left ventricular segmental dysfunction, as evidenced by greater than 85% of the left ventricular perimeter (right anterior oblique position) demonstrating no movement (akinesis) and/or paradoxical motion (dyskinesis) during systole. The ejection fraction in each patient was severely diminished to less than 15%. There were no associated mechanical defects. All 12 of these patients died in the acute phase of AMI, 11 on conventional medical therapy and one during coronary arteriography, the single catheterization-related death. Further, mortality was 100% during the acute period of AMI in the 35 patients with refractory cardiogenic shock who were not deemed suitable candidates for left heart catheterization and angiography.

In the 23 patients selected for immediate surgical treatment, the operation was performed as soon as possible, usually within 1 hour after completion of the cardiac catheterization. Operative mortality was 9/23 (39%). A variety of procedures were applied in refractory cardiogenic shock: (1) repair of ventricular septal defect with infarctectomy in six patients[124]; (2) mitral valve replacement with infarctectomy or coronary bypass grafts in five; (3) infarctectomy with coronary bypass grafts in four; and (4) infarctectomy alone in one patient. It is noted that coronary artery bypass was not performed as the sole procedure in any patient with pump failure. Employment of coronary artery bypass grafts alone was performed for threatened extension of transmural infarction. Coronary artery bypass, alone or in combination with infarctectomy, was utilized for intractable ventricular tachy-cardia-fibrillation.

Figure 8 demonstrates the pre- and postoperative left ventriculograms in the right anterior oblique view in patient A.T. who underwent successful acute infarctectomy for cardiogenic shock. The improvement in wall motion of the residual ventricle is apparent postoperatively, as well as the marked enhancement of ejection fraction.

The pre- and postoperative data from patient G.C. with cardiogenic shock due to acute ventricular septal rupture are shown in Figure 13 of Chapter 2. Operation was performed within 6 hours after admission to the Coronary Care Unit for AMI. Repair of the muscular ventricular septal defect was achieved by the new technique of sandwiching both sides of the septum with two Teflon® patches sutured together to enclose the infarcted septal area completely[124] (Figure 9). Postoperative catheterization demonstrated correction of the large left-to-right intracardiac shunt by abolition of the early reappearance phase of the presurgical indicator dye dilution curves and absence of the oxygen step-up from right atrium to right ventricle.

The duration of follow-up in the 14 patients who survived operation was 2 to 54 months (average 16 months). Late mortality occurred in one out of 23 patients (4%). Thus, there are presently 13 long term survivors with symp-

BEFORE SURGERY
Acute MI + Shock

POST-SURGERY
Acute Infarctectomy

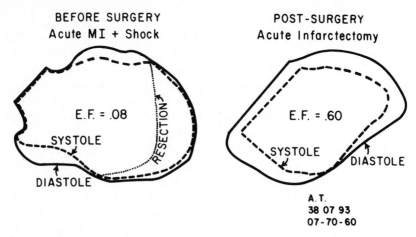

A.T.
38 07 93
07-70-60

Figure 8   Pre and postoperative left ventriculograms in right anterior oblique view in patient A.T. who underwent acute infarctectomy for cardiogenic shock. MI = myocardial infarction; EF = ejection fraction. (From Amsterdam, E.A., Miller, R.R., Hughes, J.L., et al: Emergency surgical therapy of complicated acute myocardial infarction: indications and results in cardiogenic shock, intractable ventricular tachycardia, and extending infarction. In H.I. Russek (Ed.): *Cardiovascular Problems.* University Park Press, Baltimore, 1976, pp. 447-451, with permission.)

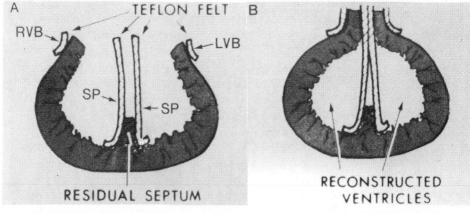

Figure 9   A: Schematic illustration demonstrating ventriculotomy of left and right ventricles with infarctectomy and septal resection. The remaining septum is sandwiched by two Teflon® patches (SP) using horizontal mattress sutures and two Teflon® rectangular bolsters placed on both free ventricular walls. RVB = right ventricular bolster; LVB = left ventricular bolster. B: Complete cardiac closure is achieved as follows: The two rectangular bolsters are placed over both ventricular walls and horizontal mattress sutures are passed through the first bolster, the left ventricle, both septal patches, the right ventricle, and right ventricular bolster so that no suture is tied in direct contact with muscle. (From Iben, A.B., Miller, R.R., Amsterdam, E.A., et al: Successful immediate repair of acquired ventricular septal defect and survival in patients with acute myocardial infarction shock using a new double patch technique. *Chest*, **66**: 665, 1974, with permission.)

tomatic performance (criteria of the New York Heart Association) of class I in two patients, II in eight, and III in three individuals. Postoperative cardiac catheterization in the eight patients in whom this procedure was performed demonstrated significant improvement in group mean values for systemic arterial pressure, left ventricular end-diastolic pressure, and cardiac index. Following operation, cardiac index rose to normal in all patients in whom it was decreased prior to surgery, and preoperatively elevated left ventricular filling pressure became normal (below or equal to 12 mm Hg) in all but one individual.

These observations indicate that, in acute myocardial infarction associated with cardiogenic shock or recurrent ventricular tachycardia-fibrillation intractable to conventional medical therapy, the procedure of left heart catheterization and angiography is both feasible and important in identifying patients with surgically approachable lesions. A relatively high proportion of AMI patients with these highly lethal complications have cardiac abnormalities which are correctable by emergency operative intervention.

In our experience, approximately one-half of patients with refractory pump failure due to AMI are appropriate candidates for complete cardiac catheterization and angiographic evaluation to assess the prospect of surgical therapy. Of these complicated AMI patients undergoing emergency catheterization, potentially correctable lesions by operation are detected in two-thirds of the individuals. In the patients thus selected for emergency surgical therapy, approximately 60% achieve long term survival following cardiac operation. Therefore, emergency cardiac catheterization and the application of immediate surgery in appropriate individuals allow chronic survival in approximately 30% of AMI patients with cardiogenic shock who would in all likelihood have succumbed with conventional medical management.

In AMI patients with primary refractory, recurrent ventricular tachycardia-fibrillation in whom rapid secondary deterioration of cardiac pump function is not a major factor, emergency angiography has afforded detection of operable defects in all of our patients. Furthermore, immediate cardiac surgery, consisting of coronary artery bypass alone or in combination with infarctectomy, has been successful in providing long term survival in this particular subset of complicated AMI patients in whom the outlook is poor with conventional pharmacological and electrical antiarrhythmic measures.

From our experience in the evaluation for, and the application of surgical intervention in complicated AMI, certain principles of clinical relevance have emerged in the management of these patients. Successful surgical intervention in acute intractable pump failure is associated with the presence of a major mechanical disturbance of ventricular performance such as ventricular septal defect, mitral regurgitation, or segmental dyssynergy potentially amenable to operative correction. Thus pump failure principally due to massive myocardial necrosis with shock wholly the result of loss of myocardial contractile units has not been reversible by coronary artery bypass as the sole procedure.

In addition, as reported previously from our institution[119], intractable pump failure is unusual with acute transmural diaphragmatic AMI alone, in the absence of old infarction. Thus the area of muscle necrosis is considerably less with diaphragmatic infarction compared to anterior wall infarction, and in the latter acute pump failure can readily occur on the basis of extensive infarction alone without associated mechanical abnormalities[125]. Therefore, the occurrence of cardiogenic shock in diaphragmatic AMI suggests the presence of an additional mechanical lesion substantially contributing to cardiac failure, the etiology of which should be carefully sought by cardiac catheterization and angiography.

It is important to emphasize that cardiac catheterization and surgical therapy for correction of complicated acute myocardial infarction require the close cooperation and expertise of a well coordinated cardiology-cardiac surgery team. In addition to the ready availability of expensive equipment for invasive evaluation and open-heart operation, considerable competence and flexibility of a relatively large number of individuals comprising the medical-surgical team are essential. In such a setting characteristic of a major medical center with sufficient experienced personnel and adequate facilities, surgically remediable lesions can be identified by cardiac catheterization with angiography, carried out at acceptable risk, and emergency heart surgery can be applied with significant benefit in reducing mortality in cardiogenic shock and intractable life-threatening arrhythmias complicating acute myocardial infarction.

CONCLUSIONS

Myocardial infarction shock is a syndrome characterized by severe impairment of circulatory function. It accounts for the major proportion of mortality in the hospital phase of acute myocardial infarction and is chiefly related to extensive loss of left ventricular muscle, although extramyocardial factors may be contributory. Quantitative hemodynamic evaluation allows accurate assessment of prognosis related to cardiac pump dysfunction in acute myocardial infarction and provides a physiologic basis for rational application of available modes of treatment. Therapy consists of pharmacologic agents, mechanical circulatory assist, and surgery to correct mechanical cardiac defects related to the infarction. The goal of treatment is to reduce myocardial ischemia, limit infarct size, and enhance circulatory function. Positive inotropic agents may increase myocardial ischemic injury because of the increase in myocardial oxygen demands which they produce in a physiologic setting in which concomitant rise in oxygen supply is precluded by coronary obstructive disease. Mechanical circulatory assist has the capacity to enhance cardiac performance while simultaneously reducing myocardial ischemia by decreasing left ventricular afterload and increasing coronary blood flow. Evaluation for surgically correctable cardiac defects is initiated in appropriate patients when shock is refractory to medical management and mechanical circulatory assist. Systematic application of a widening range of therapeutic alternatives provides the potential for prevention of myocardial infarction shock and reduction of mortality when AMI shock occurs.

Acknowledgments

The authors gratefully acknowledge the technical assistance of Robert Kleckner, Martie Wood, Robbie Brocchini, Denise Salmon, and Leslie Silvernail.

References

1. Cox, J.L., McLaughlin, V.W., Flowers, N.C., and Horan, L.G.: The ischemic zone surrounding acute myocardial infarction. Its morphology as detected by dehydrogenase staining. *Am. Heart J.*, **76**: 650, 1968.
2. Amsterdam, E.A., Massumi, R.A., Zelis, R., and Mason, D.T.: Evaluation and management of cardiogenic shock. Part II. Drug therapy. *Heart and Lung*, **1**: 663, 1972.
3. Gunnar, R.M. and Loeb, H.S.: Use of drugs in cardiogenic shock due to acute myocardial infarction. *Circulation*, **45**: 211, 1972.
4. Kuhn, L.A.: The treatment of cardiogenic shock. Part II. The use of pressor agents in the treatment of cardiogenic shock. *Am. Heart J.*, **74**: 725, 1967.
5. Kuhn, L.A.: Changing treatment of shock following acute myocardial infarction—a critical evaluation. *Am. J. Cardiol.*, **20**: 757, 1967.
6. Binder, M.J.: Effect of vasopressor drugs on circulatory dynamics in shock following myocardial infarction. *Am. J. Cardiol.*, **16**: 834, 1965.
7. Shubin, H. and Weil, M.H.: The treatment of shock complicating acute myocardial infarction. *Prog. Cardiovas. Dis.*, **10**: 30, 1967.
8. Smith, H.J., Priol, A., Morch, J., and McGregor, M.: Hemodynamic studies in cardiogenic shock: treatment with isoproterenol and metaraminol. *Circulation*, **35**: 1084, 1967.
9. Puri, P.S. and Bing, R.J.: Effect of drugs on myocardial contractility in the intact dog and in experimental myocardial infarction. *Am. J. Cardiol.*, **21**: 886, 1968.
10. Serur, J.R. and Urschel, C.W.: Attenuation of inotropic interventions by myocardial ischemia. *Cardiovas. Res.*, **7**: 458, 1973.
11. Amsterdam, E.A., Kamiyama, T., Rendig, S., and Mason, D.T.: Differential regional contractile actions of digitalis in experimental myocardial infarction. *Clin. Res.*, **22**: 257A, 1974.
12. Scheidt, S., Ascheim, R., and Killip, R.: Shock after acute myocardial infarction. *Am. J. Cardiol.*, **26**: 556, 1970.
13. Wolk, M.J., Scheidt, S., and Killip, T.: Heart failure complicating acute myocardial infarction. *Circulation*, **45**: 1125, 1972.
14. Tennant, R. and Wiggers, C.J.: The effect of coronary occlusion on myocardial contraction. *Am. J. Physiol.*, **112**: 351, 1935.
15. Tatooles, C.J. and Randal, W.C.: Local ventricular bulging after acute coronary occlusion. *Am. J. Physiol.*, **201**: 451, 1961.
16. Maroko, P.R., Kjekshus, J.K., Sobel, B.E., et al: Factors influencing infarct size following experimental coronary artery occlusions. *Circulation*, **43**: 67, 1971.
17. Maroko, P.R. and Braunwald, E.: Modification of myocardial infarction size after coronary occlusion. *Ann. Intern. Med.*, **79**: 720, 1973.

18. Braunwald, E. and Maroko, P.R.: The reduction of infarct size—an idea whose time (for testing) has come. *Circulation*, **50**: 206, 1974.
19. Sonnenblick, E.H. and Skelton, C.L.: Oxygen consumption of the heart: physiological principles and clinical implications. *Mod. Concepts Cardiovasc. Dis.*, **40**: 9, 1971.
20. Berne, R.M.: Regulation of coronary blood flow. *Physiol. Rev.*, **44**: 1, 1964.
21. Amsterdam, E.A., Williams, D.O., Caudil, C., et al: Hemodynamic effects of propranolol in acute myocardial infarction: beneficial and deleterious actions. *Clin. Res.*, **22**: 257A, 1974.
22. Braunwald, E., Maroko, P.R., and Libby, P.: Reduction of infarct size following coronary occlusion. *Circ. Res.*, **35**: suppl III: 192, 1974.
23. Mueller, H.S., Ayres, S.M., Religa, A., et al: Propranolol in the treatment of acute myocardial infarction. *Circulation*, **49**: 1078, 1974.
24. Mason, D.T., Zelis, R., and Amsterdam, E.A.: Actions of the nitrites on the peripheral circulation and myocardial oxygen consumption: significance in the relief of angina pectoris. *Chest*, **59**: 296, 1971.
25. Smith, E.R., Redwood, D.R., McCarron, W.E., et al: Coronary artery occlusion in the conscious dog. Effects of alterations in arterial pressure produced by nitroglycerin, hemorrhage, and alpha-adrenergic agonists on the degree of myocardial ischemia. *Circulation*, **47**: 51, 1973.
26. Hirschfeld, J.W., Boxer, J.S., Goldstein, R.E., et al: Reduction in severity and extent of myocardial infarction when nitroglycerin and methoxamine are administered during coronary occlusion. *Circulation*, **49**: 291, 1974.
27. Epstein, S.E., Kent, K.M., Goldstein, R.E., et al: Reduction of ischemic injury by nitroglycerin during acute myocardial infarction. *N. Engl. J. Med.*, **292**: 29, 1975.
28. Williams, D.O., Amsterdam, E.A., and Mason, D.T.: Hemodynamic effects of nitroglycerin in acute myocardial infarction: decrease in ventricular preload at the expense of cardiac output. *Circulation*, **51**: 421, 1975.
29. Capone, R., Mason, D.T., Amsterdam, E.A., et al: A comparison of the action of short and long-action nitrites on the peripheral circulation. *Clin. Res.*, **20**: 204, 1972.
30. Franciosa, J.A., Mikulic, E., Cohn, J.N., et al: Hemodynamic effects of orally administered isosorbide dinitrate in patients with congestive heart failure. *Circulation*, **50**: 1020, 1974.
31. Willis, W.H., Russell, R.O., Mantle, J.A., et al: Hemodynamic response to sublingual isosorbide dinitrate in unstable angina pectoris. *Am. J. Cardiol.*, **33**: 179, 1974.
32. Franciosa, J.A., Guiha, N.H., Limas, C.J., et al: Improved left ventricular function during nitroprusside infusion in acute myocardial infarction. *Lancet*, **1**: 650, 1972.
33. Chatterjee, K., Parmley, W.W., Ganz, W., et al: Hemodynamic and metabolic responses to vasodilator therapy in acute myocardial infarction. *Circulation*, **48**: 1183, 1973.
34. Miller, R.R., Vismara, L.A., Zelis, R., et al: Clinical use of sodium nitroprusside in chronic ischemic heart disease. *Circulation*, **51**: 328, 1975.
35. Williams, D.O., Hilliard, G.K., Cantor, S.A., et al: Comparative mechanisms of ventricular unloading by systemic vasodilator agents in therapy of cardiac failure: nitroprusside versus phentolamine. *Am. J. Cardiol.*, **35**: 177, 1975.
36. Kelley, D.T., Delgado, C.E., Taylor, D.R., et al: Use of phentolamine in acute myocardial infarction associated with hypertension and left ventricular failure. *Circulation*, **47**: 729, 1973.
37. Shell, W.E. and Sobel, B.E.: Protection of jeopardized ischemic myocardium by reduction of ventricular afterload. *N. Engl. J. Med.*, **291**: 481, 1974.
38. Redwood, D.R., Smith, E.R., and Epstein, S.E.: Coronary artery occlusion in

the conscious dog. Effects of alterations in heart rate and arterial pressure on the degree of myocardial ischemia. *Circulation*, **46**: 323, 1972.

39. Mason, D.T., Spann, J.F., and Zelis, R.: Pathogenesis and treatment of the low cardiac output syndrome. In W.W. Oaks (Ed.): *Pre- and Postoperative Management of the Cardiopulmonary Patient*. F.A. Davis, Philadelphia, 1970, p. 328.

40. Soroff, H.S., Cloutier, C.T., Birtwell, W.C., et al: External counterpulsation. *JAMA*, **229**: 1441, 1974.

41. Maroko, P.R., Bernstein, E.F., Libby, P., et al: The effects of intra-aortic balloon counterpulsation on the severity of myocardial ischemic injury following acute coronary occlusion. Counterpulsation and myocardial injury. *Circulation*, **45**: 1150, 1972.

42. DeLaria, G.A., Johnsen, K.H., Sobel, B.E., et al: Delayed evolution of myocardial ischemic injury after intra-aortic balloon counterpulsation. *Circulation*, **50** suppl. II: 242, 1974.

43. O'Rourke, M.F., Chang, V.P., Windsor, H.M., et al: Acute severe cardiac failure complicating myocardial infarction. *Brit. Heart J.*, **37**: 169, 1975.

44. Willerson, J.T., Curry, G.C., Watson, J.T., et al: Intra-aortic balloon counterpulsation in patients in cardiogenic shock, medically refractory left ventricular failure and/or recurrent ventricular tachycardia. *Am. J. Med.*, **58**: 183, 1975.

45. Maroko, P.R., Hale, S.L., and Braunwald, E.: The influence of oxygen inhalation on the severity of myocardial ischemic injury following experimental coronary occlusion. *Circulation*, **48** Suppl. IV: 128, 1973.

46. Poliwoda, H.: The thrombolytic therapy of acute myocardial infarction. *Angiology*, **17**: 528, 1966.

47. Maroko, P.R., Libby, P., Ginks, W.R., et al: Coronary artery reperfusion. I. Early effects on local myocardial function and the extent of myocardial necrosis. *J. Clin. Invest.*, **51**: 2710, 1972.

48. Ginks, W.R., Sybers, H.D., and Maroko, P.R.: Coronary artery reperfusion. II. Reduction of myocardial infarct size at one week after coronary occlusion. *J. Clin. Invest.*, **51**: 2710, 1972.

49. Libby, P., Maroko, P.R., Sobel, B.E., et al: Reduction of experimental myocardial infarct size by corticosteroid administration. *J. Clin. Invest.*, **52**: 599, 1973.

50. Maroko, P.R., Davidson, D.M., Libby, P., et al: Effects of hyaluronidase administration on myocardial ischemic injury in acute infarction. *Ann. Intern. Med.*, **82**: 516, 1975.

51. Amsterdam, E.A., Foley, D., Massumi, R.A., et al: Influence of increased glucose availability and mannitol on performance of hypoxic myocardium. *J. Clin. Invest.*, **51**: 4A, 1972.

52. Atkins, J.M., Wildenthal, K., and Horwitz, L.D.: Cardiovascular responses to hyperosmotic mannitol in anesthetized and conscious dogs. *Am. J. Physiol.*, **225**: 132, 1973.

53. Willerson, J.T., Weisfeldt, M.I., Sanders, C.A., et al: Influence of hyperosmolar agents on hypoxic cat papillary muscle function. *Cardiovasc. Res.*, **8**: 8, 1974.

54. Hutton, I., Marynick, S.P., Fixler, D.E., et al: Changes in reginal coronary blood flow with hypertonic mannitol in conscious dogs. *Cardiovasc. Res.*, **9**: 47, 1975.

55. Maroko, P.R. and Carpenter, C.B.: Reduction in infarct size following acute coronary occlusion by the administration of cobra venom factor. *Clin. Res.*, **21**: 950, 1973.

56. Maroko, P.R., Libby, P., Sobel, B.E., et al: The effect of glucose-insulin-potassium infusion on myocardial infarction following experimental coronary artery occlusion. *Circulation*, **45**: 1160, 1972.

57. Sybers, H.D., Maroko, P.R., Ashraf, M., et al: The effect of glucose-insulin-

potassium on cardiac ultrastructure following acute experimental coronary occlusion. *Am. J. Pathol.*, **70**: 401, 1973.

58. Stanley, A.W., Moraski, R.E., Russell, R.O., et al: Alteration of myocardial fuel and oxygen extraction by glucose-insulin-potassium. *Clin. Res.*, **22**: 13A, 1974.
59. Amsterdam, E.A., Foley, D., Massumi, R.A., et al: Enhancement of myocardial function during hypoxia by increased glucose availability. *Am. J. Cardiol.*, **29**: 251, 1972.
60. Amsterdam, E.A., DeMaria, A.N., Miller, R.R., et al: Intermediate coronary syndrome: clinical and angiographic considerations and results of medical versus surgical therapy. *Clin. Res.*, **23**: 76A, 1975.
61. Vatner, S.F., McRitchie, R.J., Maroko, P.R., et al: Effects of catecholamines, exercise, and nitroglycerin on the normal and ischemic myocardium in conscious dogs. *J. Clin. Invest.*, **54**: 563, 1974.
62. Amsterdam, E.A., Choquet, Y., Lenz, J., et al: Attenuation of positive inotropic action of digitalis by hypoxia and comparison with isoproterenol. *Circulation*, **46**: 124, 1972.
63. Maroko, P.R., Libby, P., and Braunwald, E.: Effect of pharmacologic agents on the function of the ischemic heart. *Am. J. Cardiol.*, **32**: 930, 1973.
64. Serur, J.R. and Urschel, C.W.: Attenuation of inotropic interventions by myocardial ischemia. *Cardiovasc. Res.*, **7**: 458, 1973.
65. Davidson, S., Maroko, P.R., and Braunwald, E.: Effects of isoproterenol on contractile function of the ischemic and anoxic heart. *Am. J. Physiol.*, **227**: 439, 1974.
66. Amsterdam, E.A., Zelis, R., Kohfeld, D.B., et al: Effect of morphine on myocardial contractility: negative inotropic action during hypoxia and reversal by isoproterenol. *Circulation*, **44**: Suppl. II: 135, 1971.
67. Maroko, P.R., Libby, P., Covell, J.W., et al: Precordial ST segment mapping: an atraumatic method for assessing alterations in the extent of myocardial ischemic injury. The effects of pharmacologic and hemodynamic interventions. *Am. J. Cardiol.*, **29**: 223, 1972.
68. Pelides, L.J., Reid, D.W., Thomas, M., et al: Inhibition by beta-blockade of the ST segment elevation after acute myocardial infarction in man. *Cardiovasc. Res.*, **6**: 295, 1972.
69. Cohn, J.N.: Blood pressure measurement in shock. Mechanisms of inaccuracy in auscultory and palpatory methods. *JAMA*, **199**: 972, 1967.
70. Cohn, J.N., Khatri, I.M., and Hamosh, P.: Bedside catheterization of the left ventricle. *Am. J. Cardiol.*, **25**: 66, 1970.
71. Swan, H.J.C., Ganz, W., Forrester, J., et al: Catheterization of the heart in man with use of a flow directed balloon-tipped catheter. *N. Engl. J. Med.*, **283**: 447, 1970.
72. Forrester, J.S., Diamond, G., McHugh, T.J., et al: Filling pressures in the right and left sides of the heart in acute myocardial infarction: a reappraisal of central venous pressure monitoring. *N. Engl. J. Med.*, **285**: 190, 1971.
73. Cohn, J.N.: Monitoring techniques in shock. *Am. J. Cardiol.*, **26**: 565, 1970.
74. Loeb, H.S., Rahimtoola, S.H., Rosen, K.M., et al: Assessment of ventricular function after acute myocardial infarction by plasma volume expansion. *Circulation*, **47**: 720, 1973.
75. Ramo, B.W., Myers, N., Wallace, A.G., et al: Hemodynamic findings in 123 patients with acute myocardial infarction in admission. *Circulation*, **42**: 567, 1970.
76. Parmley, W.W., Diamond, G., Tomoda, H., et al: Clinical evaluation of left ventricular pressures in myocardial infarction. *Circulation*, **45**: 358, 1972.
77. Weber, K.T., Ratshin, R.A., Janicki, J.S., et al: Left ventricular dysfunction

following acute myocardial infarction. *Am. J. Med.*, **54**: 697, 1973.

78. Price, J., Amsterdam, E.A., Miller, R.R., et al: Prognosis in acute myocardial infarction assessed by left heart catheterization. *Circulation*, **48**: 204, 1973.
79. DaLuz, P., Afifi, A.A., Liu, V., et al: Objective index of hemodynamic status for quantitation of severity and prognosis of shock complicating myocardial infarction. *Am. J. Cardiol.*, **29**: 259, 1972.
80. Amsterdam, E.A., DeMaria, A.N., Wood, M., et al: Accurate assessment of prognosis in acute myocardial infarction by hemodynamic evaluation. *Clin. Res.*, **23**: 170A, 1975.
81. Scheidt, S., Fillmore, S., Ascheim, R., et al: Objective assessment of prognosis after acute myocardial infarction. *Circulation*, **41**: 196, 1970.
82. Sobel, B.E., Bresnahan, G.F., Schell, W.E., et al: Estimation of infarct size in man and its relation to prognosis. *Circulation*, **46**: 640, 1972.
83. Zaret, B.L., Pitt, B., and Ross, R.S.: Determination of the site, extent and significance of regional ventricular dysfunction during acute myocardial infarction. *Circulation*, **45**: 441, 1972.
84. Allen, H.N., Danzig, R., and Swan, H.J.C.: Incidence and significance of relative hypovolemia as a cause of shock associated with acute myocardial infarction. *Circulation*, **35**: Suppl. II: 50, 1967.
85. Russell, R.O., Jr., Rackley, C.E., Pombo, J., et al: Effects of increasing left ventricular filling pressure in patients with acute myocardial infarction. *J. Clin. Invest.*, **49**: 1539, 1970.
86. Amsterdam, E.A., Massumi, R.A., Zelis, R., et al: Evaluation and management of cardiogenic shock. Part I. Approach to the patient. *Heart and Lung*, **1**: 402, 1972.
87. Crexells, C., Chatterjee, K., Forrester, J.S., et al: Optimal filling pressure in the left side of the heart in acute myocardial infarction. *N. Engl. J. Med.*, **289**: 1263, 1973.
88. Amsterdam, E.A., DeMaria, A.N., Hughes, J.L., et al: Myocardial infarction shock: mechanisms and therapy. In D.T. Mason (Ed.): *Congestive Heart Failure*, Yorke Medical Books, New York City, 1976, in press.
89. Yurchak, P.M., Rolett, E.C., Cohen, L.S., et al: Effects of norepinephrine on the coronary circulation in man. *Circulation*, **30**: 180, 1964.
90. Nies, A.S. and Melmon, K.L.: The rational management of cardiogenic shock. *Cardiovasc. Clin.*, **1**: 65, 1969.
91. Goldberg, L.I. and Talley, R.C.: Current therapy of shock. *Adv. Intern. Med.*, **17**: 363, 1971.
92. Goldberg, L.I.: Dopamine—clinical uses of an endogenous catecholamine. *N. Engl. J. Med.*, **291**: 707, 1974.
93. Amsterdam, E.A., Bonanno, J., Mansour, E., et al: Effects of dopamine on hemodynamics and myocardial metabolism in patients with coronary artery disease. *Clin. Res.*, **20**: 202, 1972.
94. Loeb, H.S., Winslow, E.B.J., Rahimtoola, S.H., et al: Acute hemodynamic effects of dopamine in patients with shock. *Circulation*, **44**: 163, 1971.
95. Krasnow, N., Rolett, E.L., Yurchak, P.M., et al: Isoproterenol and cardiovascular performance. *Am. J. Med.*, **37**: 514, 1964.
96. Smith, H.J., Oriol, A., March, J., et al: Hemodynamic studies in cardiogenic shock: treatment with isoproterenol and metaraminol. *Circulation*, **35**: 1084, 1967.
97. Mason, D.T.: Digitalis pharmacology and therapeutics: recent advances. *Ann. Intern. Med.*, **80**: 520, 1974.
98. Marano, A.J., Jr., Kline, H.J., Cestero, J., et al: Hemodynamic effects of ouabain in experimental acute myocardial infarction with shock. *Am. J. Cardiol.*, **17**: 327, 1966.

99. Malmcrona, R., Schroder, G., and Werko, L.: Haemodynamic effects of digitalis in acute myocardial infarction. *Acta Med. Scand.*, **180**: 55, 1966.
100. Balcon, R., Hoy, J., and Sowton, E.: Haemodynamic effects of rapid digitalization following acute myocardial infarction. *Brit. Heart J.*, **30**: 373, 1968.
101. Hodges, M., Friesinger, G.C., Riggins, R.C.K., et al: Effects of intravenously administered digoxin on mild left ventricular failure in acute myocardial infarction in man. *Am. J. Cardiol.*, **29**: 749, 1972.
102. Rahimtoola, S.H., Sinno, M.Z., Chuquimia, R., et al: Effects of ouabain on impaired left ventricular function in acute mycardial infarction. *N. Engl. J. Med.*, **287**: 527, 1972.
103. Amsterdam, E.A., Huffaker, H.K., DeMaria, A., et al: Hemodynamic effects of digitalis in acute myocardial infarction and comparison with furosemide. *Circulation*, **46**: 113, 1972.
104. Rahimtoola, S.H., Loeb, H.S., and Gunnar, R.M.: Digitalis in myocardial infarction. In R.M. Gunnar, H.S. Loeb, and S.H. Rahimtoola (Eds.): *Shock in Myocardial Infarction*. Grune & Stratton, Inc., New York, 1974, pp. 157-172.
105. Cohn, J.N., Tristani, F.E., and Khatri, I.M.: Cardiac and peripheral vascular effects of digitalis in clinical cardiogenic shock. *Am. Heart J.*, **78**: 318, 1969.
106. Amsterdam, E.A., Mansour, E.J., Hughes, J.L., et al: Present status of glucagon and bretylium tosylate. In H. Russek and B. Zohman (Eds.): *Changing Concepts in Cardiovascular Disease*. Williams & Wilkins Co., Baltimore, 1972, p. 215.
107. Chatterjee, K. and Swan, H.J.C.: Vasodilator therapy in acute myocardial infarction. *Mod. Concepts Cardiovasc. Dis.*, **43**: 119, 1974.
108. Miller, R.R., Vismara, L.A., Williams, D.O., et al: Comparative pharmacologic mechanisms of left ventricular unloading in clinical congestive heart failure: Differential effects of nitroprusside, phentolamine and nitroglycerin on cardiac function and peripheral circulation. *Circ. Res.*, 1976, in press.
109. Dennis, C., Carlens, E., Senning, A., et al: Clinical use of a cannula for left-heart bypass without thoracotomy: experimental protection against fibrillation by left-heart bypass. *Ann. Surg.*, **156**: 623, 1962.
110. Amsterdam, E.A., Massumi, R.A., Zelis, R., et al: Evaluation and management of cardiogenic shock. Part III. The roles of cardiac surgery and mechanical assist. *Heart and Lung*, **2**: 122, 1973.
111. Mueller, H., Giannelli, S., Jr., and Ayres, S.M.: Mechanical cardiac assistance in shock following acute myocardial infarction. In R.M. Gunner, H.S. Loeb, and S.H. Rahimtoola (Eds.): *Shock in Myocardial Infarction*, Grune & Stratton, Inc., New York, 1974, pp. 229-265.
112. Lesch, M.: Assisted circulation in the treatment of shock complicating acute myocardial infarction. *Cardiovasc. Clin.*, **3**: 22, 1971.
113. Scheidt, S., Wilner, G., Mueller, H., et al: Intra-aortic balloon counterpulsation in cardiogenic shock. *N. Engl. J. Med.*, **288**: 979, 1973.
114. Willerson, J.T., Curry, G.C., Watson, J.T., et al: Intra-aortic balloon counterpulsation in patients in cardiogenic shock, medically refractory left ventricular failure and/or recurrent ventricular tachycardia. *Am. J. Med.*, **58**: 183, 1975.
115. Leinbach, R.C., Mundth, E.D., Dinsmore, R.E., et al: Selective coronary and left ventricular cineangiography during intra-aortic balloon assist for cardiogenic shock. *Am. J. Cardiol.*, **26**: 644, 1971.
116. Leinbach, R.C., Gold, H.K., Dinsmore, R.E., et al: The role of angiography in cardiogenic shock. *Circulation*, **47**: 95, 1973.
117. Messer, J.V., Willerson, J.T., Loeb, H.S., et al: Evaluation of external pressure circulatory assist in acute myocardial infarction. *Clin. Res.*, **23**: 197A, 1975.
118. Amsterdam, E., Banas, J., Criley, M., et al: Clinical evaluation of external pressure circulatory assist in acute myocardial infarction. Submitted, *N. Engl. J. Med.*, 1976.

119. Amsterdam, E.A., Miller, R.R., and Mason, D.T.: Surgery for acute myocardial infarction. In R. M. Gunner, H.S. Loeb, and S.H. Rahimtoola (Eds.): *Shock in Myocardial Infarction.* Grune & Stratton, Inc., New York, 1974, p. 257.
120. Amsterdam, E.A., Miller, R.R., Hughes, J.L., et al: Emergency surgical therapy of complicated acute myocardial infarction: indications and results in cardiogenic shock, intractable ventricular tachycardia, and extending infarction. In H.I. Russek (Ed.): *Cardiovascular Problems.* University Park Press, Baltimore, 1976, pp. 447-451.
121. Amsterdam, E.A., Choquet, Y., Bonanno, J., et al: Correlative hemodynamics and angiography in acute coronary syndromes. *Clin. Res.,* **21**: 232, 1973.
122. Mason, D.T., Amsterdam, E.A., Miller, R.R., et al: Consideration of the therapeutic roles of pharmacologic agents, collateral circulation and saphenous vein bypass in coronary artery disease. *Am. J. Cardiol.,* **28**: 608, 1971.
123. Amsterdam, E.A., Choquet, Y., Bonanno, J.A., et al: Quantification of left ventricular function and coronary arteriography in acute coronary insufficiency, myocardial infarction and cardiogenic shock: application to therapy. *Clin. Res.,* **21**: 398, 1973.
124. Iben, A.B., Miller, R.R., Amsterdam, E.A., et al: Successful immediate repair of acquired ventricular septal defect and survival in patients with acute myocardial infarction shock using a new double patch technique. *Chest,* **66**: 665, 1974.
125. Mason, D.T., Amsterdam, E.A., Miller, R.R., et al: Recent advances in pathophysiology and therapy of myocardial infarction shock. In H. Russek (Ed.): *Cardiovascular Disease: New Concepts in Diagnosis and Therapy.* University Park Press, Baltimore, 1974, p. 143.

CHAPTER 13

Electropharmacology and Clinical Pharmacology of Antiarrhythmic Drugs*

Leonard S. Gettes, M.D.; Russell McAllister, M.D.;
Chia-Maou Chen, M.D.

This Chapter reviews the underlying electropharmacology of key anti-arrhythmic drugs with their prescribed manner of use. No other clinical intervention has proved so effective in reducing mortality and morbidity in the coronary care unit. For this reason, an in-depth discussion of major therapeutic agents is provided to help assure full and appropriate therapeutic benefit.

Many pharmacological agents are currently available for the treatment of cardiac arrhythmias[1]. Some relieve the underlying cause of arrhythmia such as potassium, oxygen, NaH_2CO_3; others act by altering autonomic tone, such as digitalis, propranolol, phenylephrine, edrophonium, and Prostigmin®. Still others act directly on the electrophysiologic properties of the individual cell. In this chapter we will consider the electrophysiologic mechanisms which may contribute to the antiarrhythmic effects of the third group of drugs and will review their clinical pharmacology. It is our conviction that a consideration of these factors is important to the proper clinical use of the drugs.

EFFECT OF DRUGS ON ELECTROPHYSIOLOGIC ABNORMALITIES RELATED TO ARRHYTHMIA GENESIS

Our present level of knowledge, while admittedly still incomplete, permits us to understand more about the possible mechanisms underlying the anti-arrhythmic effect of a given drug and in so doing provides valuable clues regarding the mechanisms underlying the arrhythmia. In a previous chapter, some of the electrophysiologic abnormalities contributing to arrhythmia genesis were discussed. In this chapter we shall consider the electrophysiologic effects of the drugs in relation to these abnormalities. The reader is also referred to the recent extensive reviews of Hoffman, Rosen,

*Some of the studies reported were supported by a grant from NIHL 5R01-HL13321-06

245

TABLE I

EFFECT OF ANTIARRHYTHMIC DRUGS ON ELECTROPHYSIOLOGIC PARAMETERS

	Quinidine Procaine Amide	Lidocaine	DPH	Verapamil	Propranolol < 0.3 μg/ml	Propranolol > 0.3 μg/ml	Bretylium
I. Spontaneous Impulse Formation							
Diastolic Depol. > -60 mV	Suppress	Suppress	Suppress	Suppress	—	Suppress	Enhance
Diastolic Depol. < -60 mV	?	—	?	Suppress	?	?	?
Transient Depol. < -60 mV	?	—	?	Suppress	?	?	?
Sinus Rate	Slow	—	Slow	Slow	Slow	Slow	Speed then Slow
II. Conduction							
Shift Steady-State (dV/dt) max Relationship	—	+	+	—	—	—	?
Prolong Recovery (dV/dt) max	—	++	+	—	—	—	?
Rate Dependent ↓ (dV/dt) max	++	+	–+	—	—	+	?
QRS Widening (Non-Premature beat)	+	—	—	—	—	?	—
HV Prolongation	+	—	—	—	—	?	—
AH Prolongation	+–	—	—	++	+	+	—
Slow Conduction in Ischemic Myocardium	+	+	+	?	—	?	?
III. Refractoriness							
Action Potential Duration (APD)	Variable	Shorten	Shorten	No Change	No Change	Shorten	Prolong
Effective Refractory Period (ERP)	Prolong	Shorten & Prolong (RMP Dependent)	Shorten	No Change	No Change	Prolong	Prolong
ERP/APD	Prolong	Prolong	Prolong	No Change	No Change	Prolong	No Change

+ = Effect

— = No Effect

? = Information Not Available

(dV/dt) max = Maximum rate of rise of the action potential upstroke.

RMP = Resting membrane potential.

and Wit concerned with the electrophysiologic mechanisms responsible for cardiac arrhythmias and for the action of antiarrhythmic drugs[2].

Spontaneous Impulse Formation

As indicated earlier, spontaneous impulse formation can be divided into two major categories: (1) that due to spontaneous depolarization throughout diastole and (2) that due to transient or after-depolarizations.

Each of these major categories can be further divided into those which occur at membrane potentials more or less negative than the threshold for the rapid sodium inward current. The ability to suppress such spontaneous activity may be accomplished by either increasing the outward current component or decreasing the inward current component of the "pacemaker currents". Spontaneous activity may also be suppressed by preventing the inward current which is itself responsible for the upstroke of the propagated action potential (either the rapid inward sodium current or the slow inward calcium dependent current).

Although the effect of each of the drugs on these parameters has not been specifically tested, partial information is available from single fiber, intact heart, and clinical studies.

Procaine amide, quinidine[3], lidocaine[4], and diphenylhydantoin[5] each suppress spontaneous diastolic depolarization in stretched Purkinje fibers or in Purkinje fibers exposed to low (less than 3 mM) concentrations of potassium. In general these spontaneous depolarizations occur at membrane potentials more negative than -60 mV. The frequency with which this type of spontaneous impulse formation is associated with arrhythmias is not known and therefore the relevence of this drug effect may be questioned. Lidocaine prevents ventricular fibrillation in isolated hearts perfused with low K solutions[6] and ventricular arrhythmias in intact animals and man due to a variety of causes[4]. However, it produces only light and transient slowing of the rate of the escape pacemaker in patients with complete AV block[7,8], perhaps the only pure examples of a spontaneously depolarizing ectopic ventricular pacemaker. Nonetheless, lidocaine is still unsafe to use in this situation because it may cause exit block[7]. In addition, clinically applicable concentrations of lidocaine do not suppress spontaneous depolarization in the -40 to -50 mV range[9] and do not slow the sinus rate[10]. These results suggest that in the clinical situation, the efficacy of lidocaine may be more likely due to the prevention of reentry rather than to suppression of spontaneous impulse formation. Similar studies have not been carried out for other drugs although all are thought contraindicated in patients with complete atrioventricular block.

Verapamil is unique in its ability to block the slow inward calcium sensitive current[11-13]. This drug does suppress spontaneous depolarizations in Purkinje fibers and in ventricular fibers depolarized to -40mV or less[9,12,14]. It also slows sinus rate[15] and prevents the transient subthreshold after depolarizations induced by digitalis[16]. However, the ability of verapamil to exert an antiarrhythmic effect by virtue of this mechanism has not been established.

Conduction

As reviewed in the earlier chapter, slowed conduction contributing to the development of unidirectional block is one of the requirements for reentry. Antiarrhythmic drugs may therefore prevent reentry by further depressing conduction and converting unidirectional into bidirectional block or by improving conduction and removing the unidirectional block (Figure 1). There is evidence to suggest that both mechanisms may be operative.

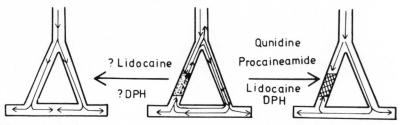

Figure 1 Schematic representation of conduction through a triangular arrangement of cardiac fibers. On the left, conduction is normal and the base of the triangular section is excited from the impulse propagating through both sides. In the center, unidirectional block is present in the left arm of the triangular section. Impulse propagates through the right arm, excites the base then passes retrogradely through the blocked section allowing reentry to occur. On the right, bidirectional block is present and reentry can not occur.

Quinidine, procaine amide, lidocaine, diphenylhydantoin, and verapamil may each depress conduction but they do so by different mechanisms and under somewhat different circumstances. As indicated above, conduction velocity is determined by steady-state and time dependent variables effecting the upstroke of the action potential[17]. The steady-state effects are voltage dependent and will be seen at all rates and in premature beats. The time dependent effects are also voltage dependent and will be seen in premature beats and when the heart rate is rapid. These time dependent effects may be due to changes in the recovery characteristics of the action potential upstroke or to changes in metabolic factors. Quinidine and procaine amide markedly alter intraventricular conduction as indicated on the ECG by QRS widening[18] in non-premature beats and on His electrograms by prolongation of HV intervals[19,20]. This conduction slowing is markedly rate dependent[21]. We attributed this rate dependent effect to metabolic factors since the drugs do not alter either the voltage dependent steady-state or recovery characteristics of the action potential upstroke[22] but do cause marked rate dependent slowing of the upstroke[23-25]. The absence of voltage related effects explains the observation that the depression of conduction induced by procaine amide is not progressively exaggerated in ischemic tissue[26].

Lidocaine does not prolong the QRS complex[18] or prolong the HV interval in non-premature beats[27] under normal conditions. In single fiber studies, lidocaine in concentrations less than 5 μg/ml, does not decrease the rate of rise of the action potentials in fibers perfused with solutions having a K^+ concentration below 3.0 mM or have a resting potential more negative than -80 mV[4,28,29]. However, lidocaine shifts the steady-state relationship between the resting potential and rapid upstroke of the action potential (Figure 2) and prolongs the recovery time of the action potential[21], i.e. the time required for the rate of rise of the upstroke to regain its steady-state value after a preceding depolarization (Figure 3). These effects are reflected in the single fiber by slowing of the action potential upstroke when the extracellular potassium is raised[21,30]. In the intact dog heart, the effects are reflected by marked slowing of conduction in non-premature beats when the serum potassium is raised (and therefore the membrane potential is decreased) causing more marked QRS widening and greater prolongation of the HV interval[31] and by progressive slowing of conduction within an ischemic zone following experimental coronary ligation[26,32]. The observation that the slowing of conduction is more marked in premature responses and at rapid rates suggests that in depressed and presumably depolarized myocardium, slow-

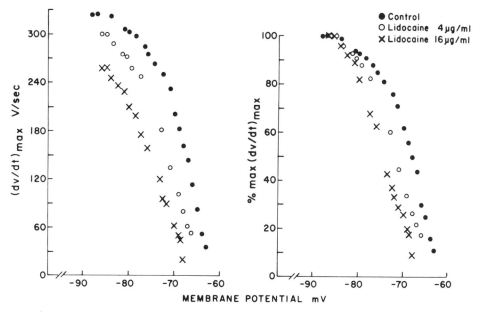

Figure 2   Effects of 4 and 16 μg/ml of lidocaine HCl on the steady-state relationship between resting membrane potential and (dV/dt) max in a fiber stimulated at 0.2/sec. Absolute values are shown in the graph on the left and normalized values in the graph on the right. Lidocaine caused a dose-dependent decrease in (dV/dt) max at all resting potential levels and shifted the normalized curves along the voltage axis in the direction of more negative membrane potentials. (From Chen, C.M., Gettes, L.S., and Katzung, B.G.: Effect of quinidine and lidocaine on steady state and recovery kinetics of (dV/dt) max. *Circ. Res.*, **37**: 20, 1975, with permission.)

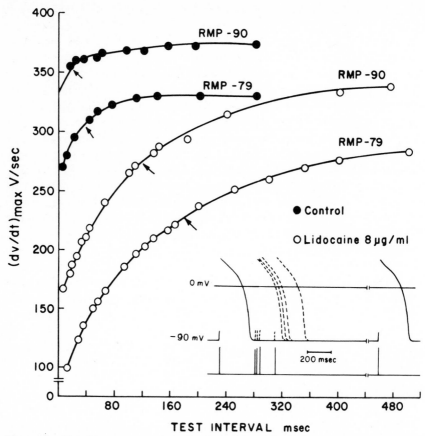

Figure 3 Graphic representation of an experiment in which the effect of lidocaine, 8 μg/ml on the recovery of (dV/dt) max was determined when the resting membrane potential (RMP) was -90 and -79 mV. The arrows indicate the time constant (τ) with which (dV/dt) max in the premature action potential regained the steady-state value. The method is illustrated in the insert. The conditioning or basic action potentials (0.2/sec) are shown by the solid lines and the premature action potentials by the broken lines; the differentiated upstroke spikes are shown below the action potentials. The test intervals were measured from the end (within 1 mV) of the conditioning action potential to the onset of the premature action potential. The figure illustrates the prolongation of recovery of (dV/dt) max induced by lidocaine. (From Chen, C.M., Gettes, L.S., and Katzung, B.G. Effect of quinidine and lidocaine on steady state and recovery kinetics of (dV/dt) max. *Circ. Res.*, **37**: 20, 1975, with permission.)

ing of conduction and the creation of bidirectional block may explain, at least in part, the antiarrhythmic effectiveness of the drug.

It is possible that in the non-depolarized myocardium, lidocaine may improve conduction in premature responses and in this way relieve unidirectional block (Figure 1). Such an effect has been demonstrated in isolated preparations of Purkinje-papillary muscle junction[33] and may be related to shortening of the action potential duration induced by the drug[28,29] (See below). Because of this factor, premature responses arising from incompletely repolarized fibers and therefore from a decreased membrane potential will, after lidocaine administration, arise from a more completely repolarized fiber and have a more rapid rate of depolarization. Lidocaine may also improve conduction by suppressing diastolic depolarization in the -80 to -60 mV range. The action potential will thereby arise from a more negative membrane potential and have a more rapid upstroke[34].

Diphenylhydantoin (DPH) shares with lidocaine the ability to shift the curve relating membrane potential to (dV/dt) max resulting in a more marked slowing of the upstroke of the action potential in partially depolarized fibers[35]. The shift in the steady-state curve would explain the observation that the drug slows the upstroke when the extracellular K is raised[30,36] (and the resting potential decreased) and would be expected to slow conduction within an ischemic (and therefore partially depolarized) zone[37].

DPH also shares with lidocaine the ability to shorten action potential duration[5]. Thus, as with lidocaine, this mechanism might improve conduction of early premature responses occurring in non-depolarized myocardium. The effects of rate on the upstroke of DPH treated fibers is not completely clear. Although no rate related effect was observed in guinea pig ventricular fibers at any resting potential[35], a rate dependent decrease in upstroke velocity has been reported in atrial fibers when the concentration of DPH exceeded 5 μg/ml and the potassium concentration exceeded 4.5 mM[36].

Verapamil does not alter the voltage dependent steady-state or recovery characteristics of the action potential upstroke in fibers whose resting membrane potential is more negative than -60 mV, i.e., the sodium dependent upstroke[35,38]. It does however, slow or prevent depolarization in fibers with resting potentials less negative than -50 mV, i.e., the calcium dependent upstroke[11,12], and in this way may induce bidirectional block and prevent reentry in severely depolarized fibers whose upstroke is dependent on the slow inward current system.

The effects of the various drugs on SA and AV conduction are complicated by: (1) their indirect effects on vagal tone and (2) the presence of both slow channel dependent and rapid channel dependent responses within the regions. For instance, quinidine and procaine amide exert anticholinergic effects and may speed AV conduction[19]. In addition, their direct effects may slow AV conduction[19,39] by affecting either or both types of responses. Lidocaine does not affect AV conduction in normal hearts[4,27] but may slow AV conduction in K$^+$ depolarized hearts[40], presumably by its effect on the fibers having depressed rapid (fast channel) responses. Dilantin may speed AV conduction[5] by unknown, possibly centrally mediated mechanisms while verapamil slows AV conduction[11], by virtue of its ability to depress slow channel responses.

Refractory Period

As indicated earlier, the refractory period is defined as the time following depolarization required for the fiber to repolarize to that membrane potential at which the recovery of the inward currents allows a second propagated depolarization to occur. This time is determined by three factors: (1) action potential duration; (2) the voltage dependent steady-state relationship between the membrane potential and the upstroke of the action potential; and (3) the recovery characteristics of the action potential upstroke (also voltage dependent). As a result of the combined effects of these factors the earliest propagated response may arise before the fiber is fully repolarized, i.e., from a membrane potential less negative than the resting potential, or may not occur until after the fiber has been completely repolarized, i.e., from the resting membrane potential (Figure 4). In the former case, refractoriness is said to be voltage dependent. In the latter, it is termed time dependent. The refractory periods of the fibers in the AV junction[41] and those surrounding the SA node[42] normally extend beyond the end of the action potential and are therefore examples of normal time dependent refractoriness. Time dependent refractoriness has also been reported in Purkinje fibers following coronary artery ligation[43].

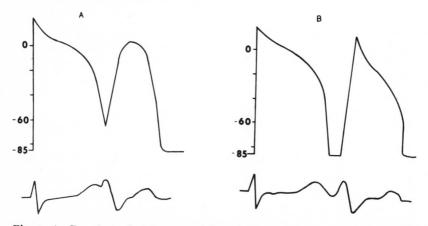

Figure 4 Drawings of action potentials and ECG's to illustrate voltage and time dependent refractoriness. In each panel, a nonpremature response and the earliest premature response are shown. On the left, the earliest premature action potential arises from an incompletely repolarized fiber and the premature QRS occurs shortly after the apex of the T wave. This represents voltage dependent refractoriness. On the right, the earliest premature action potential does not occur until the fiber is repolarized, i.e., after the end of the nonpremature action potential. The corresponding premature QRS originates after the T wave. This represents time dependent refractoriness. See Text.

The influence of the various drugs on refractoriness will reflect their differences on the parameters mentioned above. Quinidine and procaine amide have variable effects on the plateau and slow the phase of rapid repolarization resulting in variable changes in action potential duration and changes in the ST segment and T wave of the ECG[18]. Although neither drug alters the steady-state or recovery characteristics, both cause marked rate dependent effects possibly by depressing the sodium potassium ATPase system[25]. This results in a change in the membrane potential from which the earliest premature response can be evoked to more negative values. The rate dependent effect also results in a decrease in membrane responsiveness, that is, the membrane potential-(dV/dt) max relationship in premature responses. As a result of these changes the refractory period is lengthened following administration of these drugs and the refractory period duration expressed as a function of the duration of the action potential is prolonged[3].

As mentioned above, lidocaine shortens action potential duration, shifts the steady-state membrane potential (dV/dt) max curve, and prolongs the recovery characteristics of the action potential upstroke. As a result of the interplay between these factors, the effect of lidocaine on refractory period may be different at different resting membrane potentials. In fibers with a resting potential more negative than -80 mV, the shortening of the action potential may predominate and result in a shortening of the refractory period[44] although the membrane responsiveness curve will change and the refractory period duration will be prolonged relative to the action potential duration[4]. In partially depolarized fibers, the shift in the voltage dependent steady-state and recovery characteristics will predominate and the refractory period will be prolonged in spite of the shortened action potential duration. That is, time dependent refractoriness will be induced[21]. This factor, coupled with the conduction changes referred to above may explain the reported induction of infra-His AV block in patients with intraventricular conduction disturbances[45].

Diphenylhydantoin, as indicated above, shortens action potential duration and shifts the steady-state membrane potential upstroke velocity relationship but does not alter recovery characteristics and does not induce rate dependent slowing of the action potential upstroke. Thus, its actions are different from the other three drugs. The shortening of the action potential duration explains the shortening of refractory period which has been observed in man[46]. The shift in the steady-state relationship would explain the observations that refractory period is lengthened when expressed relative of action potential duration and conduction velocity is slowed in depressed myocardium[37]. Single fiber studies have demonstrated an improvement in "membrane responsiveness"[5] which cannot be explained by the effect of the drug on the parameters referred to.

Verapamil has not been shown to influence refractoriness in fibers having a membrane potential more negative than -60 mV[11]. In fibers with less negative potentials, the suppression of the slow inward current would be expected to prolong the time dependent refractoriness already present in these fibers.

Propranolol and bretylium tosylate have not been included in the above discussions because it is not yet clear as to whether their antiarrhythmic effects can be attributed to directly mediated electrophysiologic changes or to changes which result from alterations in sympathetic activity. Propranolol has been clearly shown to have effects on the single fiber which are similar to those of quinidine and procaine amide[35]. The non-beta blocking isomer of propranolol also possesses antiarrhythmic effects when tested in animals[47]. However, in clinically applicable concentrations (less than 0.3 μg/ml) propranolol does not alter the steady-state or recovery characteristics of the action potential upstroke and does not induce rate dependent slowing of the upstroke[35]. Thus, in these doses, quinidine-like effects cannot be identified. Moreover, propranolol, unlike quinidine, does not alter the QRS complex on the electrocardiogram[18] or prolong the HV interval in man[48]. Therefore, it is reasonable to attribute its effect on sinus node, AV conduction and both supra-ventricular and ventricular arrhythmias to beta adrenergic blockade[49].

Bretylium tosylate also presents difficulties in classification. The drug does not suppress spontaneous impulse formation in the single fiber or cause changes in upstroke of the action potential similar to that of any other direct acting antiarrhythmic drug. Nor does it lengthen the refractory period relative to action potential duration as do the other drugs[50]. Moreover, bretylium does not prevent ventricular fibrillation in the isolated perfused rabbit heart induced by premature stimuli or perfusion with low K solutions[6], although both types are prevented by lidocaine[6]. These results suggest that bretylium's antiarrhythmic effects are also mediated by the sympathetic nervous system. It has been postulated[51,52] that the early, acute effects of the drug may be due to the sympathetic stimulation which results from the inhibition of re-uptake and the resultant accumulation of norepinephrine at the nerve terminals, while the latter effect may be due to effective adrenergic blockade resulting from depletion of releasable norepinephrine stores.

THE CLINICAL PHARMACOLOGY OF ANTIARRHYTHMIC DRUGS

Introduction

The antiarrhythmic drugs under discussion produce toxic as well as therapeutic effects and, as a group, have a low toxic:therapeutic ratio. Since the consequences of toxicity are usually serious, and potentially lethal, it is imperative that the clinician use these agents with an understanding of the factors determining the occurrence of both beneficial and deleterious responses. This implies an appreciation for clinical pharmacokinetics—a rapidly expanding body of knowledge relating to the processes of drug absorption, distribution, biotransformation and metabolism, and elimination. Fortunately, the pharmacokinetic parameters of most antiarrhythmic drugs are reasonably well-defined, and their usefulness in guiding patient therapy may be seen without resort to either oversimplification or excessive involvement in mathematical manipulations required for other groups of drugs. In this section, we will outline several basic principles of pharmacokinetics and discuss their relevence to the use of the antiarrhythmic drugs.

Blood Level Measurements

Measurement of the concentrations of the cardiac glycosides, quinidine, procaine amide, lidocaine, diphenylhydantoin, and propranolol in the blood are becoming increasingly available, both in hospital and private commercial laboratories, and therapeutic and toxic ranges are reasonably well-established for each of these drugs. However, in order for drug blood level measurements to be clinically useful, several conditions must be satisfied[53,54].

1. *The concentration of the drug at its site of action must be accurately reflected by the concentration of drug in the blood or plasma.*

This condition, in turn, is predicated upon the assumption that the drug is acting by a reversible process. Drugs such as reserpine, which acts by irreversible binding to receptor sites, cannot be studied by blood level measurements. None of the cardio-active drugs under consideration bind irreversibly to myocardial tissue, and, therefore, each may be profitably studied by measurement of concentrations in blood.

2. *An equilibrium must have been established between the concentration of drug at its site of action and its concentration in blood.*

If a drug is administered by a single or repeated bolus, no steady-state condition between tissue and blood concentrations will be established. In this situation, blood level studies will be either useless or misleading. Under conditions of continuing administration, such as constant intravenous infusion or chronic oral dosing, some degree of equilibrium will be established between tissue and blood concentrations. In this circumstance, measurements of blood levels of the drug may be quite helpful.

3. *The clinical response to a drug must be correlated with the concentration of the drug in the blood.*

This condition implies that tissue binding is reversible and that a tissue-blood equilibrium has been established. It also requires that the substance being measured is the same as that which is producing an effect. Some drugs are partially or totally inactive themselves and depend upon biotransformation in the body to produce active metabolites. In this situation, blood level measurements of the parent compound will not be correlated with pharmacologic effect. The antiarrhythmic drugs do, in fact, produce effects which correspond relatively well to their blood concentrations, even though each one is extensively metabolized, and metabolites with pharmacologic effects similar to those of the parent drugs have been described. Furthermore, for blood levels to be meaningful, it is important that *both* therapeutic and toxic effects correlate with drug concentrations in blood. Toxicity which is idiosyncratic and non-dose related can neither be predicted nor avoided by blood level studies. Many of the deleterious effects seen with the antiarrhythmic agents under consideration are indeed related to tissue concentrations and are, therefore, often avoidable with the clinical use of blood level determinations.

There are several ways in which determinations of drug concentrations in blood can provide valuable assistance to the physician.

1. *To confirm the clinical diagnosis of drug toxicity*[55].

The physician must make certain judgments about his patient and the way in which that patient is likely to respond to a drug, based on the patient's status and on information from both clinical and laboratory studies. He then selects a dose and a dosing interval which he believes will produce a desired effect without causing toxicity. With some drugs, the therapeutic effect may be easily determined, such as the disappearance of ventricular premature beats. However, the margin of safety between therapeutic and toxic levels will remain unknown unless the toxic manifestations are correlated to drug concentrations in blood. It is important to recognize that wide variations may occur between the peak drug level in the blood after an oral dose and the trough level at the end of the dosing interval, and that these variations may extend from toxic to sub-therapeutic levels.

2. *To determine if a patient is handling a given drug as anticipated.*

The physician's initial decisions on drug dosage are based on his knowledge of how an "average" patient would react. However, many factors may complicate the manner in which a drug is handled by a patient. For instance, the rate of lidocaine metabolism may be impaired by the hepatic congestion accompanying heart failure and blood levels which are greater than anticipated from a given dose may result[56]. Quinidine excretion may be reduced if primary renal insufficiency is present, or if glomerular filtration rate is decreased, as may occur when cardiac output is reduced. In these situations, the blood and tissue levels of quinidine would be greater than expected[57]. Other factors which may alter handling of drugs include: nutritional state, degree of obesity, concurrently administered drugs, genetic factors, etc.

3. *To determine patient compliance with a prescribed regimen.*

The degree of patient adherence to a prescribed regimen varies with its complexity[58]. Since (a) most antiarrhythmic agents in chronic therapy require repeated dosing during a 24-hour period, (b) multiple cardiac drugs are often given at the same time, and (c) patients may give inaccurate drug histories, blood level determinations are often the best way to determine patient compliance.

Pharmacokinetic Principles

The methods used in pharmacokinetic analysis are designed to describe in mathematical terms the rates of drug distribution and elimination, and to provide a quantitative model from which optimal size and frequency of drug doses may be derived[59]. To the clinician without a substantial background in pharmacology, many of the analyses presented and much of the terminology employed may seem esoteric. However, there are several important pharmacologic aspects which the physician must understand in order to provide rational and effective therapy for his patients.

1. *The route(s) of drug elimination*

In the examples noted above, lidocaine, which is eliminated by hepatic metabolism, will accumulate to potentially toxic levels if the usually prescribed doses are given to patients with impaired liver function[56], while drugs handled largely by renal excretion may reach toxic concentrations in the presence of renal insufficiency[60].

2. *The two compartment model*[61]

This model assumes that the body may be viewed as a central compartment comprising the blood volume and extracellular fluid into which the drug first enters and a peripheral compartment comprising those tissues into which the drug moves from the central compartment. Drug elimination occurs only from the central compartment. Thus, that portion of drug in the peripheral compartment must move back into the central compartment before elimination can occur. Rate constants may be derived for movement between the compartments, and an elimination rate constant for movement from the central compartment can be calculated. The most useful parameter, however, is the overall elimination rate constant, which describes the combined rate of all methods of irreversible drug elimination from the body. From this elimination rate constant may be derived the *half-life of disposition for the drug*, the half-life being the time required for the concentration of drug in the central compartment to fall by 50%.

3. *First-order kinetics*

Digitalis glycosides, lidocaine, procaine amide, quinidine, and propranolol are all handled by first-order kinetics. That is, the rate at which drug elimination occurs is proportional to the drug concentration. Thus, the greater the quantity of drug in the body, the more drug will be eliminated in a given time. Stated another way, the half-life of disposition is independent of the absolute drug concentration. For drugs eliminated by first-order kinetics, the half-life may be derived simply by a semilog plot of serial blood concentrations against time.

The usefulness of the half-life concept is exemplified by digoxin. The half-life of digoxin is approximately 1.6 days. Since 50% of the drug will be eliminated in 1.6 days, 35% will be eliminated in one day (assuming normal renal function); therefore, doses given at daily intervals should approximate 35% of the estimated total amount of digoxin in the body[62]. In the absence of renal function, the half-life of digoxin is prolonged to 4.4 days[63]; the daily drug losses will then by approximately 14%, rather than the 35% seen with normal renal function, and the daily digoxin dose must be reduced by over one-half (i.e., from 35% to 14%).

The utility of the half-life constant extends to determination of proper dosing intervals. Since the level of the drug in the blood declines by 50% over the time course of a single half-life period, the degree of variation in blood level can be controlled by decreasing or increasing the dosing interval. If the physician wishes to avoid blood level fluctuations of greater than 50%, he must give the drug at intervals not greater than the drug's half-life. If the

50% variation is too great, he must give the drug more frequently. These points have considerable practical significance as, for example, in the case of procaine amide whose elimination half-life is approximately three hours, and whose therapeutic blood level range is approximately 4-8 μg/ml; a dose interval greater than a single half-life will result in either periodic toxicity or subtherapeutic blood levels. Similar analyses may be applied to all the anti-arrhythmic drugs presently under consideration. The mathematical foundation for these concepts has been well described[63,64] and may be found in standard texts[65].

4. *Volume of distribution*[66,67]

Although this is an artificial concept, it has useful clinical implications. The concept relates the concentration of a drug in the blood to the total amount of drug in the body at any given time:

Volume of Distribution (Vd) = total drug in body ÷ blood level

If the blood level of a drug is quite low at a time when a large amount of drug is known to be in the body, the volume of distribution may be many times the actual volume of the body, implying wide distribution and avid tissue uptake of the drug. In this situation, blood levels become less precise as guides to the tissue concentration at the active site. Conversely, a small value for the volume of distribution implies that the drug remains mainly in the circulating blood with little tissue distribution.

Specific Antiarrhythmic Drugs

1. Quinidine

Quinidine has many actions in common with quinine, including anti-pyretic, antimalarial, and oxytocic effects. It has distinct parasympatholytic properties[68], similar to, but less pronounced than those of atropine. Parenteral administration of quinidine regularly produces peripheral vasodilatation, a decrease in peripheral resistence, and a fall in arterial pressure[69].

In addition to the electrophysiologic effects of quinidine reviewed above, the drug exerts a depressant effect on myocardial contractility[70], although it is generally believed to be minimal. Nonetheless, in the presence of previously abnormal myocardial function, this effect may become significant even at blood levels below the usual toxic range.

Clinical pharmacology. Quinidine is rapidly and virtually completely absorbed from the stomach. After entry into the central compartment, the drug is approximately 80% bound by plasma proteins in the albumin fraction[71]. It is rapidly distributed to the tissues (peripheral compartment) where, except in the brain, uptake is rapid, resulting in a high volume of distribution[72,73].

After tissue distribution, quinidine undergoes extensive biotransformation, primarily in the liver. The major degradation products are hydroxylated derivatives[74,75] which have less cardiac activity than the parent com-

TABLE II

CLINICAL PHARMACOLOGY OF ANTIARRHYTHMIC DRUGS

Drug	Oral Absorption	T/2	V_d	Route of Elimination	Serum Protein Binding	Therapeutic Levels in Plasma	Suggested Dosage Regimens
Quinidine	95-100%	3-4 hr	High	Liver	80%	2-8 μg/ml	IV: Not recommended PO: 200-400 mg q4h (quinidine sulfate) 325-650 mg q8-12h (quinidine gluconate)
Procaine Amide	75-95%	3 hr	High	Kidney (60%) Liver (40%)	15%	4-8 μg/ml	IV: 25-50 mg/min, to total of 12 mg/kg, as loading dose 6 mg/kg q3hr as maintenance PO: 250-500 mg q3h
Lidocaine	< 50%	Alpha: 8-10′ Beta: 108′	High	Liver	60-70%	1.5-6 μg/ml	IM: 200-250 mg IV: 50-100 mg as loading dose at 25-50 mg/min; 1-4 mg/min as maintenance
Propranolol	Probably complete; active hepatic extraction from portal blood	IV: 2.5 hr PO: 3-6 hr (depending upon duration of Rx)	High	Liver	90-95%	Varies: Probably > 30 ng/ml	IV: 1-2 mg/min PO: Varies (above 30 mg/day)
DPH	Varies (entero-hepatic recycling)	20 hr	High (zero-order kinetics)	Liver	93%	10-20 μg/ml	IV: 1000 mg as loading dose at 100 mg/5 min PO: 1000 mg as loading dose with 300 mg/d maintenance
Verapamil (data from dog studies)	?	IV: 40 min	? High	Liver	?	50-300 ng/ml	?

pound[72]. It is of some interest that quinidine has been shown to inhibit the hepatic microsomal metabolism of pentobarbital[76] and perhaps propranolol[77], thereby revealing a potential for drug interaction which has not been well studied in human subjects.

The half-life of orally administered quinidine sulfate in normal subjects is about three to four hours. Peak levels in blood occur within one to two hours following oral ingestion[78], and blood concentrations are higher if the drug is given in the fasting state[79].

There is considerable evidence that quinidine blood levels correlate meaningfully with its cardiac effects[72,80,84]. Conversion of atrial fibrillation will occur in most patients likely to respond to the drug at blood levels less than $8\,\mu g/ml$, the average conversion level being $5.9\,\mu g/ml$ in the study by Socolow and Edgar[84]. The therapeutic range of blood levels is generally held to be 2-8 $\mu g/ml$[85], with toxic effects occurring at higher levels. Toxicity however, may occur in patients with drug levels well within the therapeutic range[86]. The primary usefulness of quinidine blood levels will be (1) to show that a patient does, in fact, have sufficient drug in the central compartment to produce an effect upon the heart, and (2) to discourage dose increases in patients with blood levels at the upper portion of the therapeutic range.

Both quinidine and its metabolites are excreted into the urine and it has been reported that impairment in renal function decreases quinidine excretion and causes higher serum drug levels[57,87]. However, this contention was recently challenged by Kessler et al[88] who found similar ranges of half-life values in a group of azotemic patients as in the normal controls.

The half-life of only 3-4 hours for quinidine sulfate necessitates frequent daily dosing to avoid blood levels greater than $6\text{-}8\,\mu g/ml$, which may be toxic, or less than $2\,\mu g/ml$ which may be subtherapeutic. Six hourly dosing schedule used by most physicians may thus be expected to result in either subtherapeutic or toxic drug levels or both.

An alternate approach has involved the development of quinidine preparations with a more prolonged duration of action than the monosulfate salt. The gluconate salt gives peak blood levels on an average of five hours after a dose, and effective blood levels in the therapeutic range are present up to 10 hours after dosing. The use of quinidine gluconate, therefore, allows drug administration two or three times daily, while maintaining therapeutic levels.

The parenteral use of quinidine has been discouraged by most authors, because of hypotension and depressed myocardial contractility[78].

Toxicity. The toxic reactions to quinidine fall into three categories: (1) hypersensitivity reactions, including hematologic abnormalities (leukopenia, anemia, and thrombocytopenia), skin rash, and anaphylaxis[72]; (2) general toxic reactions, including gastrointestinal disturbances, abnormalities of central nervous system function such as tinnitus and confusion (cinchonism), drug fever[89] and very rarely—hepatotoxicity[90,91]; (3) cardiovascular toxicity, manifested by hypotension and/or various arrhythmias, including atrioventricular and intraventricular conduction block and ventricular arrhythmias and fibrillation. Because of the marked depression in conduction induced by the drug, it should be used with great caution in patients with pre-existing conduction abnormalities such as AV or bundle branch block.

2. *Procaine Amide*

As indicated above, the electrophysiologic effects of procaine amide are similar to those discussed earlier for quinidine. In addition, procaine amide, like quinidine, depresses myocardial contractility and decreases peripheral vascular resistance[92,93].

Clinical pharmacology. Absorption of procaine amide after oral doses may be quite variable, contrary to previously held opinion. In normal fasting subjects, this drug is retained in the stomach for 15-30 minutes. It is then from 75-95% absorbed within about one hour[94]. In patients with an acute myocardial infarction, however, considerable variation in the amount and rate of absorption has been observed with some subjects absorbing less than 50% of a given dose and having delays in peak blood levels for five hours. These findings prompted Koch-Weser to suggest that initial parenteral administration was preferable to oral dosing in all patients[94,95].

After intramuscular administration, absorption of procaine amide is complete. The drug is in the blood within two minutes and peak levels are achieved within 30 minutes[95,96]. However, distribution of the drug may be incomplete during rapid absorption from an injection site[96] and therefore intravenous dosing is preferable in patients requiring parenteral therapy.

After entry into the central compartment, procaine amide is about 15% bound to plasma proteins. As with quinidine, procaine amide has a high volume of distribution (above 150L) and is rapidly distributed to the tissues (peripheral compartment); the highest tissue concentrations are found in heart, liver and kidney and are four to five times the drug's concentration in plasma[97].

The elimination of procaine amide from the blood follows first-order kinetics at all concentration ranges studied and the half-life of elimination averages three hours in normal subjects[95,98,99]. In patients with normal renal function, more than half of the drug is excreted unchanged into the urine[94,95], the excretion rate being directly related to creatinine clearance[98]. Alterations in urinary pH can affect procaine amide elimination and the excretion rate increases when the urine is acid[98]. In addition, procaine amide is metabolized by the hepatic enzyme N-acetyltransferase producing N-acetyl-procaineamide which has recently been shown to have only slightly less antiarrhythmic potency than that of the parent compound[100]. As might be anticipated, the elimination rate is slowed in patients having primary renal disease, diminished renal blood flow due to congestive heart failure, or hepatic dysfunction[98]. A drug half-life of eleven hours has been reported in patients with end-stage renal insufficiency[101] and the drug is readily dialyzable[101].

Koch-Weser has coordinated a series of studies[94,95,96,102,103] which have established a strong correlation between the serum concentration of procaine amide and its therapeutic and toxic effects. The generally effective therapeutic range for procaine amide is 4-8 μg/ml, with an occasional patient requiring higher levels for effect. These findings were confirmed by Gey et al[104].

In addition, plasma levels above 12 μg/ml were almost never effective if lower levels were not[108]. Thus, there appears to be a clearer dividing line between therapeutic and toxic effects with procaine amide than with quinidine.

Since the half-life of procaine amide in patients with normal renal function is approximately three hours, three hour dosing intervals are required if fluctuations of plasma levels of greater than 50% are to be prevented. Greater degrees of plasma level variation will assure either subtherapeutic or toxic levels during some period in the dose interval. For this reason, six hourly dose intervals are inappropriate for effective therapy[95,102]. Sustained released preparations of procaine amide in use in Europe produce therapeutic blood levels when administered every eight hours[81].

Procaine amide can be safely administered intravenously if given no more rapidly than 25-50 mg/min, with a total loading dose of 12 mg/kg and maintenance therapy of 5 mg/kg every three hours[78,102]; or 100 mg intravenously over a two-minute period, repeated every five minutes until abolition of the arrhythmia, the development of toxicity (see below), or a total dose of 1000 mg[105].

Toxicity. Toxicity from procaine amide is well correlated to blood levels over 8 μg/ml. Cardiac toxicity is usually the result of conduction slowing producing AV and intraventricular conduction blocks. However, the drug has been safely used in patients with intraventricular conduction disturbances[106]. The non-cardiac manifestations of toxicity include various gastrointestinal problems, central nervous system effects (including weakness, depression, hallucination, and abnormalities in gustatory sensation), and hematologic abnormalities including agranulocytosis and hypersensitivity reactions.

In chronic use, procaine amide may induce a clinical syndrome resembling systemic lupus erythematosus, including the presence of LE cells and antinuclear antibody[107-110], but excluding renal involvement[108] and lowered serum complement[109]. The occurrence of polyarthralgias, myalgias, fever, and serositis is preceded by the development of antinuclear antibody titers and appears to be independent of the dose of procaine amide, the duration of therapy, or the age of the patient[110]. In a prospective study, approximately 50% of patients who had received procaine amide for six months developed antinuclear antibody[111], although the incidence of patients with clinical symptoms was lower. Both the symptoms and the presence of antinuclear antibodies usually regress after the drug is discontinued[108].

3. *Lidocaine*

Clinical pharmacology. The oral administration of lidocaine has not proved practical, because doses which produce therapeutic blood levels also produce symptoms of central nervous system toxicity[112,113]. Since less than half of an oral dose of lidocaine reaches the systemic circulation, it appears likely that the drug is rapidly metabolized on the first pass through the liver, with accumulated metabolites producing the toxic manifestations[114-116].

The intramuscular administration of 200-250 mg lidocaine results in therapeutic blood concentrations within 15 minutes which persist for an hour or more[113,117,118]. Absorption from the site of injection is proportional to blood flow through the site. Therefore, injection into the deltoid musculature produces higher plasma levels than injection into the thigh or buttock[119]. The concentration of injected solution also affects absorption rate, and effective blood levels are achieved more slowly when the solutions are hypertonic[119]. Because therapeutic blood levels of lidocaine can be achieved by intramuscular injection, this mode of therapy has been proposed as a prophylactic measure for patients in the pre-hospital phase of acute myocardial infarction[120,121].

When lidocaine is given intravenously, its disposition follows the first-order kinetics and can be readily described by the two-compartment model[122,123]. After a single intravenous dose, blood levels decline rapidly during the initial, or alpha phase of distribution, with a half-life of 8-10 minutes. This correlates well with the clinical observations that the antiarrhythmic effect of a bolus injection lasts for 15-20 minutes[124]. The second, or beta phase of blood level decline represents elimination from the body and has a half-life of approximately 108 minutes[122]. The elimination half-life describes the disposition kinetics during constant intravenous infusion. Since approximately three to four half-lives are necessary to achieve 90 percent of steady-state blood levels, lidocaine given by constant intravenous infusion without a bolus, or priming, dose will require over five hours to reach the desired, or equilibrium blood level[125]. For this reason, lidocaine should be administered as a bolus dose of 1-1.5 mg/kg followed by a constant infusion of 1-4 mg/min for maintenance of the initial therapeutic blood level.

Lidocaine is 60-70 percent bound to plasma proteins and is avidly taken up by heart, kidney, and brain. At steady-state, only six percent of the total quantity of lidocaine in the body can be found in the central compartment[124]. As anticipated, the volume of distribution is high, averaging about 100 L during equilibrium and 40 L during the initial distribution decline phase[122,124]. Since the required bolus dose may be calculated as the product of the volume of distribution times the desired initial blood level, a therapeutic concentration of 2μg/ml requires a bolus dose of approximately 80-100 mg. The proper infusion rate into the central compartment is determined by the total body elimination rate constant, which in turn is related to the beta phase half-life, the volume of distribution at steady-state, and the desired blood level. To maintain a concentration of 2μg/ml (after bolus dosing), therefore, an infusion rate of 1-2 mg/min is required[126]. Thus, the empirically determined bolus dose and infusion rate appears to be pharmacokinetically appropriate.

Elimination of lidocaine from the body is primarily accomplished by hepatic metabolism[127-129], with only about ten percent of the drug removed by renal excretion[130]. The rate of removal of lidocaine by the liver is rapid and is a function of total liver blood flow[131]. In patients with circulatory depression or with intrinsic liver disease, hepatic blood flow is reduced; lidocaine clearance and rate of elimination are thereby diminished, and drug accumulation to toxic levels may occur[56]. In such patients, the bolus dose and infusion rate should be reduced. Furthermore, the concurrent administration of drugs such as propranolol which decrease liver blood flow will decrease the rate of lidocaine elimination[132]. It is clear that altered patterns of blood flow may affect lidocaine clearance from the body[133,134]. Many patients who require lidocaine therapy may have disturbances in normal hemodynamic parameters resulting in hepatic congestion or decreased hepatic blood flow and may be receiving other cardioactive drugs. For this reason, the kinetics of lidocaine elimination, as determined in normal subjects, must be viewed only as useful guides in fashioning a therapeutic program.

Under steady-state conditions, blood concentrations of lidocaine correlate well with both therapeutic efficacy and the development of toxicity. The usual range of blood levels effective against arrhythmias is $1.5-6\mu g/ml$, with toxicity occurring at higher blood levels. Occasionally, lidocaine toxicity may occur at lower drug concentrations, possibly due to the accumulation of toxic degradation products[116].

Toxicity. Lidocaine's popularity may be attributed not only to its clinical efficacy[135-137], but also to its lack of significant cardiac toxicity[138-140]. The most common manifestation of toxicity from lidocaine is disturbed central nervous system function. Findings range from mild symptoms, including dizziness, paresthesias, alterations of mood, confusion, speech disturbances, and fasciculations, to grand mal seizures[124,141].

In patients with pre-existing impairment of intramyocardial conduction, lidocaine, even in low doses, may transiently induce more pronounced conduction disturbances including atrioventricular block[45].

4. *Diphenylhydantoin (Phenytoin, DPH)*

Clinical pharmacology. Diphenylhydantoin like bretylium and verapamil, differs from the conventional antiarrhythmic agents considered in this chapter in that its kinetics cannot be adequately described by a first-order model. The clinical use of DPH has been, in the past, largely empiric and only recently have studies begun to adequately explain the complex disposition patterns of this drug.

After intravenous administration, DPH is rather slowly distributed to its various peripheral compartments[142]. For this reason, rapid intravenous administration may produce excessively high blood levels and substantial toxicity. Bigger et al[143] have described an approach to intravenous therapy which appears to produce appropriate drug blood levels and to avoid significant complications. DPH is given in 100 mg increments at five-minute intervals until the desired therapeutic effect is seen, clinical toxicity (i.e., nystagmus, etc.) becomes evident, or a total of 1000 mg has been given. This method was developed after the observation that about 90% of the arrhythmias responsive to DPH were abolished at plasma levels below 18 μg/ml, and that little therapeutic effect could be seen at levels below 10 μg/ml; indeed, in many patients, a critical blood concentration can be shown, below which the arrhythmia will recur[144]. Effective therapy with DPH, therefore, depends upon achieving and maintaining effective blood levels of the drug.

Intramuscular DPH administration, although widely used, is generally an ineffective method to rapidly achieve desirable blood levels, since the drug concentrations produced are erratic and low[145]. The intramuscular route, however, offers the advantages of less frequent administration, greater convenience, and increased safety, when compared to intravenous use. In a recent study, Kostenbauder et al[146] showed that absorption of DPH from an injection site was initially rapid (22% of the dose absorbed during the first 30 minutes) but then became very slow (only 50% of the total dose absorbed during the first 24 hours). Up to five days were required for complete drug absorption from the injection site, leading to the conclusion that DPH precipitates in tissues after intramuscular injection and requires redissolution for continuing absorption.

With oral DPH administration, absorption occurs only after gastric emptying into the small bowel, and peak plasma levels are not usually achieved for four to six hours[147]. Once the drug appears in the blood, levels are sustained for several hours. There is inferential evidence suggesting that enterohepatic cycling may be responsible for continuing drug absorption. This factor complicates kinetic analysis after oral drug use[147,148]. Because of the sustained blood levels, a single daily dose of DPH has been shown sufficient to maintain effective concentrations during chronic therapy[149].

The half-life of DPH varies with the drug blood levels produced. Most kinetic studies report a half-life of 18-20 hours, provided levels above 10 μg/ml are not achieved[146,150]. When therapeutic levels are produced, i.e., 10-20 μg/ml, half-life statements become less meaningful. DPH is transformed by hepatic microsomal metabolism into the parahydroxylated derivative, and this enzymatic process appears to become saturated at drug blood concentrations exceeding 10 μg/ml[151]. Wheras other antiarrhythmic drugs disappear at a rate proportional to their concentration in the body (first-order kinetics), DPH elimination—when blood levels are above 10 g/ml—occurs at a constant rate, independent of blood levels (zero-order kinetics). Therefore, at high concentrations, DPH blood levels decline more slowly than at concentrations below 10 μg/ml.

To further complicate the kinetic picture, individuals vary markedly in their intrinsic ability to metabolize DPH. In the absence of overt hepatic dysfunction, this seems to be genetically determined and correlates well with an individual's ability to metabolize isoniazid[152]. In addition to the innate variability in metabolic capacity, a number of other drugs may effect the elimination rate for DPH. When hepatic microsomal enzyme activity is increased by inducing agents, such as phenobarbital, elimination of DPH occurs at a faster rate, and clinical effects may be diminished[153]. Other drugs, such as isoniazid, appear to decrease the metabolism of DPH when administered concurrently[154].

When one considers the many factors affecting the disposition kinetics of DPH, including the zero-order elimination pattern, enterohepatic recycling, genetic variation in enzymatic capacity, and the potential for interaction with other drugs, it becomes apparent that prediction of the DPH blood levels is unreliable. Therefore, blood level monitoring is essential to avoid toxicity, and to assure maintenance of blood levels in the desired range.

Toxicity. Toxicity resulting from the use of DPH in acute antiarrhythmic therapy has been reported to include local venous thrombosis and ventricular fibrillation[155]. Although a negative inotropic effect regularly occurs after rapid intravenous administration[156,157], hypotension may be seen even with slow infusions[158]. Some of these effects seen may be due to the diluent used in the commercial preparation[156]. Although the incidence of AV block following DPH use is low, this phenomenon may occur especially during treatment of patients with supraventricular tachyarrhythmias[159,160]. Damato has attributed this effect to the enhanced entry of stimuli into the atrio-ventricular junction with decremental conduction[161].

During chronic administration, non-cardiac toxicity occurs. The central nervous system effects include: nystagmus, diplopia, blurring of vision, dysarthria, and ataxia. Other toxic reactions include the drug interactions noted above, skin rash, gingival hyperplasia, and induction of folic acid deficiency[162].

5. Verapamil

Clinical pharmacology. Verapamil was first introduced as a coronary vasodilator in 1962[163]. Since 1966, it has been used outside of the United States as an antiarrhythmic agent and has been very effective in the treatment of the reentrant AV junctional tachyarrhythmias both with and without WPW[164-167]. However, little information is available concerning its clinical pharmacology.

A small series of studies on experimental animals have suggested that verapamil is well absorbed from the upper gastrointestinal tract, metabolized in the liver, and its major degradation products excreted in the bile and urine[168,169]. In the dog, verapamil binds "significantly" to serum proteins and disappears with a half-life of 70 minutes[169]. The half-life of the metabolites of verapamil may be as long as 10 hours[169].

Recent studies in our laboratory[170] have utilized a fluorometric assay for verapamil in plasmas and tissues which is capable of reliably measuring drug concentrations as low as 10 ng/ml. After intravenous administration in dogs, fluorescent verapamil disappears with a half-life of approximately 45 minutes and a volume of distribution of about 90 liters, indicating a high degree of tissue binding. Its elimination is almost entirely by hepatic metabolism and may be complex[171].

Clinical observations in human subjects given verapamil intravenously have demonstrated an onset of effect within one to two minutes, and maximal activity 10-15 minutes after injection. Drug effects may be detected as long as six hours later. After oral administration, clinical effect can be seen within 30 minutes, and last up to six hours[172].

The ability of verapamil to antagonize the calcium inward current not only causes slowing of AV conduction and slowing of the sinus rate, but also blocks excitation-contraction coupling[173] and induces a negative inotropic effect[174,175].

Toxicity. Toxicity resulting from verapamil can be the result of its effects on sinus rate, AV conduction, and/or contractility. Transient asystole[176], bradycardia[167], and hypotension[177] have occurred. The administration of verapamil after prior treatment with beta-adrenergic blockers appears to be especially hazardous[165], resulting in profound depression of ventricular function. Verapamil may also be dangerous to administer to patients with the "sick-sinus syndrome"[165,178].

Our current studies suggest that the effects of verapamil on the various parameters of electrophysiologic and contractile activity may be reflected in and predicted by drug plasma levels[171]. This observation implies that blood level monitoring may be useful in order to avoid the depression of cardiac contractility seen at higher blood levels. Such results, if confirmed in human studies, would considerably expand the potential usefulness of verapamil as an antiarrhythmic drug.

6. *Propranolol*

Although many beta receptor blocking agents other than propranolol have been developed and studied within the last 10 years[179,180], propranolol remains the only beta-adrenergic blocker available for clinical use in the United States.

Clinical pharmacology. After intravenous administration, the elimination of propranolol follows first-order kinetics with a half-life of 2-3 hours[181-183]. It is 90-95% bound to plasma proteins[184] and is widely distributed in tissues with an apparent volume of distribution of 150-250 L[181,182]. Propranolol is rapidly removed from the systemic circulation by an hepatic uptake process which, as with lidocaine, is a function of hepatic blood flow[185]. If the beta blocking effect of propranolol reduces cardiac output, liver blood flow will be lowered and the elimination of the drug correspondingly decreased[186]. The elimination half-life is not significantly altered in severe renal failure[187,188].

After oral administration the kinetics of propranolol become more complex. Although absorption from the gut is virtually complete, hepatic extraction removes a large fraction of the drug from the portal venous blood, (pre-systemic extraction), resulting in low bio-availability and blood concentration after small oral doses[189]. With single oral doses over 30 mg, or with continuing oral administration, the removal process becomes saturated and hepatic extraction falls[190]. During continued oral administration on a six hourly dose regimen, the half-life ranges from three to six hours, the extraction process remains saturated, and drug accumulation continues until a steady-state is reached within about 36-48 hours. The degree of pre-systemic extraction varies widely between patients, accounting for a 20 fold variation in blood concentrations of the drug in individuals receiving the same oral dose (see Figure 5). It is therefore impossible to predict accurately the blood

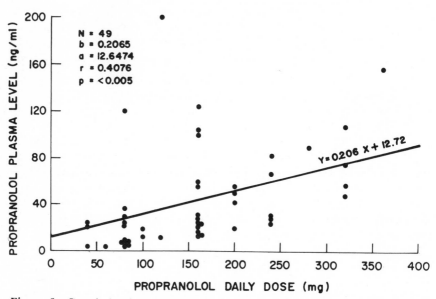

CORRELATION BETWEEN ORAL PROPRANOLOL DOSE AND PLASMA LEVEL (4-6 HRS. p̄ DOSE)

Figure 5 Correlation between oral propranolol dose and plasma level 4-6 hours later. Propranolol levels were drawn at the end of the dosing interval in 49 patients who had received the indicated dose for a minimum of 2 weeks.

levels of propranolol in a given individual on any chronic oral dose regimen. In addition, an active metabolite, 4-hydroxy propranolol, with active beta blocking properties, is produced after initial oral dosing[191]. This metabolite is not detectable after five days of oral therapy[192] and is not observed after intravenous drug use. The relationship between propranolol blood concentrations and effects is affected by the degree of resting sympathetic tone. When parameters of beta adrenergic activity are examined in a particular subject, such as the chronotropic response to infused isoproterenol or treadmill exercise, there is a clear correlation between the plasma propranolol concentration and the effects measured[192,193]. There is, however, considerable variation between individuals in the blood levels required to produce a given effect[194]. Nies and Shand have suggested that differences in drug binding to plasma proteins might explain the variability[181], since a change of only five percent in the amount of bound drug will double the quantity of free drug available to receptor sites. For the above reasons, a physiologic evaluation of the extent of beta blockade induced by propranolol therapy, such as blockade of exercise tachycardia, is of greater clinical usefulness than blood level studies. It is possible that, in the future, a more consistent correlation between blood concentration and effect will be described.

Toxicity. A report from the Boston Collaborative Drug Surveillance Program revealed a 9.3% incidence of adverse reactions to propranolol in hospitalized patients[195]. Of these, one-third were considered serious. Minor reactions included asymptomatic bradycardia, central nervous system disturbances (drowsiness, fatigue, dizziness, blurring of vision), hypotension, and second degree block. Serious problems included complete AV block, congestive heart failure, and bradycardia with angina pectoris. This high incidence may be due in large part to inadequate patient evaluation prior to propranolol therapy. It should also be remembered that the effects of propranolol on the SA node and AV junction will be additive to the vagal enhancement induced by digitalis. This may result in SA and/or AV block (See Chapter 4; Figure 9).

Absolute contraindications to propranolol include poorly compensated or overt left ventricular failure due to impaired ventricular function, bronchospastic disorders, and the higher degrees of heart block. Most complications during propranolol administration are not dose-related but occur very early after treatment has been initiated. If a patient tolerates small doses without difficulty, dosage can usually be increased without fear of subsequent dramatic toxicity.

7. Bretylium

Clinical pharmacology. Bretylium tosylate is a quarternary ammonium compound which accululates selectively in sympathetic ganglia and post-ganglionic nerves and results in inhibition of neurotransmitter release, similar to the effects of guanethidine[196,197]. Hemodynamic studies in patients given bretylium revealed a dose related depression of blood pressure, an increase in resting cardiac output, and blockade of the cold pressor response[199].

Bretylium is poorly absorbed after oral administration, but well absorbed after intramuscular administration, with 70-80% of the drug being excreted in the urine during the first 24 hours[200]. Since the drug is removed by renal filtration, the rate of excretion is decreased in patients with impaired renal function[199,200]. The disposition kinetics have been found to be complex and do not follow a first-order pattern, suggesting a multicompartmental system[201]. A similar model has recently been described for guanethidine, which is also selectively accumulated in adrenergic tissues[202].

Parenteral bretylium has been shown to increase myocardial contractility[203]. In low doses this effect requires the presence of intact sympathetic nerve endings, indicating that the drug acts by causing release of norepinephrine. In high doses, the increased contractility appears to be a direct effect, probably through stimulation of beta adrenergic receptors[204,205].

Unlike guanethidine, bretylium inhibits intraneuronal monoamine oxidase[206]. This may account for the absence of myocardial depression even with chronic use of bretylium[207].

Toxicity. No distinct toxicity results from the drug other than that predictable from its known pharmacologic activity. Because of its sympatholytic activity, which reduces peripheral vascular resistance, bretylium may produce disturbing hypotension in patients treated for arrhythmias, especially those with acute myocardial infarction[208].

Clinical Aspects of Antiarrhythmic Therapy

The specific clinical indications for the antiarrhythmic drugs are discussed elsewhere in this book. However, a few general remarks outlining our thoughts about the approach to arrhythmia management may be pertinent.

1. The underlying cause(s) of the arrhythmia should be sought and if possible, treated. Examples of readily remediable underlying causes include: hypoxia, acidosis, abnormalities in serum potassium, digitalis excess, quinidine or procaine amide toxicity, congestive heart failure, thyrotoxicosis, and bradycardia such as associated with sinus node disease or AV block. Underlying causes which may be more difficult to remedy include: myocardial or valvular disease, myocardial ischemia or infarction, ventricular aneurysm, and the various AV junctional bypass tracts.

2. Supraventricular tachycardias usually respond to drugs which increase the effects of acetylcholine either by stimulating vagal discharge, slowing the metabolism of acetylcholine, or removing the opposing effects of sympathetic stimulation. Moreover, the long term ambulatory use of drugs which accomplish these aims, such as digitalis and propranolol, is often effective in preventing the recurrence of these tachycardias[209] or in slowing the ventricular response to them. However, in certain situations, the additional use of direct acting drugs is useful. For example, quinidine may be used to prevent the atrial premature beats which usually initiate repetitive supraventricular tachycardias. Verapamil, although not currently available for use in the United States, has also proved to be extremely effective in the treatment of repetitive supraventricular tachycardias most likely by virtue of its direct effect on the slow channel responses which characterize the AV junction (See Chapter 4). Quinidine or procaine amide may also be used to prolong the refractory period and slow conduction in AV junctional bypass pathways[210] in patients with WPW syndrome. Furthermore, quinidine and procaine amide are effective in converting atrial fibrillation and flutter to sinus rhythm, whereas the vagally mediated drugs are more useful in slowing the ventricular response to these arrhythmias by increasing AV block.

3. For reasons which are not well understood, lidocaine and DPH are usually not effective in the management of supraventricular arrhythmias[4,5]. This limited usefulness may reflect: (a) the critical role of the AV junction in repetitive supraventricular tachycardias and the inability of lidocaine and DPH to influence significantly AV conduction due to their lack of effect on

"slow channel" responses and (b) the less marked rate dependent effect of lidocaine and DPH than of quinidine on action potential upstroke in fibers with normal resting potentials. This may explain why lidocaine and DPH are not useful in converting atrial fibrillation and flutter to normal sinus rhythm whereas quinidine may be.

4. Each of the direct acting drugs may be effective in the treatment of ventricular arrhythmias in a variety of situations. However, none will be successful in all situations. This is probably due to an inability to combine our understanding of the electrophysiologic effects of the drug with our understanding of factors responsible for the arrhythmia. It is possible that this tailoring of antiarrhythmic drug thereapy may become possible as sophisticated electrophysiological studies are employed more often to define the pathophysiology of the arrhythmia and the effects of the drugs. However, at the present time, such studies are limited to only a few centers. This fact coupled with the urgency with which it is often necessary to treat ventricular tachyarrhythmias necessitates an empirical approach to the use of the drugs, once causative or contributing factors have been identified and treated. The use of lidocaine as the initial drug in the treatment of serious ventricular tachyarrhythmias is recommended because of its rapid onset, its lack of cardiac toxicity, and its proven efficacy. However, the need to achieve effective plasma concentrations must be kept in mind. If lidocaine therapy is unsuccessful, it is reasonable to add other drugs. Indeed, the difference in the electrophysiologic properties of the various drugs provide a rationale for their combined use. Frequently, such utilization may prove beneficial when each drug alone has proved ineffective.

5. Unfortunately, the ability of the currently available direct acting drugs to provide long term ambulatory suppression of ventricular arrhythmias has been disappointing[211]. The possible exceptions are the exercise related tachyarrhythmias which may be suppressed by propranolol[49]. In this situation, propranolol may act in two ways: (a) to block the effects of beta sympathetic stimulation induced by exercise or (b) to lessen exercise induced myocardial ischemia. In both situations, propranolol is more likely to act by preventing the cause rather than by exerting a direct electrophysiologic change in the cardiac fibers.

CONCLUSION

In this chapter we have reviewed the electropharmacology and pharmacokinetics of the more frequently used antiarrhythmic drugs. However, we have not dealt in depth with specific treatment programs. The use of new drugs currently under investigation in the United States and other countries, and the development of other drugs would render such programs obsolete in the near future. Moreover, the status of bretylium, which may have the unique ability to interrupt ventricular fibrillation and to achieve the long term suppression of refractory ventricular arrhythmias[212], and of verapamil in arrhythmias other than supraventricular tachycardia is not clear. Furthermore, the increased use of ventricular pacing and of cardiac surgery in the treatment of refractory ventricular tachyarrhythmias may lead to significant modifications in our approach to this problem. However, regardless of the methods or drugs in vogue at any given time, the successful management of cardiac arrhythmias will require an understanding of the pathogenesis of the arrhythmias, the mode(s) of action of the therapy employed, and the clinical pharmacology of the drugs administered.

References

1. Gettes, L.S.: The electrophysiologic effects of antiarrhythmic drugs. *Am. J. Cardiol.*, **28**: 526, 1971.
2. Rosen, M.R., Hoffman, B.F., and Wit, A.L.: Electrophysiology and pharmacology. V. VI. VII. VIII. IX. X. *Am. Heart J.*, **89**: 526, 665, 804, 808; **90**: 117, 265, 397, 521, 665, 1975.
3. Hoffman, B.F., Rosen, M.R., and Wit, A.L.: Electrophysiology and pharmacology of cardiac arrhythmias. VII. Cardiac effects of quinidine and procaine amide. B. *Am. Heart J.* **90**: 117, 1975.
4. Rosen, M.R., Hoffman, B.F., and Wit, A.L.: Electrophysiology and pharmacology of cardiac arrhythmias. V. Cardiac antiarrhythmic effects of lidocaine. *Am. Heart J.*, **89**: 526, 1975.
5. Wit, A.L., Rosen, M.R., and Hoffman, B.F.: Electrophysiology and pharmacology of cardiac arrhythmias. VIII. Cardiac effects of diphenylhydantoin. B. *Am. Heart J.*, **90**: 397, 1975.
6. Aravindakshen, V. and Gettes, L.S.: Effect of bretylium tosylate and lidocaine in experimentally induced ventricular fibrillation in isolated rabbit hearts. *Cardiovasc. Res.*, **9**: 19, 1975.
7. Aravindakshan, V. and Gettes, L.S.: Unpublished Observation.
8. Ross, J.C. and Dunning, A.J.: Effect of lidocaine on impulse formation and conduction defects in man. *Am. Heart J.*, **89**: 686, 1975.
9. Imanishi, S. and Surawicz, B.: Lidocaine-resistant automaticity in depolarized guinea pig ventricular myocardium. *Circulation*, **50** Suppl. III: 145, 1974.
10. Mandel, W.J. and Bigger, J.T.: Electrophysiologic effects of lidocaine on isolated canine and rabbit atrial tissue. *J. Pharmacol. Exp. Ther.*, **178**: 81, 1971.
11. Rosen, M.R., Wit, A.L., and Hoffman, B.F.: Electrophysiology and pharmacology of cardiac arrhythmias. VI. Cardiac effects of verapamil. *Am. Heart J.*, **89**: 665, 1975.
12. Cranefield, P.F. *The Conduction of the Cardiac Impulse: The Slow Response and Cardiac Arrhythmias.* Futura Publishing Company, New York, 1975.
13. Kohlhardt, M., Bauer, B., Krausse, H., and Fleckenstein, A.: New selective inhibitors of the transmembrane Ca conductivity in mammalian myocardial fibres. *Experientia*, **15**: 288, 1972.
14. Cranefield, P.F., Aronson, R.S., and Wit, A.L.: Effect of verapamil on the normal action potential and on a calcium dependent slow response of canine cardiac Purkinje fibers. *Circ. Res.*, **34**: 204, 1974.
15. Zipes, D.P. and Fischer, J.C.: Effects of agents which inhibit the slow channel on sinus node automaticity and atrioventricular conduction in the dog. *Circ. Res.*, **34**: 184, 1974.
16. Ferrier, G.R., Saunders, J.H., and Mendez, C.: A cellular mechanism for the generation of ventricular arrhythmias by acetylstrophanthidin. *Circ. Res.*, **32**: 600, 1973.
17. Gettes, L.S. and Reuter, H.: Slow recovery from inactivation of inward currents in mammalian myocardial fibres. *J. Physiol.*, **240**: 703, 1974.

18. Surawicz, B. and Lasseter, K.C.: Effect of drugs on the electrocardiogram. *Prog. Cardiovasc. Dis.*, **13**: 26, 1970.
19. Josephson, M.E., Seides, S.F., Batsford, W.P., Weisfogel, G.M., Akhtar, M., Caracta, A.R., Lau, S.H., and Damato, A.N.: The electrophysiological effects of intramuscular quinidine on the atrioventricular conducting system in man. *Am. Heart J.*, **78**: 55, 1974.
20. Josephson, M.E., Caracta, A.R., Ricciutti, M.A., Lau, S.H., and Damato, A.N.: Electrophysiologic properties of procaine amide in man. *Am. J. Cardiol.*, **33**: 596, 1974.
21. Wallace, A.G., Cline, R.E., Sealy, W.C., Young, W.G., and Troyer, W.C.: Electrophysiologic effect of quinidine: studies using chronically implanted electrode in awake dogs with and without cardiac denervation. *Circ. Res.*, **19**: 960, 1966.
22. Chen, C.M., Gettes, L.S., and Katzung, B.G.: Effect of quinidine and lidocaine on steady-state and recovery kinetics of (dV/dt) max. *Circ. Res.*, **37**: 20, 1975.
23. Johnson, E.A. and McKinnon, M.G.: The differential effect of quinidine and pyrilamine on the myocardial action potential at various rates of stimulation. *J. Pharmacol. Exp. Ther.*, **120**: 460, 1957.
24. Heistracher, P.: Mechanism of action of antifibrillatory drugs. *Naunyn-Schmiedebergs Arch. Pharmak.*, **269**: 199, 1971.
25. Chen, C.M. and Gettes, L.S.: Combined effects of rate, membrane potential and drugs on (dV/dt) max. Submitted to *Circ. Res.*
26. Hope, R.R., Williams, D.O., El-Sherif, N., Lazzara, R., and Scherlag, B.J.: The efficacy of antiarrhythmic agents during acute myocardial ischemia and the role of heart rate. *Circulation*, **50**: 507, 1974.
27. Rosen, M.R., Lau, S.H., Weiss, M.B., and Damato, A.N.: The effect of lidocaine on atrioventricular and intraventricular conduction in man. *Am. J. Cardiol.*, **25**: 1, 1970.
28. Davis, L.D. and Temte, J.V.: Electrophysiological actions of lidocaine on canine ventricular muscle and Purkinje fibers. *Circ. Res.*, **24**: 639, 1969.
29. Bigger, J.T. and Mandel, W.J.: Effect of lidocaine on transmembrane potentials of ventricular muscle and Purkinje fibers. *J. Clin. Invest.*, **49**: 63, 1970.
30. Singh, B.N. and Vaughan Williams, E.M.: Effects of altering potassium concentration on the action of lidocaine and diphenylhydantoin on rabbit atrial and ventricular muscle. *Circ. Res.*, **29**: 286, 1971.
31. Saito, S., Chen, C.M., and Gettes, L.S.: Effect of lidocaine on intraventricular conduction in dog heart at various K level. *Circulation*, **52** Suppl. V: 85, 1975.
32. Kupersmith, J., Antman, E.M., and Hoffman, B.F.: In vivo electrophysiologic effects of lidocaine in canine acute myocardial infarction. *Circ. Res.* In Press.
33. Bigger, J.T. and Mandel, W.J.: Effect of lidocaine on canine Purkinje fibers and at the ventricular muscle Purkinje fiber junction. *J. Pharmacol. Exp. Ther.*, **172**: 239, 1970.
34. Singer, D.H., Lazzara, R., and Hoffman, B.F.: Interrelationship between automaticity and conduction in Purkinje fibers. *Circ. Res.*, **21**: 537, 1967.
35. Chen, C.M. and Gettes, L.S.: Comparison of antiarrhythmic drug effect on the determinants of (dV/dt) max. *Federation Proceedings*, **34** (No. 3): 775, 1975.
36. Jensen, R.A. and Katzung, B.G.: Electrophysiological actions of diphenylhydantoin of rabbit atria. *Circ. Res.*, **26**: 17, 1970.
37. Wald, R.W., Downar, E., and Waxman, M.B.: The effect of antiarrhythmic drugs on unidirectional conduction in Purkinje fibers. *Circulation*, **52** Suppl. II: 84, 1975.
38. Rosen, M.R., Ilvento, J.P., Gelband, H., and Merker, C.: Effects of verapamil on electrophysiologic properties of canine cardiac Purkinje fibers. *J. Pharmacol. Exp. Ther.*, **189**: 414, 1974.

39. Hoffman, B.F., Rosen, M.R., and Wit, A.L.: Electrophysiology and pharamcology of cardiac arrhythmias. VII. Cardiac effects of quinidine and procaine amide. *Am. Heart J.*, **89**: 804, 1975.
40. Saito, S., Chen, C.M., and Gettes, L.S.: Unpublished Observation.
41. Merideth, J., Mendez, C., Mueller, W.J., and moe, G.K.: Electrical excitability of atrioventricular nodal cells. *Circ. Res.*, **23**: 69, 1968.
42. Strauss, H.C. and Bigger, J.T.: Electrophysiological properties of the rabbit sinoatrial perinodal fibers. *Circ. Res.*, **31**: 490, 1972.
43. Lazzara, R., El-Sherif, N., and Scherlag, B.J.: Disorders of cellular electrophysiology produced by ischemia of the canine His bundle. *Circ. Res.*, **36**: 444, 1975.
44. Josephson, M.R., Caracta, A.R., Lau, S.H., and Gallagher, J.J.: Effects of lidocaine on refractory periods in man. *Am. Heart J.*, **84**: 778, 1972.
45. Gupta, P.K., Lichstein, E., and Dhadda, K.D.: Lidocaine induced heart block in patients with bundle branch block. *Am. J. Cardiol.*, **33**: 487, 1974.
46. Bissett, J.K., DeSoyza, N.D., Kane, J.J., and Murphy, M.L.: Improved intraventricular conduction of premature beats after diphenylhydantoin. *Am. J. Cardiol.*, **33**: 493, 1974.
47. Barrett, A.M. and Collum, V.A.: The biological properties of the optical isomers of propranolol and their effects on cardiac arhythmias. *Brit. J. Pharmacol.*, **34**: 43, 1968.
48. Seides, S.F., Josephson, M.E., Batsford, W.P., Weisfogel, G.M., Lau, S.H., and Damato, A.N.: The electrophysiology of propranolol in man. *Am. Heart J.*, **88**: 733, 1974.
49. Gettes, L.S.: Beta adrenergic blocking drugs in the treatment of cardiac arrhythmia. *Cardiovasc. Clinics*, **2**: 212, 1970.
50. Bigger, J.T. and Jaffe, C.C.: The effect of bretylium tosylate on the electrophysiologic properties of ventricular muscle and Purkinje fibers. *Am. J. Cardiol.*, **27**: 82, 1971.
51. Bassett, A.L. and Hoffman, B.F.: Antiarrhythmic drugs: electrophysiological actions. *Ann. Review of Pharmacol.*, **2**: 143, 1971.
52. Bernstein, J.G. and Koch-Weser, J.: Effectiveness of bretylium tosylate against refractory ventricular arrhythmias. *Circulation*, **45**: 1024, 1972.
53. Brodie, B.B. and Mitchell, J.R.: The value of correlating biological effects of drugs with plasma concentrations. In D.S. Davies and B.N.C. Pritchard (Eds.): *Biological Effects of Drugs in Relation to their Plasma Concentrations.* University Park Press, Baltimore, 1973.
54. Koch-Weser, J.: Serum drug concentrations as therapeutic guides. *N. Engl. J. Med.*, **287**: 227, 1972.
55. Prescott, L.F., Roscoe, P., and Forrest, J.A.H.: Plasma concentrations and drug toxicity in man. In D.S. Davies and B.N.C. Pritchard (Eds.): *Biological Effects of Drugs in Relation to their Plasma Concentrations.* University Park Press, Baltimore, 1973.
56. Thompson, P.D., Rowland, M., and Melmon, K.L.: The influence of heart failure, liver disease, and renal failure on the disposition of lidocaine in man. *Am. Heart J.*, **82**: 417, 1971.
57. Bellet, S., Roman, L.R., and Boza, A.: Relation between serum quinidine levels and renal function: studies in normal subjects and patients with congestive failure and renal insufficiency. *Am. J. Cardiol.*, **27**: 368, 1971.
58. Blackwell, B., Patient compliance. *N. Engl. J. Med.*, **289**: 249, 1973.
59. Greenblatt, D.J. and Koch-Weser, J.: Clinical pharmacokinetics. *N. Engl. J. Med.*, **293**: 702, 1975.
60. Tozer, T.N.: Nomogram for modification of dosage regimens in patients with chronic renal function impairment. *J. Pharmocokin. Biopharmaceut.*, **2**: 13, 1974.

61. Riegelman, S., Loo, J.C.K., and Rowland, M.: Shortcomings in pharmaco-kinetic analysis by conceiving the body to exhibit properties of a single compartment. *J. Pharm. Sci.*, **57**: 117, 1968.

62. Jelliffe, R.W.: An improved method of digoxin therapy. *Ann. Intern. Med.*, **69**: 703, 1968.

63. Jelliffe, R.W.: A mathematical analysis of digitalis kinetics in patients with normal and reduced renal function. *Math. Biosci.*, **1**: 305, 1967.

64. Kruger-Thiemer, E.: Formal theory of drug dosage regimens. *J. Theor. Biol.*, **13**: 212, 1966.

65. Melmon, K.L. and Morrelli, K.F. (Eds.): *Clinical Pharmacology: Basic Principles in Therapeutics.* The MacMillan Co., New York, 1972.

66. Riegelman, S., Loo, J.C.K., and Rowland, M.: Concept of a volume of distribution and possible errors in evaluation of this parameter. *J. Pharm. Sci.*, **57**: 128, 1968.

67. Gibaldi, M., Nagashima, R., and Levy, G.: Relationship between drug concentration in plasma or serum and amount of drug in the body. *J. Pharm. Sci.*, **58**: 193, 1969.

68. Hiatt, E., Brown, D., Quinn, G., and McDuffie, K.: The blocking action of the cinchona alkaloids and certain related compounds of the cardio-inhibitory vagus endings of the dog. *J. Pharmacol. Exp. Ther.*, **85**: 55, 1945.

69. Ferrer, M.I., Harvey, R.M., Werko, L., Dresdale, D.T., Cournand, A., and Richards, D.W.: Some effects of quinidine sulfate on the heart and circulation in man. *Am. Heart J.*, **36**: 816, 1948.

70. Angelakos, E.T. and Hastings, E.P.: The influence of quinidine and procaine amide on myocardial contractivity in vivo. *Am. J. Cardiol.*, **5**: 791, 1960.

71. Conn, H.L. and Luchi, R.J.: Some quantitative aspects of the binding of quinidine and related quinoline compounds by human serum albumin. *J. Clin. Invest.*, **40**: 509, 1961.

72. Conn, H.L.: Quinidine as an antiarrhythmic agent. In *Advances in Cardio-pulmonary Diseases*, Vol. 2. Year Book Medical Publishers, Chicago, 1964.

73. Moe, G.K. and Abildskov, J.A.: Antiarrhythmic drugs. In L.S. Goodman and A. Gilman (Eds.): *The Pharmacological Basis of Therapeutics*, 3rd Edition. The MacMillan Company, New York, 1966.

74. Palmer, K.H., Martin, B., Baggett, B., and Wall, M.E.: The metabolic fate of orally-administered quinidine gluconate in humans. *Biochem. Pharmacol.*, **18**: 1845, 1969.

75. Brodie, B.B., Baer, J.E., and Craig, L.C.: Metabolic products of the cinchona alkaloids in human urine. *J. Biol. Chem.*, **188**: 567, 1951.

76. Boulos, B.M., Short, C.R., and Davis, L.E.: Quinine and quinidine inhibition of pentobarbital metabolism. *Biochem. Pharmacol.*, **19**: 723, 1970.

77. McAllister, R.G., Shand, D.G., and Oates, J.A.: The interaction of quinidine and propranolol: metabolic effects. Manuscript in preparation.

78. Sokolow, M. and Perloff, D.B.: The clinical pharmacology and use of quinidine in heart disease. *Prog. Cardiovasc. Dis.*, **3**: 316, 1960.

79. Ditlefsen, E.L.: Concentrations of quinidine in blood following oral, parenteral, and rectal administration. *Acta Med. Scand.*, **146**: 81, 1953.

80. Wegria, R. and Boyle, M.N.: Correlation between the effect of quinidine sulfate on the heart and its concentration in the blood plasma. *Am. J. Med.*, **4**: 373, 1948.

81. Edwards, I.R., Hancock, B.W., and Saynor, R.: Correlation between plasma quinidine and cardiac effect. *Brit. J. Clin. Pharmacol.*, **1**: 455, 1974.

82. Sokolow, M. and Ball, R.E.: Factors influencing conversion of chronic atrial fibrillation with special reference to serum quinidine concentration. *Circulation*, **14**: 568, 1956.

83. Cho, Y.W.: Quantitative correlation of plasma and myocardial quinidine concentrations with biochemical and electrocardiographic changes. *Am. Heart J.*, **85**: 648, 1973.

84. Sokolow, M. and Edgar, A.L.: Blood quinidine concentrations as a guide in the treatment of cardiac arrhythmias. *Circulation*, **1**: 576, 1950.

85. Atkinson, A.J.: Clinical use of blood levels of cardiac drugs. *Mod. Concepts Cardiovasc. Dis.*, **42**: 1, 1973.

86. Selzer, A. and Wray, H.W.: Quinidine syncope: paroxysmal ventricular fibrillation occurring during treatment of chronic atrial arrhythmias. *Circulation*, **30**: 17, 1964.

87. Gibson, T.P., Sawin, L.L., and DiBona, G.F.: Quinidine handling in renal insufficiency. *Clin. Res.*, **20**: 722, 1972.

88. Kessler, K.M., Lowenthal, D.I., Warner, H., Gibson, T., Briggs, W., and Reidenberg, M.M.: Quinidine elimination in patients with congestive heart failure or poor renal function. *N. Engl. J. Med.*, **290**: 706, 1974.

89. Schlutz, M., Zinneman, H.H., and Hall, W.H.: Drug fever caused by quinine and quinidine. *Minn. Med.*, **56**: 668, 1973.

90. Colding, H.: Et tilfoelde af kinidirallergi med feber og leverpavirkning. *Ugeskr. Laeg.*, **131**: 1657, 1969.

91. Deisseroth, A., Morganroth, J., and Winokur, S.: Quinidine induced liver disease. *Ann. Intern. Med.*, **77**: 595, 1972.

92. Zapata, D.J., Cabreva, E., and Mendez, R.: An experimental and clinical study on the effects of procaine amide (Pronestyl) on the heart. *Am. Heart J.* **43**: 854, 1952.

93. Kayden, H.J., Bordie, B.B., and Steele, J.M.: Procaine amide: a review. *Circulation*, **15**: 118, 1957.

94. Koch-Weser, J.: Pharmacokinetics of procaine amide in man. *Ann. N.Y. Acad. Sci.*, **179**: 370, 1971.

95. Koch-Weser, J. and Klein, S.W.: Procaine amide dosage schedules, plasma concentrations, and clinical effects. *JAMA*, **215**: 1454, 1971.

96. Koch-Weser, J.: Antiarrhythmic prophylaxis in ambulatory patients with coronary heart disease. *Arch. Intern. Med.*, **129**: 763, 1972.

97. Mark, L.C., Kayden, H.J., Steele, J.M., et al: The physiologic disposition and cardiac effects of procaine amide. *J. Pharmacol. Exp. Ther.*, **102**: 5, 1951.

98. Weily, H.S. and Genton, E.: Pharmacokinetics of procaine amide. *Arch. Intern. Med.*, **130**: 366, 1972.

99. Dreyfuss, J., Bigger, J.T., Cohen, A.I., and Schreiber, E.C.: Metabolism of procaine amide in rhesus monkey and man. *Clin. Pharmacol. Ther.*, **13**: 366, 1972.

100. Elson, J., Strong, J.M., Lee, W.K., and Atkinson, A.J.: Antiarrhythmic potency of N-acetylprocainamide. *Clin. Pharmacol. Ther.*, **17**: 134, 1975.

101. Gibson, T.P., Lowenthal, D.T., Nelson, H.A., and Briggs, W.A.: Elimination of procaine amide in end-stage renal failure. *Clin. Pharmacol. Ther.*, **17**: 321, 1975.

102. Koch-Weser, J.: Clinical application of the pharmacokinetics of procaine amide. *Cardiovasc. Clin.*, **6**: 63, 1974.

103. Koch-Weser, J., Klein, S.W., Foo-Canto, L.L., Kastor, J.A., and DeSanctis, R.W.: Antiarrhythmic prophylaxis with procaine amide in acute myocardial infarction. *N. Engl. J. Med.*, **281**: 1253, 1969.

104. Gey, G.O., Levy, R.H., Fisher, L., Pettet, G., and Bruce, R.A.: Plasma concentration of procaine amide and prevalence of exertional arrhythmias. *Ann. Intern. Med.*, **80**: 718, 1974.

105. Giardina, E.V., Heissenbuttel, R.H., and Bigger, J.T.: Intermittent intravenous procaine amide to treat ventricular arrhythmias. *Ann. Intern. Med.*, **78**: 183, 1973.

106. Scheinman, M.M., Weiss, A.N., Shafton, E., Benowitz, N., and Rowland, M.: Electrophysiologic effects of procaine amide in patients with intraventricular conduction delay. *Circulation*, **49**: 522, 1974.

107. Ladd, A.T.: Procaine amide induced lupus erythematosus. *N. Engl. J. Med.*, **267**: 1357, 1962.

108. Dubois, E.L.: Procaine amide induction of a systemic lupus erythematosus-like syndrome. *Medicine*, **48**: 217, 1969.

109. Blomgren, S.E., Condemi, J.L., and Vaughan, J.H.: Procaine amide induced lupus erythematosus. *Am. J. Med.*, **52**: 338, 1972.

110. Whittingham, S., Mackay, I.R., Whitworth, H.A., and Sloman, G.: Antinuclear antibody response to procaine amide in man and laboratory animals. *Am. Heart J.*, **84**: 228, 1972.

111. Blomgren, S.E., Condemi, J.L., Bignall, M.C., et al: Antinuclear antibody induced by procaine amide: a prospective study. *N. Eng. J. Med.*, **281**: 64, 1969.

112. Scott, D.B., Jebson, P.J., Godman, M.J., et al: Oral ignocaine. *Lancet*, **1**: 93, 1970.

113. Fehmers, M.C.O. and Dunning, A.J.: Intramuscularly and orally administered lidocaine in the treatment of ventricular arrhythmias in acute myocardial infarction. *Am. J. Cardiol.*, **29**: 514, 1972.

114. Boyes, R.N., Adams, H.J., and Duce, B.R.: Oral absorption and disposition kinetics of lidocaine hydrochloride in dogs. *J. Pharmacol. Exp. Ther.*, **174**: 1, 1970.

115. Smith, E.R. and Duce, B.R.: The acute antiarrhythmic and toxic effects in mice and dogs of 2-ethylamino-2', 6'acetoxylidine (L-86), a metabolite of lidocaine. *J. Pharmacol. Exp. Ther.*, **179**: 580, 1971.

116. Strong, J.M., Parker, M., and Atkinson, A.J.: Identification of glycinexylidide in patients treated with intravenous lidocaine. *Clin. Pharmacol. Ther.*, **14**: 67, 1973.

117. Bellet, S., Roman, L., Kostis, J.B., and Fleischmann, D.: Intramuscular lidocaine in the therapy of ventricular arrhythmias. *Am. J. Cardiol.*, **27**: 291, 1971.

118. Bernstein, V., Berstein, B., Briffiths, J., and Peretz, D.I.: Lidocaine intramuscularly in acute myocardial infarction. *JAMA*, **219**: 1027, 1972.

119. Cohen, L.S., Rosenthal, J.E., Horner, D.W., Atkins, J.M., Matthews, O.A., and Sarnoff, S.J.: Plasma levels of lidocaine after intramuscular administration. *Am. J. Cardiol.*, **29**: 520, 1972.

120. Valentine, P.A., Frew, J.L., Mashford, M.L., and Sloman, J.G.: Lidocaine in the prevention of sudden death in the pre-hospital phase of acute infarction: a double-blind study. *N. Engl. J. Med.*, **291**: 1327, 1974.

121. Valentine, P.A., Sloman, J.F., and McIntyre, M.: A double blind trial of lidocaine in acute cardiac infarction. In D.B. Scott and D.G. Julian (Eds.): *Lidocaine in the Treatment of Ventricular Arrhythmias.* E and S Livingstone, Edinburgh, 1971.

122. Rowland, M., Thomson, P.D., Guichard, A., and Melmon, K.L.: Disposition kinetics of lidocaine in normal subjects. *Ann. N.Y. Acad. Sci.*, **179**: 383, 1971.

123. Boyes, R.N., Scott, D.B., Jebson, P.J., Godman, M.J., and Julian, D.G.: Pharmacokinetics of lidocaine in man. *Clin. Pharmacol. Ther.*, **12**: 105, 1972.

124. Benowitz, N.L.: Clinical applications of the pharmacokinetics of lidocaine. *Cardiovasc. Clin.*, **6**: 77, 1974.

125. Bassan, M.M., Weinstein, S.R., and Mandel, W.J.: Use of lidocaine by continuous infusion. *Am. Heart J.*, **87**: 302, 1974.

126. Goldstein, A., Aronow, L., and Kalman, S.M.: *Principles of Drug Action: The Basis of Pharmacology*, 2nd Edition. John Wiley & Sons, New York, 1974.

127. Sung, C.Y. and Truant, A.P.: Physiological disposition of lidocaine and its

comparison in some respects with procaine. *J. Pharmacol. Exp. Ther.*, **112**: 432, 1954.

128. Hollinger, G.: On the metabolism of lidocaine. II. The biotransformation of lidocaine. *Acta Pharmacol. et Toxicol.*, **17**: 365, 1960.
129. Mather, L.E. and Thomas, J.: Metabolism of lidocaine in man. *Life Sci.*, **11**: 915, 1972.
130. Beckett, A.H., Boyes, R.N., and Appleton, P.J.: The metabolism and excretion of lignocaine in man. *J. Pharm. Pharmacol.*, **18** (Suppl): 765, 1966.
131. Stenson, R.E., Constantino, E.C., and Harrison, D.C.: Interrelationships of hepatic blood flow, cardiac output, and blood levels of lidocaine in man. *Circulation*, **43**: 205, 1971.
132. Branch, R.A., Shand, D.G., Wilkinson, G.R., and Nies, A.S.: The reduction of lidocaine clearance by dl-propranolol: an example of hemodynamic drug interaction. *J. Pharmacol. Exp. Ther.*, **184**: 515, 1973.
133. Benowitz, N., Rowland, M., Forsyth, R.P., and Melmon, K.L.: Circulatory influences on lidocaine disposition. *Clin. Res.*, **21**: 235, 1973.
134. Benowitz, N., Forsyth, R.P., Melmon, K.L., and Rowland, M.: Lidocaine disposition kinetics in monkey and man. II. Effects of hemorrhage and sympathomimetic drug administration. *Clin. Pharmacol. Ther.*, **16**: 99, 1974.
135. Gianelly, R., von der Groeben, J.O., Spivack, A.P., and Harrison, D.C.: Effect of lidocaine on ventricular arrhythmias in patients with coronary heart disease. *N. Engl. J. Med.*, **277**: 1215, 1967.
136. Myman, M.G. and Hammersmith, L.: Comprehensive treatment plan for the prevention of primary ventricular fibrillation in acute myocardial infarction. *Am. J. Cardiol.*, **33**: 661, 1974.
137. Pitt, A., Lipp, H., and Anderson, S.T.: Lidocaine given prophylactically to patients with acute myocardial infarction. *Lancet*, **1**: 612, 1971.
138. Harrison, D.C., Sprouse, J.H., and Morrow, A.G.: The antiarrhythmic properties of lidocaine and procaine amide: clinical and physiologic studies of their cardiovascular effects in man. *Circulation*, **28**: 486, 1963.
139. Bullhed, I.: Hemodynamic effect of lidocaine. *Acta Med. Scan.*, **186**: 53, 1969.
140. Lieberman, N.A., Harris, R.S., Katz, R.I., Lipschutz, H.M., Dolgin, M., and Fisher, V.J.: The effects of lidocaine on the electrical and mechanical activity of the heart. *Am. J. Cardiol.*, **22**: 375, 1968.
141. Boston Collaborative Drug Surveillance Program: Drug-induced convulsions. *Lancet*, **2**: 677, 1972.
142. Atkinson, A.J. and Davison, R.: Diphenylhydantoin as an antiarrhythmic drug. *Ann. Rev. Med.*, **25**: 99, 1974.
143. Bigger, J.T., Schmidt, D.H., and Kutt, H.: A method for estimation of plasma diphenylhydantoin concentration. *Am. Heart J.*, **77**: 572, 1969.
144. Bigger, J.T., Schmidt, D.H., and Kutt, H.: Relationship between the plasma level of diphenylhydantoin and its cardiac antiarrhythmic effects. *Circulation*, **38**: 363, 1968.
145. Wilensky, A.J. and Lowden, J.A.: Inadequate serum levels after intramuscular administration of diphenylhydantoin. *Neurology*, **23**: 318, 1973.
146. Kostenbauder, H.B., Rapp, R.P., McGovren, J.P., Foster, T.S., Perrier, D.G., Blacker, H.M., Hulon, W.C., and Kinkel, A.W.: Bioavailability and single-dose pharmacokinetics of intramuscular phenytoin. *Clin. Pharmacol. Ther.*, **18**: 449, 1975.
147. Albert, K.S., Sakmar, E., Hallmark, M.R., Weidler, D.J., and Wagner, J.G.: Bioavailability of diphenylhydantoin. *Clin. Pharmacol. Ther.*, **16**: 727, 1974.
148. Glazko, A.J.: Diphenylhydantoin. *Pharmacol.*, **8**: 163, 1972.
149. Haerer, A.F. and Buchanan, R.Z.: Effectiveness of single daily doses of diphenylhydantoin. *Neurology*, **22**: 1021, 1972.

150. Gerber, N. and Wagner, J.F.: Explanation of dose-dependent decline of diphenylhydantoin plasma levels by fitting to the integrated form of the Michaelis-Menten equation. *Res. Commun. Chem. Pathol. Pharmacol.*, **3**: 455, 1972.

151. Gerber, N., Lynn, R., and Oates, J.: Acute intoxication with 5,5-diphenylhydantoin (Dilantin) associated with impairment of biotransformation. *Ann. Intern. Med.*, **77**: 765, 1972.

152. Brennan, R.W., Dehejia, H., Kutt, H., Verebely, K., and McDowell, F.: Diphenylhydantoin intoxication attendant to slow inactivation of isoniazid. *Neurology*, **20**: 687, 1970.

153. Cucinell, S.A., Conney, A.H., Sansur, M., and Burns, J.J.: Drug interactions in man. I. Lowering effect of phenobarbital on plasma levels of bishydroxycoumarin (Dicumarol) and diphenylhydantoin (Dilantin). *Clin. Pharmacol. Ther.*, **6**: 420, 1965.

154. Kutt, H., Winters, W., and McDowell, R.H.: Depression of parahydroxylation of diphenylhydantoin by antituberculosis chemotherapy. *Neurology*, **16**: 594, 1966.

155. Mercer, E.N. and Osborne, J.A.: The current status of diphenylhydantoin in heart disease. *Ann. Intern. Med.*, **67**: 1084, 1967.

156. Louis, S., Kutt, H., and McDowell, F.: The cardiocirculatory changes caused by intravenous Dilantin and its solvent. *Amer. Heart J.*, **74**: 523, 1967.

157. Lieberson, A.D., Schumacher, R.R., Childress, R.H., Boyd, D.L., and Williams, J.F.: Effects of diphenylhydantoin on left ventricular function in patients with heart disease. *Circulation*, **36**: 692, 1967.

158. Karliner, J.S.: Intravenous diphenylhydantoin sodium (Dilantin) in cardiac arrhythmias. *Dis. Chest.*, **51**: 256, 1967.

159. Conn, R.D.: Diphenylhydantoin sodium in cardiac arrhythmias. *N. Engl. J. Med.*, **272**: 277, 1965.

160. Rosen, M., Lisak, R., and Rubin, I.L.: Diphenylhydantoin in cardiac arrhythmias. *Am. J. Cardiol.*, **20**: 674, 1967.

161. Damato, A.N.: Diphenylhydantoin: pharmacological and clinical use. *Prog. Cardiovasc. Dis.*, **12**: 1, 1969.

162. Toman, J.E.P.: Drugs effective in convulsive disorders. In L.S. Goodman and A. Gilman (Eds.): *The Pharmacological Basis of Therapeutics*. 3rd Edition. The MacMillan Company, New York, 1965.

163. Haas, H. and Hartfelder, G.: Alpha-isopropyl-alpha-(N-methyl-N-homoveratryl-delta-aminopropyl)-3,-4,-dimethoxyphenyl-acetonitril, eine Substanz mit coronargefaberweiternden Eigenshaften. *Arzneimittel Forsch*, **12**: 549, 1962.

164. Schamroth, L., Krikler, D.M., and Garrett, C.: Immediate effects of intravenous verapamil in cardiac arrhythmias. *Brit. Med. J.*, **1**: 660, 1972.

165. Kirkler, D. and Spurrell, R.: Verapamil in the treatment of paroxysmal supraventricular tachycardia. *Postgrad. Med. J.*, **50**: 446, 1974.

166. Spurrell, R.A.J., Kirkler, D.M., and Sowton, E.: Effects of verapamil on electrophysiological properties of anomalous atrioventricular connexion in Wolff-Parkinson-White syndrome. *Brit. Heart J.*, **36**: 256, 1974.

167. Gotsman, M.S., Lewis, B.S., Bakst, A., and Mitha, A.S.: Verapamil in life threatening tachyarrhythmias. *S. Afr. Med. J.*, **46**: 2017, 1972.

168. Belz, G.G. and Bender, F.: *Therapie der Herzrhythmusstorungen mit Verapamil*. Gustav Fisher Verlag, Stuttgart, 1974.

169. McIlhenny, H.M.: Metabolism of 14 C-Verapamil. *J. Med. Chem.*, **14**: 1178, 1971.

170. McAllister, R.G. and Howell, S.M.: Fluorometric assay of verapamil in biological fluids and tissues. *J. Pharm. Sci.*, **65**: 431, 1976.

171. McAllister, R.G.: Unpublished Observations.
172. Peuch, P.: Dissection de la conduction sinoventriculaire pour l'etude du Verapamil injectable. Centre Hospitalier, Montpellier, 1972.
173. Fleckenstein, A., Doring, H.J., and Kammermeier, K.: Einfluss von Beta-Receptorenblockern und verwandten Substanzen auf Erregung. Kontraktion und Energiestoffwechsel der Myokardfaser. *Klin. Wschr.*, **46**: 343, 1968.
174. Nayler, W.G. and Szeta, J.: Effect of verapamil on contractibility, oxygen utilization, and calcium exchangeability on mammalian heart muscle. *Cardiovasc. Res.*, **6**: 120, 1972.
175. Ross, G. and Jorgensen, C.R.: Cardiovascular actions of iproveratril. *J. Pharmacol. Exp. Ther.*, **158**: 504, 1967.
176. Rickless, J.P.D. and Gilchrise, W.S.L.: An antidysrhythmic agent. *Brit. Med. J.*, **4**: 429, 1971.
177. Filias, N. and Zanoni, G.: Klinische Analyse der antiarrhythmischen Wirkung des Verapamils. *Schweiz med. Wschr.*, **102**: 406, 1972.
178. Husaini, M.H., Kvasnicka, J., Pyden, L., and Holmberg, S.: Action of verapamil in sinus node, atrioventricular, and intraventricular conduction. *Brit. Heart J.*, **35**: 734, 1973.
179. Dollery, C.T., Paterson, J.W., and Conolly, M.E.: Clinical pharmacology of beta receptor blocking drugs. *Clin. Pharmacol. Ther.*, **10**: 765, 1969.
180. Fitzgerald, J.D.: Perspectives in adrenergic beta-receptor blockade. *Clin. Pharmacol. Ther.*, **10**: 292, 1969.
181. Nies, A.S. and Shand, D.G.: Clinical pharmacology of propranolol. *Circulation*, **52**: 6, 1975.
182. Shand, D.G.: Drug therapy: propranolol. *N. Engl. J. Med.*, **293**: 280, 1975.
183. Shand, D.G., Nuckills, E.M., and Oates, J.A.: Plasma propranolol levels in adults with observations in four children. *Clin. Pharmacol. Ther.*, **11**: 112, 1970.
184. Evans, G.H. and Shand, D.G.: Disposition of propranolol. VI. Independent variation in steady state circulating drug concentration and half-life as a result of plasma drug binding in man. *Clin. Pharmacol. Ther.*, **14**: 494, 1973.
185. Shand, D.G., Evans, G.H., and Nies, A.S.: The almost complete hepatic extraction of propranolol during intravenous administration in the dog. *Life Sci.*, **10**: 417, 1971.
186. Nies, A.S., Evans, G.H., and Shand, D.G.: The hemodynamic effects of beta-adrenergic blockade on the flow-dependent hepatic clearance of propranolol. *J. Pharmacol. Exp. Ther.*, **184**: 716, 1973.
187. Lowenthal, D.T., Briggs, W.A., Gibson, T.P., Nelson, H., and Cirksena, W.J.: Pharmacokinetics of propranolol in chronic renal disease. *Clin. Pharmacol. Ther.*, **16**: 761, 1974.
188. Thompson, F.D., Joekes, A.M., and Foulkes, D.M.: Pharmacodynamics of propranolol in renal failure. *Brit. Med. J.*, **2**: 434, 1972.
189. Shand, D.G., Rangno, R.E., and Evans, G.H.: The disposition of propranolol. II. Hepatic elimination in the rat. *Pharmacology*, **8**: 344, 1972.
190. Shand, D.G. and Rangno, R.E.: The disposition of propranolol. Elimination during oral absorption in man. *Pharmacology*, **7**: 159, 1972.
191. Paterson, J.W., Conolly, M.E., and Dollery, C.T.: The pharmacodynamics and metabolism of propranolol in man. *Pharmacologia Clinica*, **2**: 127, 1970.
192. Cleaveland, C.R. and Shand, D.G.: Effect of route of administration on the relationship between beta-adrenergic blockade and plasma propranolol level. *Clin. Pharmacol. Ther.*, **13**: 181, 1972.
193. Coltart, D.J. and Shand, D.G.: Plasma propranolol levels in the quantitative assessment of beta-adrenergic blockade in man. *Brit. Med. J.*, **3**: 731, 1970.
194. Zacest, R. and Koch-Weser, J.: Relation of propranolol plasma level to beta-blockade during oral therapy. *Pharmacology*, **7**: 178, 1972.

195. Greenblatt, D.J. and Koch-Weser, J.: Adverse reactions to propranolol in hospitalized medical patients: a report from the Boston Collaborative Drug Surveillance Program. *Am. Heart J.*, **86**: 478, 1973.
196. Boura, A.L.A., Copp, F.C., Duncombe, W.G., Green, A.F., and McCoubrey, A.: The selective accumulation of bretylium in sympathetic ganglia and their postganglionic nerves. *Brit. J. Pharmacol.*, **15**: 265, 1960.
197. Green, A.F.: Antihypertensive drugs. In *Advances in Pharmacology*, Vol. I. Academic Press, New York, 1962.
198. Taylor, S.H. and Donald, K.W.: The circulatory effects of bretylium in man. *Brit. Heart J.*, **22**: 588, 1960.
199. Dollery, C.T., Emslie-Smith, D., and McMichael, J.: Bretylium tosylate in the treatment of hypertension. *Lancet*, **1**: 296, 1960.
200. Kuntzman, R., Tsai, I., Chang, R., and Conney, A.A.: Disposition of bretylium in man and rat. *Clin. Pharmacol. Ther.*, **11**: 829, 1970.
201. Duncombe, W.G. and McCoubrey, A.: The excretion and stability to metabolism of bretylium. *Brit. J. Pharmacol.*, **15**: 260, 1960.
202. Oates, J.A., Mitchell, J.R., Feagin, O.T., Kaufmann, J.S., and Shand, D.G.: Distribution of guanidinium antihypertensives—mechanism of their selective action. *Ann. N.Y. Acad. Sci.*, **179**: 302, 1971.
203. Gaffney, T.E., Braunwald, E., and Cooper, T.: Analysis of the acute circulatory effects of guanethidine and bretylium. *Circ. Res.*, **10**: 83, 1962.
204. Priola, D.V., Spurgeon, H.A., Blauw, A.S., Cannon, W.B., and Dong, E.: The mechanisms of the inotropic action of bretylium tosylate on the heart. *J. Pharmacol. Exp. Ther.*, **187**: 121, 1973.
205. Graham, J.D. and Chandler, B.M.: The effects of lidocaine, propranolol, procaine amide, and bretylium tosylate on the contractility of isolated cat papillary muscles. *Canad. J. Physiol. Pharmacol.*, **51**: 763, 1973.
206. Maines, J.E. and Williams, R.L.: Contrasting effects of bretylium and guanethidine on renal function. *Arch. Int. Pharmacodyn.*, **205**: 94, 1973.
207. MacAlpin, R.N., Salis, E.G., and Kivowitz, C.F.: Prevention of recurrent ventricular tachycardia with oral bretylium tosylate. *Ann. Intern. Med.*, **72**: 909, 1970.
208. Luomanmake, K., Heikkila, J., and Hartel, G.: Bretylium tosylate. Adverse effects in acute myocardial infarction. *Arch. Intern. Med.*, **135**: 515, 1975.
209. Gettes, L.S. and Yoshonis, K.F.: Rapidly recurring supraventricular tachycardia: a manifestation of reciprocating tachycardia and an indication for propranolol therapy. *Circulation*, **41**: 689, 1970.
210. Wellens, Hein J.J. and Durrer, D.: Effect of procaine amide, and quinidine in the Wolff-Parkinson-White syndrome. *Circulation*, **50**: 114, 1974.
211. Jelinek, M.V., Lohrbauer, L., and Lown, B.: Antiarrhythmic drug therapy for sporadic ventricular ectopic arrhythmias. *Circulation*, **49**: 659, 1974.
212. Sanna, G. and Archidiacono, R.: Chemical ventricular defibrillation of the human heart with bretylium tosylate. *Am. J. Cardiol.*, **32**: 982, 1973.

CHAPTER 14
Management of Tachyarrhythmias

James R. Morgan, M.D.; Barry Dzindzio, M.D.;
Helen Starke, M.D.; Alan D. Forker, M.D.

Identification and control of tachyarrhythmias are essential to reducing morbidity and mortality. This Chapter defines the underlying mechanisms, diagnostic criteria, and modes of management available for their control. Fundamental to effective therapy is the establishment of an accurate diagnosis. Effective antiarrhythmic management is frequently precluded by difficulty in differentiating one arrhythmia from others. To assist in better management, clinical electrocardiographic clues to diagnostic pitfalls are also well defined herein.

The purpose of this chapter is to provide a practical guide for the primary care physician in the management of the common tachyarrhythmias. Bradyarrhythmias and heart block are covered in other chapters. The tachyarrhythmias to be discussed include: (1) sinus tachycardia, (2) atrial tachycardia, (3) atrial tachycardia with (atrioventricular) AV block, (4) atrial flutter, (5) atrial fibrillation, (6) multifocal atrial tachycardia, (7) AV junctional tachycardia, (8) ventricular tachycardia, and (9) ventricular fibrillation.

Tachyarrhythmias are common and are likely to be encountered in any emergency room, hospital room, or physician's office. When confronted with an arrhythmia problem, three questions always need to be answered: (1) What is the diagnosis and etiology of the arrhythmia? (2) What treatment is needed? (3) How fast is treatment needed? In any arrhythmia situation, the old adage, "treat the patient and not the arrhythmia" still stands.

HEMODYNAMIC CONSEQUENCES OF THE TACHYARRHYTHMIAS

With the exception of ventricular fibrillation, the tachyarrhythmias occur in a broad spectrum of symptomatic and hemodynamic severity. Depending on the type and severity of the underlying heart disease, co-existent noncardiac disease, and the state of the compensatory mechanisms, the patient may be completely asymptomatic or totally incapacitated with any of these arrhythmias. For example, a young adult with atrial tachycardia of several days duration may be asymptomatic or have only mild fatigue; but a patient with ischemic heart disease may develop angina pectoris secondary to sinus tachycardia of only 120 beats per minute.

The urgency of treatment depends primarily upon the hemodynamic consequences of the tachycardia. The normal heart can maintain an appropriate stroke volume, cardiac output, and blood pressure over a wide range of heart rates. However, above 160 beats per minute, diastolic filling time is shortened sufficiently to compromise the stroke volume, and therefore cardiac output and blood pressure fall[1].

Tachyarrhythmias that are associated with a loss of properly timed atrial contraction have another cause of decreased cardiac output—the loss of atrial systole[2]. These rhythms include atrial fibrillation, AV dissociation, AV junctional rhythm, and ventricular tachycardia. In normal hearts, loss of atrial systole causes a temporary drop in cardiac output of around 15%; but compensatory mechanisms, such as increased heart rate, decreased peripheral resistance, and increased contractility, may return the cardiac output to normal[3]. In mitral stenosis, atrial systole takes on added importance since early diastolic flow is delayed and atrial contraction must contribute a larger percentage of the diastolic load. Loss of atrial systole in mitral stenosis may decrease the cardiac output by as much as 30-50%[4]. In patients with a poorly compliant left ventricle, such as aortic stenosis or idiopathic hypertrophic subaortic stenosis (IHSS), atrial systole is crucial for added ventricular filling. Loss of atrial contraction may cause a precipitous drop in cardiac output, leading to overt heart failure[5].

The sequence of ventricular activation may also alter the hemodynamic consequences of a tachycardia. Although this may not be a factor in the supraventricular tachycardias, it may be a significant variable in patients with ventricular tachycardia. Patterns of ventricular activation that change patterns of ventricular contraction will lead to variations in cardiac output. Experimental pacing of either the left or right ventricle produces a variable cardiac output response[6]. This may, in part, explain why some patients with ventricular tachycardia are capable of maintaining a reasonable cardiac output while others are not.

Cardiac work and myocardial oxygen requirements are directly proportional to heart rate. The normal heart has a cardiac output reserve sufficient to supply the increased needs of the myocardium to a heart rate of at least 160 beats per minute. When cardiac reserve is inadequate, heart failure may occur even at lower rates. Cardiac reserve may be insufficient because of inadequate supply of oxygen to a normal myocardial mass, as in coronary heart disease, anemia, abnormal hemoglobins, or lung disease, all of which limit oxygen delivery. On the other hand, a normal oxygen delivery may be insufficient to meet the increased demands of an enlarged myocardial mass, such as seen in left ventricular hypertrophy due to aortic stenosis.

Coronary blood flow, especially important in ischemic heart disease, can be significantly decreased by arrhythmias. Frequent premature ventricular contractions can decrease coronary blood flow as much as 25%, rapid supraventricular tachycardias by as much as 35%, and ventricular tachycardias up to 60%[7]. In ventricular fibrillation coronary blood flow drops to zero.

POTENTIAL CORRECTABLE FACTORS IN THE GENESIS OF ARRHYTHMIAS

It is important to emphasize potentially correctable etiologic factors, since the treatment of arrhythmias without correction of underlying causes will be less successful. The electrophysiology of cardiac arrhythmias is covered in Chapter 4.

Frequently multiple factors are responsible for an arrhythmia. If such is the case, then each one must be corrected while directing therapy at the secondary arrhythmia. Many times correction of the precipitating factor will lead to termination of the arrhythmia. Directing therapy at the arrhythmia rather than at the underlying cause is frequently futile, often leading to patient discomfort, expense, and risk.

DeSanctis et al conveniently divided the causes of tachyarrhythmias into five broad and overlapping categories: metabolic, anatomic, autonomic, hemodynamic, and iatrogenic[8]. Table I lists some of the common arrhythmogenic factors that are encountered in our practice.

SINUS TACHYCARDIA

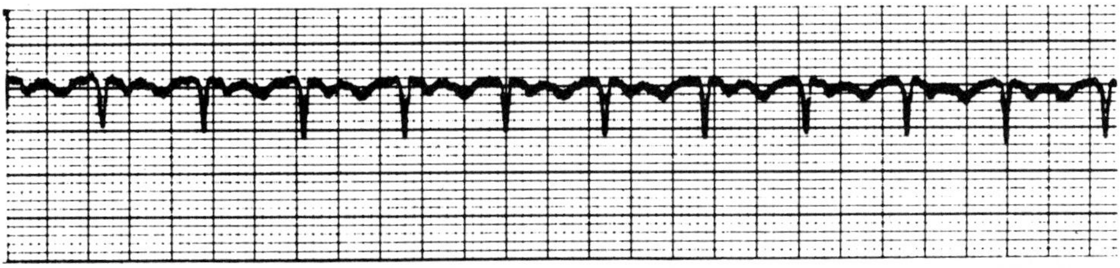

Figure 1   Sinus tachycardia with regular atrial rate, ventricular rate, and P-R intervals; and a ventricular response of 130 beats per minute.

Sinus tachycardia is defined as a regular sinus mechanism at a rate of 100-150 beats per minute. It is a normal response to emotional stress, excitement, and many other life events. Unexplained sinus tachycardia in a resting patient should provoke a search for etiologic factors, such as decreased blood volume, hypoxemia, peripheral AV shunt, hyperthyroidism, anemia, infection and fever, heart failure, or anxiety. It is unusual for a patient to have a resting sinus tachycardia above 140 beats per minute, so one should exclude the possibility of another arrhythmia in this situation. Sinus tachycardia itself does not require treatment, but the situation producing it should be sought for and corrected.

ATRIAL TACHYCARDIA

Paroxysmal atrial tachycardia (PAT) is the most common paroxysmal tachycardia in children and young adults. The ECG diagnosis depends

TABLE I
COMMON CORRECTABLE ARRHYTHMOGENIC FACTORS

A. Metabolic
1. Electrolyte imbalance
2. Acid-base imbalance
3. Hypoxia
4. Hypercarbia
5. Thyroid disease

B. Anatomic
1. SA node ischemia
2. AV node ischemia
3. Pericardial irritation
4. Cardiac trauma

C. Autonomic
1. Increased vagal tone
   a. Pain
   b. Acute inferior wall infarction
   c. Vagotonic drugs
2. Increased catecholamines
   a. Emotional stress
   b. Pheocheomocytoma
   c. Sympathomimetic drugs
   d. Central nervous system insult

D. Hemodynamic
1. Mitral valve disease
2. Left ventricular failure
3. Systemic hypertension
4. Hypotension
5. Pulmonary emboli

E. Iatrogenic
1. Digitalis
2. Diuretics
3. Morphine
4. Thyroid preparations
5. Anorexants
6. Decongestants
7. Antidepressants
8. Sedatives
9. Cordicosteroids
10. Bronchodilators

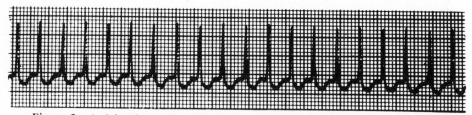

Figure 2 Atrial tachycardia with the P waves visible at the end of the T wave, especially in the mid portion of the rhythm strip, and a P-R interval of 0.06 seconds.

upon regular but abnormally shaped P waves followed by an identical ventricular rate of 150-250 beats per minute. With rates above 200 per minute, there is frequently some degree of AV block and this will be discussed later. PAT is generally thought to be caused by a reentry mechanism[9]. In

PAT complicating the Wolff-Parkinson-White (WPW) syndrome, there is strong histological and electrophysiological evidence of reentry by way of an accessory conduction pathway[10]. In the absence of the WPW syndrome, the evidence for reentry mechanism is less conclusive but generally accepted. In some experimental models, PAT has been caused by a rapid unifocal atrial focus[11], but this seems less unlikely in the usual clinical situation.

The clinical setting for PAT can be quite varied. By far the most common presentation is the older child or young adult without any cardiovascular disease. The rate is usually 160-180 beats per minute and the symptoms are usually limited to palpitations and a feeling of fatigue. The patient can frequently give a history of abrupt onset. If several episodes have occurred in the past, the patient may relate a history of abrupt termination, either spontaneously or following various therapeutic maneuvers.

In older adults, where underlying heart disease is more common, patients present more frequently with ischemic chest pain, hypotension, heart failure, or even shock. With these complications, immediate electrical cardioversion is indicated. When there is no underlying heart disease, the patient usually is not in serious hemodynamic difficulty. This allows plenty of time for the clinician to plan a series of therapeutic maneuvers which will usually revert the arrhythmia to a normal sinus mechanism (Table II).

TABLE II
TREATMENT OF PAT

1. Carotid sinus massage
2. Valsalva Maneuver
3. Sedation — IV Valium®
4. + Tensilon®
5. Raise systolic pressure
6. Propranolol — if hypotension, heart failure, AV block, or acute bronchospasm absent
7. Digoxin vs electrical cardioversion

The primary objective of therapy is to create increased vagal tone in order to inhibit conduction through the AV junctional tissues and prevent reentry. The first maneuver to try is carotid sinus massage. After making sure that the patient has no carotid bruits, and no history, signs, or symptoms of a transient ischemic attack are present, moderately heavy massage over first the right and then the left carotid sinus should be performed. The pressure should be maintained for five to ten seconds under constant ECG monitoring. Either no effect or abrupt termination of the arrhythmia will occur. Only one carotid sinus should be massaged at a time.

A second therapeutic maneuver that can be applied is the Valsalva maneuver. The patient is asked to take in a deep breath and then bear down with a closed epiglottis, as if having a bowel movement. This should be held for a minimum of ten seconds. This maneuver creates an abrupt fall in cardiac output and blood pressure, with a secondary increase in heart rate and peripheral vascular resistance by reflex sympathetic stimulation. On sudden release of the increased intrathoracic pressure, the cardiac output returns to normal. In the face of increased peripheral vascular resistance from increased sympathetic tone, an overshoot phenomenon occurs with an increased blood pressure[12], and a reflex bradycardia that is vagally mediated. It is at this time (during the reflex bradycardia) that the arrhythmia is converted. Carotid sinus massage can be added to the Valsalva maneuver, especially during the time of blood pressure overshoot.

Another interesting method employed to increase vagal tone is the so-called diving reflex—the patient immerses his face in cold water. This again brings on an increased sympathetic tone, which causes a reflex bradycardia. Although sometimes effective, it is attended by a moderate amount of patient discomfort and we do not use it for this reason. We also do not recommend eyeball pressure, since it is potentially dangerous, especially in the elderly, and furthermore it is rarely effective.

Mild sedation should be considered in any patient who is extremely anxious. Diazepam (Valium®) is effective at a dose of 5-10 mg intravenously. Diazepam should be injected directly intravenously rather than through intravenous tubing, since it tends to adhere to the plastic tubing, and it tends to precipitate in 5% dextrose and water.

Tensilon® may be tried because of its anticholinesterase effect and ability to chemically increase vagal tone. This drug allows a buildup of acetylcholine at nerve endings. It is recommended to first start with a test done of 1 mg IV; after waiting one minute, follow with the intravenous injection of up to 10 mg IV slowly. Occasionally, cholinergic side effects will require the use of atropine to counteract their unpleasantness. If Tensilon® by itself is unsuccessful, it may be administered in combination with carotid sinus massage and the Valsalva maneuver to increase its therapeutic efficacy.

If the above maneuvers have not been successful in converting PAT, a very successful approach to increasing vagal tone is to provoke a small rise in the systolic blood pressure[13]. The aim is to raise systolic pressure 30-40 mg Hg above baseline systolic pressures. This maneuver should not be used if the baseline systolic pressure is above 160-180 mm Hg. By increasing systolic pressure, one is in effect performing carotid sinus massage intravascularly. It is most effective in patients who have a low baseline pressure. Phenylephrine (Neo-Synephrine) 1 mg diluted up to 10 cc's with saline, can be given slowly over two-three minutes intravenously, stopping when the optimum blood pressure response is obtained. At the time of peak blood pressure response, a mild headache may develop; if the arrhythmia is not converted spontaneously, carotid sinus massage should be repeated with peak pressure response.

An alternative to phenylephrine is metaraminol (Aramine®), which is prepared by diluting 100 mg of drug in 250 cc's of intravenous fluid, and infused at a rate sufficient to maintain the desirable blood pressure elevation. This offers the advantage of better control of the blood pressure response. If patients are in overt congestive heart failure and/or have significant mitral valve disease, acute blood pressure elevation may be dangerous and put them into acute pulmonary edema.

If the patient does not respond to the above maneuvers, then propranolol (Inderal®) 1 mg IV every five minutes to a total dose of 5 mg, may be considered. This is particularly excellent in PAT complicating thyrotoxicosis. In the presence of congestive heart failure or asthma, propranolol can be disastrous. Care should always be exercised in administration of propranolol to a patient with left ventricular dysfunction. If propranolol does not immediately terminate the arrhythmia, worse pump failure may ensue[14].

If the patient has not converted to sinus rhythm with these therapies, and especially if this is the first episode, the patient should be hospitalized in the critical care unit, and considered for either electrical cardioversion or digitalization. Past medical history is critical at this point, since if previous cardioversion has been unsuccessful or only transiently successful, repeat cardioversion would not be indicated. On the other hand, if this is the first or second episode, cardioversion might be tried.

With a patient in the critical care unit, we generally prefer digoxin (Lanoxin®) via the intravenous route. The administration of a digitalizing dose of digoxin based on body weight (generally 0.75 mg in an adult) over a 24-hour period will frequently restore sinus rhythm. It may be helpful to repeat carotid sinus massage an hour or so after administration of the first dose of intravenous digoxin.

Followup for recurrent episodes of PAT will depend upon the frequency of attacks and the severity of symptoms. Oral digoxin continues to be the backbone of maintenance therapy. If dogoxin has been unsuccessful alone, then oral digoxin and quinidine, and/or digoxin-quinidine-propranolol combination can be tried.

ATRIAL TACHYCARDIA WITH AV BLOCK

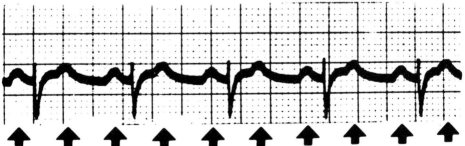

Figure 3 Atrial tachycardia with 2:1 AV block. The large arrows at the bottom indicate the P waves. The P-P and P-R intervals are constant, with an isoelectric line between each P wave.

Atrial tachycardia with AV block usually occurs in two different circumstances: (1) a physiologic block, where the atrial rate is in excess of that which can be transmitted by the AV junctional tissues. This is not uncommon in patient with atrial rates in excess of 200 beats per minute. (2) A pathological block, which occurs at slower atrial rates which should allow normal AV junctional transmission. Under these circumstances, atrial tachycardia with AV block suggests AV junctional disease, and is usually due to digitalis excess.

In the face of this arrhythmia, digitalis toxicity must always be excluded. Digitalis preparations have the ability to increase atrial automaticity, thus predisposing to rapid atrial tachycardias. Also, digitalis has the ability to increase the refractory period of the AV junctional tissues, either by vagatonic effects or by its direct effect on the AV junctional tissues[15]. The treatment of choice is removal of digitalis, correction of hypokalemia, and observation of the patient in the hospital for more serious signs of digitalis toxicity, such as ventricular arrhythmias. However, it is unusual for any further therapeutic measures to be needed.

ATRIAL FLUTTER

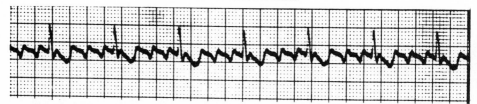

Figure 4 Atrial flutter with the typical "saw tooth" oscillation seen in lead II. A consistent 4:1 AV conduction is present.

The electrocardiographic diagnosis of atrial flutter is based upon continuous baseline "sawtooth" oscillations in the inferior leads. If just lead V_1 is observed, atrial flutter may be confused with atrial tachycardia with AV block. However, atrial flutter generally has a faster atrial rate of 250-350 beats per minute; and atrial tachycardia with AV block does not show the "sawtooth" pattern in the inferior leads of the ECG. The ventricular response in atrial flutter may be regular or variable, depending upon a constant or irregular degree of AV block. The most common ventricular rate is 150 beats per minute with 2-to-1 AV conduction. This response is so common that any time the ventricular rate is exactly 150 beats per minute, atrial flutter must be excluded. With carotid sinus massage, 2-to-1 AV block may change to a higher degree of AV block, thereby abruptly dropping the ventricular rate from 150 to 75 beats per minute or less. This will allow one to better visualize the flutter waves. With the release of carotid sinus massage, the original degree of AV block will usually return, and the arrhythmia will rarely be interrupted. An esophageal or right atrial lead may occasionally be necessary for exact diagnosis when lesser degrees of AV block are present.

Atrial flutter is generally seen in patients with significant underlying heart disease, such as rheumatic valvular disease, ischemic heart disease, or chronic pulmonary disease[10]. It may be associated with more transient causes such as acute pericarditis, pulmonary embolism, or thyrotoxicosis.

Atrial flutter is especially common in postoperative patients who may be more responsive to medical treatment[10].

Synchronized DC cardioversion is the treatment of choice for atrial flutter[17]. In the absence of digitalis therapy and with a normal serum potassium, cardioversion is a safe and highly effective mode of treatment. Atrial flutter is very responsive often requiring delivered energies of only 25-50 watt seconds[18].

If the etiology for atrial flutter is expected to be transient and the patient is hemodynamically stable, medical therapy may be tried first. The objective of therapy is to depress AV conduction and the ventricular response, and hopefully convert to sinus rhythm. Medical therapy will be most effective in the patient with pulmonary embolism and postoperative cardiac surgery[16]. Digoxin is generally the drug we would try first. However, atrial flutter is frequently refractory to pharmacologic agents and larger doses of digitalis may be required than for other atrial arrhythmias. This is the main rationale for more frequent use of electrical cardioversion in these patients.

Quinidine should not be used initially in atrial flutter, as it decreases the atrial rate and facilitates AV conduction, with the danger of producing an abrupt change to 1-to-1 AV conduction. This rapid ventricular response may be poorly tolerated. Therefore, pretreatment with digoxin is recommended before starting quinidine. Finally, the combination of digoxin and propranolol, or digoxin-quinidine-propranolol may be necessary for medical conversion to sinus rhythm and/or maintenance therapy.

Rarely, a patient may present in severe hemodynamic trouble secondary to a very rapid ventricular response from atrial flutter, and yet already be on digitalis therapy. In this situation, cardioversion has increased risk. Rapid atrial stimulation by a pacemaker catheter tip in the right atrium has been tried with some success in this situation. Although we have no extensive experience with this procedure, it has been reported to be safe and effective[19,20]. Rapid atrial stimulation will either convert the atrial flutter to sinus rhythm, convert it to atrial fibrillation, or will have no effect.

ATRIAL FIBRILLATION

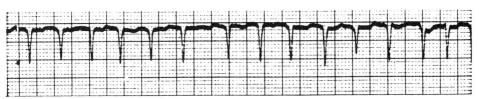

Figure 5   Atrial fibrillation with no visible atrial activity present, and irregularly irregular ventricular rate.

Atrial fibrillation is characterized by absence of discrete P wave activity and an irregularly irregular ventricular response. Fibrillatory waves are either fine or coarse, and occur at a rate greater than 400 beats per minute. Atrial fibrillation can be either paroxysmal or sustained. Paroxysmal atrial fibrillation can occur in a normal heart, especially in the younger age group and when the atria are of normal size. On the other hand, sustained atrial fibrillation is usually associated with underlying heart disease. In a large autopsy study, sustained atrial fibrillation was found prior to death in 50% of patients dying of rheumatic heart disease, 25% of patients dying of hypertensive vascular disease, and 20% of patients dying of ischemic heart disease[21]. In chronic mitral valve disease, the atria are larger and the fibrillatory waves tend to be more coarse.

In atrial fibrillation with a rapid ventricular response, the therapeutic goal is to slow AV conduction and the ventricular response, and/or to convert to sinus rhythm. Digitalis remains the drug of choice. In the absence of complicating factors, such as anemia, volume depletion, thyrotoxicosis, infection or hypoxemia, the ventricular rate can be readily controlled with digitalis. This is one of the few times that an objective end point is available for evaluation of the therapeutic efficacy of digitalis. If the patient has associated congestive heart failure, this should be treated simultaneously by the usual methods. An urgent need for emergency electrical cardioversion of atrial fibrillation is rarely seen.

If a patient has not been receiving digitalis, we prefer to initially administer digoxin intravenously. The first dose of digoxin, 0.5 mg, is given with an additional 0.25 mg intravenous dose in about 3-6 hours. This will usually decrease the ventricular rate to a reasonable value. The onset of action of intravenous digoxin is usually 15-30 minutes with the maximum effect at two hours[15]. Maximum drug concentration in the myocardium usually occurs at about six hours, at which time the incidence of toxic arrhythmias is the highest. Since the dose required for digitalization is primarily a function of body weight, the total dose for the first 24-hour period should not exceed 0.01 mg/kg[22].

However, there are some individuals that may require more or less than this suggested dose to control the ventricular response. The maintenance dose is calculated on the basis of the renal function. Jelliffe et al have reported a practical nomogram for calculating the maintenance dose based upon sex, body size, and renal function[22]. There is direct correlation between renal function and digoxin dosage. If there is difficulty controlling the ventricular response in the face of adequate digoxin doses, propranolol in small intravenous doses of 1 mg every five minutes may be added to further slow the ventricular response by depressing AV conduction. The precautions with propranolol therapy pertain here also, since mild congestive heart failure can be turned into severe failure or pulmonary edema when given to the wrong patient.

Electrical cardioversion of artrial fibrillation is usually employed under two circumstances: (1) an emergency procedure in a patient who is acutely ill from the deleterious hemodynamic effects of a rapid ventricular response, and (2) an elective procedure, in which synchronized DC cardioversion is performed in a patient who is hemodynamically stable.

When patients present to an emergency room physician with atrial fibrillation, rapid ventricular response, and deteriorating cardiac function, synchronized cardioversion during the acute presentation is indicated. The use of anesthesia depends upon the level of consciousness of the patient. If the patient is in severe hemodynamic distress, maximum dosage in this situation would be used up to 400 watt seconds with the first discharge. If the urgency is not that great, but the clinical situation suggests that deterioration may be imminent, one should start as a lower energy level, such as 100 watt seconds.

The indications for elective cardioversion of atrial fibrillation have been well described[17,23]. We feel it is easier to understand the contraindications to elective cardioversion of atrial fibrillation than to list indications. Our major contraindications are summarized in Table III. The procedure for electrical cardioversion is given in Table IV.

TABLE III

MAJOR CONTRAINDICATIONS FOR ELECTIVE CARDIOVERSION FOR ATRIAL FIBRILLATION

1. Long standing (A.F. >3 years duration), especially with chronic valvular disease, cardiomegaly and considerable left atrial enlargement.
2. Slow ventricular response in absence of therapy.
3. On digitalis with an HR > 60/min.
4. Patient is not able to maintain sinus rhythm even with quinidine therapy.
5. The patient receives no hemodynamic benefit from sinus rhythm.
6. Pheochromocytoma

TABLE IV

TECHNIQUE OF ELECTIVE CARDIOVERSION

1. Hold digoxin 36-48 hours or digitoxin 5-7 days prior to cardioversion.
2. Admit to ICU or CCU where equipment and personnel experienced in CPR are available.
3. Start oral quinidine 24-48 hours prior.
4. If a history of prior embolic phenomena is present, then the patient should be anticoagulated for two weeks.
5. The patient may need pre-cardioversion sedation.
6. A good IV route should be available (not a needle).
7. An anesthetic should be administered.
8. Always synchronize the shock with the R wave.
9. Start at low energy levels (50 W/S) since most complications occur at high energy levels.
10. The anteroposterior route is preferred, since less energy is usually required for cardioversion.
11. Monitor the patient in the special care area for 24 hours post-cardioversion.

All elective cardioversions should be conducted in a coronary care unit where cardiopulmonary resuscitation equipment is immediately available and the personnel are knowledgeable in its use. Digoxin preparations are withheld for 36 hours and digitoxin for five days[24]. Cardioversion in the presence of digitalis has a greater chance of producing ventricular arrhythmias[25]. If the ventricular response is below 60 beats per minute, we would delay until the rate has increased.

Pre-shock sedation is necessary for elective cardioversion. We use either intravenous diazepam or pentobarbital, the latter with the help of an anesthetist or anesthesiologist. A good intravenous route is a must. This should be via an intracath rather than a needle, since needles tend to be precarious due to the jerking of extremities following countershock.

We do not anticoagulate all patients prior to cardioversion. If a history of prior embolic phenomena is present, the patient should be anticoagulated for two weeks prior to cardioversion. Anticoagulation should be continued for at least one month following cardioversion, since many patients will revert back to atrial fibrillation within that period of time[23].

The defibrillator is synchronized with the peak of the R wave and tested to be sure that synchronization is correct. We start at low energy levels, usually at 50 watt seconds, and progress upwards to 50-100-200-300 watt seconds. We do not utilize energies in excess of 300 watt seconds, since this exposes the patient to an increased risk of complications, and the success rate of maintaining normal sinus rhythm with greater dosage is extremely low[23]. The patient is monitored in the coronary care unit for the remainder of that day, because many of the complications will occur within the subsequent six hours. The patient can be discharged on the following day.

The initial success rate is approximately 90%[23]. Most of the patients that revert back to atrial fibrillation do so within the first 24 hours. There is a 50% success rate at one month. The greater the cardiomegaly, especially left atrial enlargement, the longer the history of atrial fibrillation, and the greater degree of untreatable progressive heart disease, the more prone the patient will be to revert back to atrial fibrillation. With adequate prophylaxis using either quinidine or procainamide, approximately 40% of the patients successfully cardioverted can be maintained in sinus rhythm for one year. In the absence of adequate prophylaxis, this percentage drops to around 10%[23].

Some patients have no significant increase in cardiac output post-cardioversion[26]. The result occurs in approximately 45%. In the other 55%, there is a significant increase in cardiac index of 0.5 L/min/m^2 or greater. In the second group the average increase in cardiac index is about 35% but this varies greatly from 10-70%, depending upon the type of heart disease, size of the atria, and compliance of the left ventricle. If no hemodynamic benefit is obtained from conversion to sinus rhythm, repeat cardioversion is not indicated. Recently echocardiography has been shown to have prognostic value[27]. Patients with a good prognosis of maintaining sinus rhythm develop a significant A wave on the anterior leaf of the mitral valve, as visualized by echocardiography. Patients with a poor prognosis of maintaining sinus rhythm develop an insignificant A wave.

MULTIFOCAL ATRIAL TACHYCARDIA

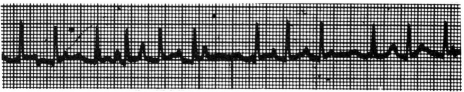

Figure 6 Multifocal atrial tachycardia with choatic atrial activity manifested by variable P wave contour, variable P-P intervals, and variable R-R intervals.

Multifocal atrial tachycardia is defined as a supraventricular arrhythmia with an atrial rate greater than 100 beats per minute and at least three separate P wave morphologies visualized. The P to P, P to R, and R to R intervals are irregularly irregular, and there may or may not be intermittent aberrant ventricular conduction.

This arrhythmia is almost found in patients with chronic obstructive pulmonary disease, although it can be found in some instances of congestive heart failure and acute myocarcial infarction[28]. Mortality rate is quite high, approaching 20%, and this is primarily due to the severity of the underlying cardiovascular disease rather than the arrhythmia itself.

Antiarrhythmic medications are generally ineffective[28]. It is extremely important to treat the underlying problem vigorously with meticulous control of hypoxia, carbon dioxide narcosis, and acid-base imbalance.

AV JUNCTIONAL TACHYCARDIA

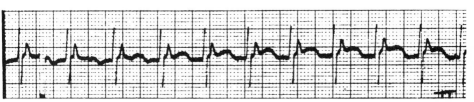

Figure 7 AV junctional tachycardia with inverted P waves preceding the normal QRS complexes by 0.08 seconds.

AV junctional tachycardia is defined as three or more consecutive premature beats of AV junctional origin with a rate greater than 70 beats per minute. It may be paroxysmal, with an abrupt termination, or it may be nonparoxysmal. These two subcategories of AV junctional tachycardia are compared in Table V[29].

Paroxysmal junctional tachycardia resembles PAT at the bedside[30]. The ventricular rate is generally 160-200 beats per minute with a precisely regular response. Carotid sinus massage either abruptly aborts the arrhythmia or has no effect. The P waves are constantly related to the QRS complex, and occur either before or after the R wave, or no P waves at all are seen since they are buried in the QRS complex. As with PAT, there fre-

TABLE V
AV JUNCTIONAL TACHYCARDIA

		Paroxysmal	Non-Paroxysmal
1.	Onset and Termination:	Sudden	Gradual
2.	Rate:	160-250/Min	70-130/Min
3.	Regularity:	Precisely Regular	± Regular (Tends to Fluctuate with Vagotonia)
4.	Carotid Sinus Massage:	Abrupt Termination or Nil	Nil
5.	QRS Contour and Duration:	Usually Normal	Usually Normal
6.	P Wave Contour:	Frequent Retrograde P'	Infrequent
7.	AV Dissociation	Uncommon (JR = AR)	Common (JR Frequently Greater AR, with Frequent Sinus Capture)
8.	Etiology:	Normals, WPW	Usually Heart Dis.—Digitalis, Acute M.I., Carditis, Post-Cardiac Surgery

JR = junctional rate
AR = atrial rate

quently is no underlying heart disease, and the therapy is identical to that outlined previously for PAT

Nonparoxysmal junctional tachycardia (NJT) has a gradual onset and termination[29,30]. A slower ventricular rate from 70-130 beats per minute is present, and there is generally no response to carotid sinus massage. AV dissociation is frequently present with a junctional rate faster than the atrial rate and no constant relationship of atrial activity to the R wave.

Nonparoxysmal junctional tachycardia (NJT) is usually an escape rhythm, secondary to bradyarrhythmias such as sinus bradycardia, sinoatrial block, or AV block. Circumstances commonly associated with NJT include digitalis toxicity, acute rheumatic fever, postoperative surgical patient, and early acute myocardial infarction. In the absence of acute myocardial infarction this arrhythmia is usually of little hemodynamic significance, so that specific antiarrhytmic treatment is rarely needed. When treatment is needed, it should be directed at the primary cause rather than towards the secondary NJT. In the presence of acute myocardial infarction, two papers have emphasized the increased mortality and poor prognosis of NJT, especially in the presence of anterior wall infarction and faster ventricular rates[31,32]. If the infarction is localized to the inferior wall, Fishenfeld et al reported a much lower mortality since 23 of 24 patients survived[32]. If a patient with chronic atrial fibrillation on digitalis therapy presents with a regular ventricular rate, AV junctional rhythm is a strong possibility. Therefore, not only is a slow ventricular response less than 60 per minute a sign of digitalis excess in atrial fibrillation, but the clinician should also be on the alert for regularization of the ventricular rate.

VENTRICULAR TACHYCARDIA

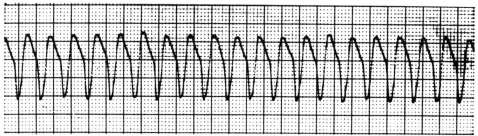

Figure 8   Ventricular tachycardia taken from a coronary care unit monitored strip. Wide QRS complexes are seen without visible atrial activity. Although a supraventricular tachycardia with aberrant ventricular conduction cannot be excluded, the patient promptly responded to intravenous lidocaine therapy, plus the QRS contour was the same as previous isolated premature ventricular contractions.

Ventricular tachycardia is defined as three or more successive beats of ventricular origin at a rate greater than 100 beats per minute. The ECG diagnosis of ventricular tachycardia is based upon: (1) wide QRS complexes equal or greater than 0.12 seconds; (2) AV dissociation, although discrete atrial activity is frequently not discernible; and (3) the presence of capture and/or fusion beats[10,33]. The ventricular rate is usually 150-200 beats per minute. Fusion beats are uncommon unless the ventricular rate is less than 150 per minute[34].

As emphasized by Schamroth, a purist can never make the diagnosis of ventricular tachycardia[10]. An argument can be brought against every diagnostic criterion. One of the most difficult problems in electrocardiographic diagnosis is the separation of ventricular tachycardia from supraventricular tachycardia with aberrant ventricular conduction. Table VI lists some helpful guidelines in this differential diagnosis[34-37].

Physical examination may assist in the diagnosis of ventricular tachycardia[34]. With complete AV dissociation, which occurs around 80% of the time, inspection of the neck veins may reveal intermittent cannon waves. Auscultation may give the impression of multiple sounds, due to wide splitting of heart sounds plus the presence of gallop sounds. Variable intensity of the first heart sound and a variable blood pressure by cuff measurement may be present. Ventricular tachycardia has no response to vagal stimulation, such as from carotid sinus massage.

Treatment of ventricular tachycardia depends upon the hemodynamic condition of the patient. Our overall approach to the treatment of ventricular tachycardia is outlined in Table VII. Generally the patient with

TABLE VI
FAVORING ABERRANT CONDUCTION

1. Preceding P wave
2. RBBB pattern
3. A triphasic rsR in lead V_1
4. Initial QRS vector looks like normally conducted beats
5. A good R in V_6 with qRs complex
6. Knowledge of pre-existing bundle branch block or WPW

FAVORING VENTRICULAR ECTOPY

1. Monophasic R in Lead V_1 or Diphasic R in V_1 with RR
2. rS or QS in V_6
3. Either all negative or all positive QRS complexes from V_1-V_6
4. Different initial QRS vector for PVC and normally conducted beats
5. Bigeminy with fixed coupling
6. Fusion beats
7. Escape beats
8. Parasystole

ventricular tachycardia is in serious hemodynamic straits and needs immediate electrical defibrillation. If the patient is in minimal distress, a trial of intravenous lidocaine is indicated[33]. A lidocaine bolus of 50-100 mg should be given IV, followed by a bolus of 100 mg every 5-10 minutes to a total of approximately 450 mg in the first hour. Successful conversion with lidocaine should be followed by an intravenous drip of 1-4 mg per minute. Oral suppressive therapy with procainamide or quinidine should also be introduced, with a plan to eventually discontinue intravenous medication. medication.

TABLE VII
TREATMENT OF VENTRICULAR TACHYCARDIA

1. Unstable patient—defibrillate immediately
2. Lidocaine: 1 mg/kg IV push
3. Procainamide: 100 mg IV slowly, repeat every 5 min., to maximum dose 1.0 gm.
4. Potassium: 1-4 mEq/min. IV (primarily postop cardiac patients with intracardiac pacemaker)
5. Dilantin®: 200-250 mg IV slowly
6. Propranolol: 1-5 mg IV slowly
7. (Bretylium — not available for use in U.S.A.)
8. Transvenous pacemaker: overdrive suppression
9. Exclude contributory correctable causes, such as ventricular aneurysm, digitalis excess, hypokalemia, etc.

If intravenous lidocaine is unsuccessful, procainamide should next be tried. This is given as a slow 100 mg bolus, followed by repetitive doses up to a maximum dose of 1.0 gm[38]. We do not recommend the intravenous use of quinidine. Intravenous Dilantin® is rarely successful unless digitalis intoxication is present. If there is reason to suspect excessive digitalis, then an intravenous potassium infusion should be started, and intravenous Dilantin® 200-250 mg given slowly may be successful. Intravenous propranolol up to a maximum dose of 5 mg may also be useful, either with or without digitalis toxicity. Bretylium still has not been approved by the Federal Drug Administration for clinical use. If the patient is unresponsive to all the above medications, then a therapeutic trial of overdrive suppression with an artificial pacemaker is indicated[33,39]. The lower the rate of the artificial pacemaker required to suppress the arrhythmia, the better the prognosis. If the patient does not respond to attempted overdrive suppression, the prognosis is grim. An aggressive evaluation with left heart catheterization and left ventriculography may be indicated to exclude a potential source for the intractable ventricular tachycardia, such as a left ventricular aneurysm. Resection of a left ventricular aneurysm for intractable ventricular tachycardia has had variable success, but potentially may be curable[40,41].

A patient presenting with ventricular tachycardia deserves a thorough evaluation following stabilization. When ventricular tachycardia is present, the patients almost always have significantly diseased hearts, with 75% being secondary to ischemic heart disease and 15% associated with rheumatic heart disease. The remaining 10% encompass a wide variety of cardiac conditions, including even apparent perfect health[42,43].

For the maintenance therapy of ventricular tachycardia, we generally prefer oral quinidine over procainamide. The two drugs have identical electrophysiologic effects, but we are more concerned about the potential side effect of procainamide-induced lupus syndrome[44], especially if used on a long term basis. If the patient has presented with acute myocardial infarction and ventricular tachycardia or fibrillation, we would continue the oral quinidine for a minimum of three months as an outpatient. At that point a complete reevaluation would be necessary including a treadmill exercise test and Holter monitoring[33]. If the Holter monitor documents recurrent ventricular irritability and/or the treadmill precipitates excessive ventricular irritability, then oral suppressive therapy should be maintained indefinitely.

Extrasystolic ventricular tachycardia is the most common form of ventricular tachycardia. The discussion to this point has primarily pertained to extrasystolic form. However, two other forms of ventricular tachycardia are possible: parasystolic ventricular tachycardia and accelerated ventricular rhythm[10]. Parasystolic ventricular tachycardia is much less common than the extrasystolic variety. The parasystolic focus is notoriously difficult to treat, has a slower ventricular response, and causes less severe hemodynamic derangement.

Accelerated ventricular rhythm has a gradual onset and offset of the arrhythmia with a rate of 60-100 beats per minute[45]. Frequent ventricular fusion beats are seen and the duration is frequently quite brief, i.e., 4-30 beats. Usually the vital signs are unchanged and this arrhythmia is seen most commonly in a stable patient with acute inferior wall myocardial infarction. The patient is frequently doing well clinically and there is no need to use suppressive therapy with intravenous lidocaine or defibrillation. Usually the arrhythmia will disappear spontaneously, although the patient should have continued cautious observation[46].

VENTRICULAR FIBRILLATION

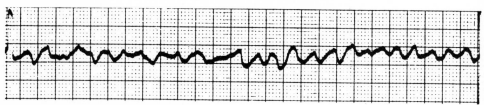

Figure 9 Ventricular fibrillation.

Ventricular fibrillation occurring in the absence of terminal heart disease can be treated with good results. Unlike previous arrhythmias there is no spectrum to this disease. The chaotic wavering baseline seen on the ECG accurately reflects the random firing of small areas of myocardium. Without rapid intervention it is uniformly fatal. Cardiopulmonary resuscitation and electrical defibrillation should be initiated immediately. Prognosis is directly proportional to the skill and speed of the cardiopulmonary resuscitation team.

Because of the frequency of encounters with tachyarrhythmias, descriptions of the most commonly seen tachyarrhythmias and the clinical approaches for the treatment of patients with these conditions have been considered here for easy reference by the busy physician.

References

1. Hurst, J.W., Logue, R.B., Schlant, R.C., and Wenger, N.K.: *The Heart.* McGraw-Hill Book Co., New York, 1974.
2. McIntosh, H.D. and Morris, J.J.: The hemodynamic consequences of arrhythmias. *Prog. Cardiovasc. Dis.,* **8**: 330, 1966.
3. Skinner, N.S., Mitchell, J.H., Wallace, A.G., and Sarnoff, S.J.: Hemodynamic effects of altering the timing of atrial systole. *Am. J. Physiol.,* **205**: 499, 1963.
4. Graettinger, J.S., Carleton, R.A., and Muenster, J.J.: Circulatory consequences of changes in cardiac rhythm produced in patients by transthoracic direct-current shock. *J. Clin. Invest.,* **43**: 2290, 1964.
5. Oram, S., Davis, J.P.M., Weinbren, L., Taggert, P., and Kitchen, L.D.: Conversion of atrial fibrillation to sinus rhythm by direct-current shock. *Lancet,* **2**: 159, 1963.
6. Lister, J.W., Klotz, D.H., Jomain, S.L., et al: Effect of pacemaker site on cardiac output and ventricular activation in dogs with complete heart block. *Am. J. Cardiol.,* **14**: 494, 1964.
7. Corday, E. and Irving, D.W.: *Disturbances in Heart Rate, Rhythm and Conduction.* W.B. Saunders Co., Philadelphia, 1964.
8. DeSanctis, R.W., Block, P., and Hutter, A.M.: Tachyarrhythmias in myocardial infarction. *Circulation,* **45**: 681, 1972.
9. Bigger, J.T. and Goldreyer, B.N.: The mechanism of supraventricular tachycardia. *Circulation,* **42**: 673, 1970.

10. Schamroth, L.: *The Disorders of Heart Rhythm*. Blackwell Scientific Publications, London, 1971.
11. Scherf, D.: Studies on auricular tachycardia caused by aconitine administration. *Proc. Exper. Biol. Med.*, **64**: 233, 1947.
12. Marshall, R.J. and Shepard, J.T.: *Cardiac Function in Health and Disease*. W.B. Saunders Co., Philadelphia, 1968, p. 110.
13. Friedberg, C.K.: *Diseases of the Heart*, 3rd Edition. W.B. Saunders Co., Philadelphia, 1966, p. 520.
14. Forker, A.D. and Wilson, C.S.: Congestive heart failure: a new iatrogenic epidemic propranolol induced. *J. Kansas Med. Soc.*, Feb. 1974, p. 33.
15. Smith, T.W. and Haber, E.: Digitalis. *N. Engl. J. Med.*, **289**: 945, 1010, 1063, 1125, 1973.
16. Lindsay, J. and Hurst, J.W.: The clinical features of atrial flutter and their therapeutic implications. *Chest*, **66**: 114, 1974.
17. Zipes, D.P.: The clinical application of cardioversion. In *Cardiovascular Clinics: Arrhythmias*. F.A. Davis, Philadelphia, 1970, p. 248.
18. Castellanos, A., Gosselin, A., and Fonseca, E.J.: Evaluation of countershock treatment of atrial flutter, with special reference to arrhythmias related to this procedure. *Arch. Intern. Med.*, **115**: 426, 1965.
19. Zeft, H.J., Cobb, F.R., Waxman, M.B., Hunt, N.C., and Morris, J.J.: Right atrial stimulation in the treatment of atrial flutter. *Ann. Intern. Med.*, **70**: 447, 1969.
20. DeSanctis, R.W.: Diagnostic and therapeutic uses of atrial pacing. *Circulation*, **43**: 748, 1971.
21. Nohara, Y.: The basic diseases underlying arrhythmias with special reference to its pathogenesis. *Jap. Circ. J.*, **26**: 203, 1962.
22. Jelliffe, R.W. and Brooker, G.: A nomogram for digoxin therapy. *Am. J. Med.*, **57**: 63, 1974.
23. Resnekov, L.: Present status of electroversion in the management of cardiac dysrhythmias. *Circulation*, **47**: 1356, 1973.
24. Doherty, J.E.: Digitalis glycosides: pharmacokinetics and their clinical implications. *Ann. Intern. Med.*, **79**: 229, 1973.
25. Lown, B., Kleiger, L., and Williams, J.: Cardioversion and digitalis drugs: changed threshold to electric shock in digitalized animals. *Circ. Res.*, **17**: 519, 1965.
26. Corliss, R.J. et al: Hemodynamic effects after conversion of arrhythmias. *J. Clin. Invest.*, **47**: 1779, 1968.
27. DeMaria, A.N., Lies, J.E., King, J.F., Muller, R.R., Amsterdam, E.A., and Mason, D.T.: Echocardiographic assessment of atrial transport, mitral movement, and ventricular performance following electroversion of supraventricular arrhythmias. *Circulation*, **51**: 273, 1975.
28. Shine, K.I., Kastor, J.A., and Yurchak, P.M.: Multifocal atrial tachycardia. Clinical and electrical cardiographic features in 32 patients. *N. Engl. J. Med.*, **279**: 344, 1968.
29. Rothfeld, E.L. and Voorman, D.M.: The ailing A-V junction. *Heart and Lung*, **4**: 909, 1975.
30. Rosen, K.M.: Junctional tachycardia. Mechanisms, differential diagnosis, and management. *Circulation*, **47**: 654, 1973.
31. Konecke, L.L. and Knoebel, S.B.: Nonparoxysmal junctional tachycardia complicating acute myocardial infarction. *Circulation*, **45**: 367, 1972.
32. Fishenfeld, J., Desser, K.B., and Benchimol, A.: Nonparoxysmal A-V junctional tachycardia associated with acute myocardial infarction. *Am. Heart J.*, **86**: 754, 1973.
33. Lown, B., Temte, J.V., and Arter, W.J.: Ventricular tachyarrhythmias: clinical aspects. *Circulation*, **47**: 1364, 1973.

34. Marriott, H.J.L. and Myerburg, R.J.: Recognition and treatment of cardiac arrhythmias and conduction disturbances. In J.W. Hurst and R.B. Logue (Eds.): *The Heart*, 3rd Edition. McGraw-Hill, New York, 1974, p. 532.
35. Sandler, I.A. and Marriott, H.J.L.: The differential morphology of anomalous ventricular complexes of RBBB-Type in lead V_1. Ventricular ectopy v.s. aberration. *Circulation*, **31**: 551, 1965.
36. Marriott, H.J.L. and Sandler, I.A.: Criteria, old and new, for differentiating between ectopic ventricular beats and aberrant ventricular conduction in the presence of atrial fibrillation. *Prog. Cardiovasc. Dis.*, **9**: 18, 1966.
37. Zipes, D.P. and Fisch, C.: Superventricular arrhythmia with abnormal QRS complex. *Arch. Intern. Med.*, **129**: 993, 1972.
38. Giardina, E.V., Heissenbuttel, R.H., and Bigger, J.T.: Intermittent intravenous procaine amide to treat ventricular arrhythmias. *Ann. Intern. Med.*, **78**: 183, 1973.
39. Zipes, D.P. and Nicoll, A.: Therapeutic approach to the patient with a hard to control ventricular arrhythmia. *Heart and Lung*, **3**: 57, 1974.
40. Graham, A.F., Miller, D.C., Stinson, E.B., Daily, P.O., Fogarty, T.J., and Harrison, D.C.: Surgical treatment of refractory life-threatening ventricular tachycardia. *Am. J. Cardiol.*, **32**: 909, 1973.
41. Kenaan, G., Mendez, A.M., Zubiate, P., Gray, R., and Kay, J.H.: Surgery for ventricular tachycardia unresponsive to medical treatment. *Chest*, **64**: 574, 1973.
42. Lesch, M., Lewis, E., Humphries, J.O., and Ross, R.S.: Paroxysmal ventricular tachycardia in the absence of organic heart disease. *Ann. Intern. Med.*, **66**: 950, 1967.
43. Forker, A., Wilson, C., and Weaver, W.: Exercise-induced "benign" paroxysmal ventricular tachycardia with normal coronary arteries. *Nebraska Med. J.*, October, 1973.
44. Donlan, J. and Forker, A.: Cardiac tamponade in procaine amide-induced lupus erythematosus. *Chest*, **61**: 685, 1972.
45. Rothfeld, E.L., Zucker, I.R., Parsonnet, V., and Alinsonorin, C.A.: Idioventricular rhythm in acute myocardial infarction. *Circulation*, **37**: 203, 1968.
46. Soyza, N., Bissett, J.K., Kane, J.J., Murphy, M.L., and Doherty, J.E.: Association of accelerated idioventricular rhythm and paroxysmal ventricular tachycardia in acute myocardial infarction. *Am. J. Cardiol.*, **34**: 667, 1974.

CHAPTER 15

Diagnostic and Therapeutic Uses for Cardiac Pacing (Bradyarrhythmias and Heart Block)

Helen Starke, M.D.; William P. Nelson, M.D.;
Robert S. Eliot, M.D.

Bradyarrhythmias, tachyarrhythmias, and conduction disturbances cause many unnecessary deaths. Their control has been immeasurably assisted by the development of electrical pacing systems that can be implanted temporarily or permanently. In addition, the use of pacing to assess the potential instabilities of electrical impulse formation and conduction has helped to prevent recurrent cardiac disasters and has led to new prophylactic clinical capabilities. This chapter reviews the circumstances in which the diagnostic and therapeutic applications of pacemakers may be beneficial.

Although experiments concerning electrical stimulation of the heart date to 1884, the first application was not until 1952. Clinical use of pacemakers began in 1960 when implantable forms became available. The procedure is now widely available and insertion is relatively easily and quickly accomplished. In most centers transvenous introduction of a pacing catheter with endocardial stimulation has removed the need for thoracotomy and epicardial electrode placement. Engineering advances have increased the electrical safety, potential utility, and projected life of the units. Early problems with battery and component failure of the power generator, and with fracture of the leads, have largely been eliminated. Additional experience and improved techniques of insertion have minimized the complications of infection, pacing catheter dislodgement, and cardiac perforation.

When serious disturbances of electrical impulse formation and/or conduction occur, pacemakers have been convincingly demonstrated to:

1. save lives in the acute situation,
2. prolong life in chronic circumstances,
3. enhance the quality of life and improve organ function.

Their use may be *temporary* or *permanent*. Power generators may have a *fixed* discharge rate or, more frequently, be designed to function *"on demand"* when critical rate slowing occurs and to be *"reset"* when ectopic activity disrupts a regular mechanism.

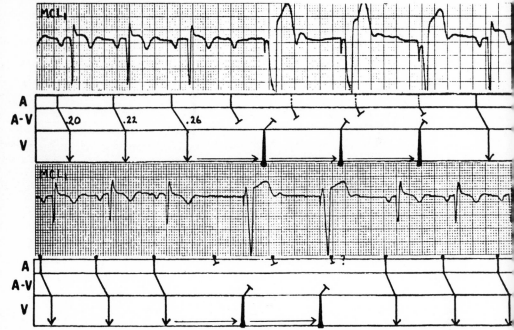

Figure 1 The function of a "demand" pacemaker is illustrated. Its "escape interval" has been set at 1.20 seconds and delays in ventricular activation greater than this interval will allow the electronic pacemaker to function. In the top rhythm strip its emergence is prompted by disturbed impulse *conduction* (Wenckebach (Type I) AV block); and in the lower strip by abnormal impulse *formation* (sinoatrial arrest or exit block).

Electrical pacemakers may be utilized for diagnostic purposes or to achieve predictable stimulation when there is default of intrinsic impulse formation or disturbed conduction. Indications for their use can be grouped as follows:

I. *Diagnostic pacing*
    1. Pacemaker stress testing for ischemic heart disease and evaluation of left ventricular dysfunction;
    2. His bundle electrography;
    3. Right atrial pacing to determine AV junction, bundle branch, and sinoatrial (SA) node disease;
    4. Evaluation of the preexcitation syndrome;
    5. Assessment of remaining conduction pathways in the presence of bilateral bundle branch block.

II. *Therapeutic pacing*
    1. Bradyarrhythmias with intact atrioventricular conduction;
        A. Sinus bradycardia
        B. Sinus arrest or block
        C. "Bradycardia-tachycardia syndrome"
        D. During coronary angiography

2. AV block;
   A. First degree AV block
   B. Second degree AV block
      i. Wenkebach (type I) AV block
      ii. Mobitz (type II) AV block
   C. Third degree AV block
   D. High grade AV block

3. Fascicular blocks;
   A. Acute bifascicular block during myocardial infarction
   B. Incomplete or intermittent trifascicular block

4. Tachyarrhythmias;
   A. Atrial tachycardia and atrial flutter
   B. Ventricular premature beats and recurrent ventricular tachycardia

Most emergency applications entail "therapy" rather than "diagnosis" and only brief mention will be made of their use for the latter indication. However, since cardiac pacing may help clarify situations likely to eventuate in sudden and serious dysrhythmias, it is relevant to have some understanding of its use in diagnosis.

I. *Diagnostic pacing*

1. *Pacemaker stress testing for ischemic heart disease and evaluation of left ventricular dysfunction.* Atrial pacing is a means of "stress testing" for ischemic heart disease. The increase in heart rate increases the myocardial oxygen demand and at the same time decreases the diastolic interlude for coronary artery perfusion of the myocardium. The pacing catheter is positioned high in the right atrium and the rate is increased in increments of 10 beats per minute every 3 minutes. Shifts of the ST segment, chest pain, or both may develop; the pacing can be terminated abruptly if this occurs. Electrocardiographic evaluation is similar to that used in exercise stress testing. The immediate slowing of the heart rate by turning off the pacemaker is an advantage that exercise stress testing does not offer. Cardiovascular physiology occurring in atrial pacing is not the same as in exercise however, and the technique has limited applications. When there is impaired left ventricular function, pacing to faster rates may demonstrate this by causing an elevation in left ventricular diastolic pressure or left atrial pressure. This can occur in patients with coronary artery disease or primary myocardial disease.

2. *His bundle electrography.* His bundle electrograms, in conjunction with atrial pacing, have diagnostic value and are of clinical, therapeutic, and prognostic significance. In general, abnormalities in the AV node have a better prognosis than those below the His bundle in the His-Purkinje system.

A multipolar catheter is inserted across the tricuspid valve and multiple intervals are measured. (A second catheter is placed in the low right atrium if PA and AH intervals are to be recorded or pacing studies are to be undertaken.)

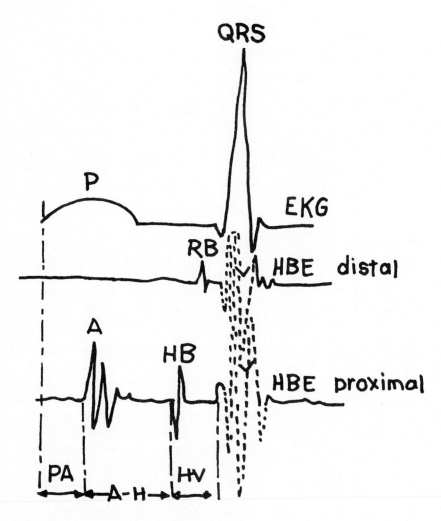

Figure 2 His Bundle Recording (See Text).

The PA interval represents the time of conduction from the high right atrium (P) to the low right atrium (A). The normal range is 25-56 msec.

The AH interval is the time from the first rapid deflection of (A) to that of the His bundle (H). It represents conduction time from the low right atrium to the His bundle. The normal range is 60-140 msec.

The HV time is the interval from the His bundle deflection to the earliest onset of ventricular depolarization (V). It represents conduction time from the His bundle, through the Purkinje system, to the ventricles. The normal range varies from 35 to 55 msec.

Sometimes the RBV interval (right bundle branch to ventricular activation) can be obtained. The normal range is 20-25 msec. In order not to confuse H and RB recordings, it is desirable to pace through the electrode recording the spike between atrial and ventricular potentials. If the QRS complexes assume the configuration of LBBB, the right bundle branch is being paced and, therefore, the RB deflection is being recorded.

Utilization of His bundle studies is referred to throughout subsequent sections in this chapter where this procedure has been found helpful. In brief, recording of His bundle electrograms may be warranted in the following situations:

1. Second degree, or complete AV block,
2. Intraventricular conduction defects (bifascicular and trifascicular blocks especially when accompanied by first degree AV block),
3. AV block or intraventricular conduction defects in acute myocardial infarction,
4. Preexcitation syndrome.

Only those situations that require relatively prompt evaluations are discussed.

3. *Right atrial pacing to determine AV junction, bundle branch, and sinoatrial (SA) node disease.* Sometimes right atrial pacing is carried out while His bundle recordings are being made in order to test the integrity of the conduction system between the atria and ventricles. Normally with increasing rates of atrial pacing, the AH time prolongs and Wenckebach AV block may occur. But with a pathologic AV junction, conduction time prolongs excessively and AV block may result above the His bundle at slower rates and will not improve with atropine.

Pacing may rarely produce prolongation of HV time in patients with latent or overt bundle branch disease, or may induce 2° or 3° AV block.

Pacing also permits evaluation of the SA node recovery time. Pacing at 120 beats/minute for three minutes produces overdrive suppression of the SA node. When pacing ceases, the SA node function should resume at an interval less than 550 msec plus the inherent prepacing interval. Failure to do this implies an abnormality of SA node automaticity or conduction to the atrium (provided that drug effects and autonomic nervous system factors are ruled out).

4. *Evaluation of the preexcitation syndrome.* Right atrial pacing is sometimes used when a patient has had recurrent bouts of paroxysmal atrial tachycardia and has a normal electrocardiogram. As the rate of pacing is increased there is prolongation of AV conduction time (AH), but the conduction time through an accessory pathway may not be similarly affected and the QRS abnormality of WPW may then become apparent.

5. *Assessment of remaining conduction pathways in the presence of bilateral bundle*

branch block. In patients who have bifascicular block, the integrity of the third fascicle can be tested by pacing the right atrium at rapid rates. (For example, a patient who has RBBB and left anterior fascicular block may, with such a rate challenge, develop complete block distal to the His bundle spike.) Any *symptomatic* patient (with lightheadedness, syncope, convulsions, etc.) with bifascicular block or unifascicular block and first degree AV block deserves His bundle and right atrial pacing studies.

II. *Therapeutic pacing*

Pacing for disturbed impulse formation or conduction can be either temporary or permanent. The choice of cardiac chamber to be paced depends upon the integrity of both the AV node and the infranodal conduction system. Pacing may be carried out for bradyarrhythmias or tachyarrhythmias.

1. *Bradyarrhythmias with intact AV conduction.* "Sick sinus node syndrome" is a term that includes symptomatic sinus bradycardia, sinoatrial block or arrest, and "the bradycardia-tachycardia syndrome."

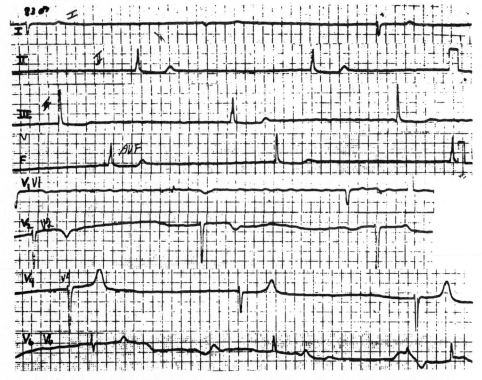

Figure 3 A striking example of a "sick sinus node syndrome". No atrial activity is demonstrable and the patient's average heart rate is 17 beats per minute. The lack of an adequate "escape" focus in the AV junction or ventricle is evident. Insertion of a permanent transvenous electronic pacemaker allowed this elderly man to resume his normal life and he is asymptomatic and active 3 years later.

A. *Sinus bradycardia.* Permanent pacing should be considered in a *symptomatic* patient with a heart rate below 60/min. The indication for pacing is often based on the clinical estimation of the patient's intolerance to a slow heart rate. Sinus node dysfunction is associated with an increased incidence of frequent premature contractions, dizziness, cardiac decompensation, syncope, and hypotension. Tape-recording monitoring is particularly helpful in correlating symptoms with ECG abnormalities. Atrial pacing for SA node recovery time may be helpful in clarifying the diagnosis and in evaluating AV conduction. Many patients with SA node disease have associated problems with AV junctional conduction and/or automaticity. If a disturbance in AV conduction is demonstrated, ventricular pacing in the demand mode is indicated; if AV conduction is normal, atrial pacing may be considered in preference to ventricular pacing. (Note: few centers have been successful with secure placement of the transvenous catheter in the atrium.)

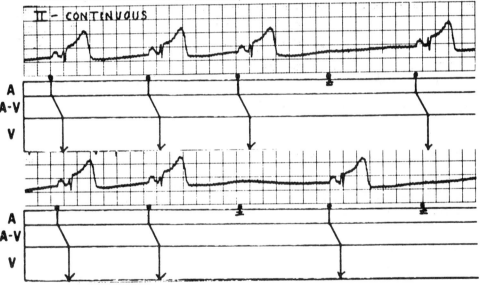

Figure 4 The ladder diagram depicts the electrocardiographic events in a young patient with an acute inferior wall myocardial infarction. Sinus bradycardia of 40 per minute is interrupted by two episodes of "sinoatrial exit-block" resulting in lengthy pauses. The sudden decrease in heart rate caused hypotension and recurrence of chest pain and justified the insertion of a temporary transvenous pacemaker.

B. *Sinoatrial arrest or block.* The symptoms of sinoatrial arrest or block are essentially the same as those due to sinus bradycardia. SA block may occur abruptly without emergence of a satisfactory "escape" pacemaker, resulting in marked bradycardia or lengthly periods of asystole. Insertion of a permanent demand type pacemaker is indicated.

C. *"Bradycardia-tachycardia syndrome"*. Sinus node dysfunction produces the bradycardia and sets the stage for the appearance of supraventricular

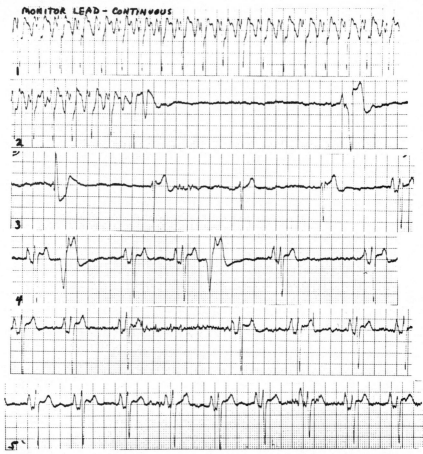

Figure 5 The problems for the patient with the "tachycardia-bradycardia syndrome" is evident in this continuous recording. The burden of a super-ventricular tachycardia in the top strip abruptly ceases and is exchanged for a marked bradycardia with the emergence of both unpredictable "escape" foci and premature ectopic depolarizations. Ultimately, a satisfactory atrial pacemaker appears, but the marked rate fluctuations provoked marked symptoms and many syncopal episodes.

tachyarrhythmias. Syncope is a common presenting complaint, but exercise intolerance, palpitations, and heart failure can also result when heart rates alternate between "too slow" and "too fast". Drug therapy alone has infrequently been successful in those patients. Management consists of the insertion of a permanent demand type pacemaker to control bradycardia and drug therapy to manage the tachyarrhythmias. While atrial pacing might be desirable, there is usually AV junctional disease present and ventricular pacing in the demand mode is recommended.

   D. *During coronary angiography.* A demand type temporary pacemaker is commonly used during coronary angiography because marked sinus bradycardia or even asystole may occur during the injection of contrast material. This is more apt to occur on injection of the right coronary artery since it supplies the SA node in 60% of subjects.

2. *Atrioventricular block.* Atrioventricular block may be caused by intrinsic disease of the conduction system or may be associated with drug therapy. It may be temporary or permanent, complete or incomplete. It may occur at different sites: (a) in the atrium, (b) in the region of the AV node, (c) in the His bundle, (d) in the bundle branches or, (e) the Purkinje system.

A. *First degree AV block.* Isolated prolongation of the PR interval does not require pacemaker therapy.

B. *Second degree AV block.*

1. Wenckebach (type I) AV block is generally a temporary phenomenon. It frequently occurs during the early stages of acute inferior wall myocardial infarction. Digitalis or quinidine excess is a frequent cause. The block is usually above the His bundle (so that narrow QRS complexes are seen) and is accompanied by a reasonably reliable junctional escape rhythm. It is often related to excessive vagal tone and may be responsive to atropine or isoproterenol. In a setting of myocardial infarction, Wenckebach block may require temporary pacing if it has prompted hypotension, low cardiac output, or heart failure, and if atropine or isoproterenol have not been effective.

2. Mobitz (type II) AV block, in contrast, occurs without the alert provided by progressive prolongation of PR intervals and thus is more treacherous than Wenckebach block. The block is usually below the His bundle and conducted impulses show a wide QRS complex. (Occasionally the block is in the His bundle and a narrow QRS complex is present.) When a beat is not conducted, transient complete bilateral bundle branch block may be implied. Subsidiary escape pacemakers are from slow idioventricular foci and are not dependable. Type II block frequently is associated with anterior wall myocardial infarction and, in this setting, should prompt insertion of a temporary pacemaker. If the patient resumes normal AV conduction, there is still debate as to the advisability of inserting a permanent pacemaker. We believe that a prolonged HV interval documented by His bundle electrogram before the patient is released from the hospital is an indication for permanent pacing. If type II AV block occurs in a *symptomatic* patient who is not having an acute myocardial infarction, a permanent demand type ventricular pacemaker is indicated. Because Mobitz block tends to be unstable with appreciable risk of asystole we recommend (as others do) that even the asymptomatic person should have a permanent pacemaker. However, hard data to support this position are not available.

C. *Third degree AV block*. In the setting of established complete AV
block, indications for pacemaker insertion include:
1. syncope,
2. heart failure,
3. low cardiac output which may be manifested by excessive fatigue,
   impaired cerebration (forgetfulness, etc.) or prerenal azotemia,
4. palpitations indicating instability of the escape pacemaker or the
   presence of competing ectopic foci. These frequently herald serious
   ventricular tachyarrhythmias.

Since the heart rate is constant and slow there is an increase in stroke
volume to achieve adequate cardiac output at rest; however, there is little
reserve and output cannot be appreciably augmented during physical activity. The majority of patients (about 80%) with *acquired* third degree AV
block have wide QRS complexes and the block is below the level of the His
bundle in most cases. In contrast patients with *congenital* AV block without
associated cardiac abnormalities usually have narrow QRS complexes and
the block is above the His bundle. Moreover, these patients frequently accelerate their ventricular rate by 20 or more beats per minute on exercise.
They rarely require pacing.

In general, it would seem that nearly all patients with chronic third degree
AV block should have a permanent demand type ventricular pacemaker.
Frequently "asymptomatic" older subjects find that their effort tolerance
improves and they are more mentally alert when paced.

During myocardial infarction complete heart block complicates about 8%
of inferior wall and 2% of anterior wall infarctions. In *inferior* wall myocardial
infarction the level of block is usually in the AV node and the heart is driven
by an escape focus in the lower AV node or His bundle. The QRS is narrow
unless coexistent fascicular disease is present; the ventricular rate is 40-70
beats per minute; the pacemaker focus is stable; the block is usually temporary; and it is often preceded by first degree AV block and type I second
degree AV block so that its onset occurs gradually. The mortality in this setting is usually about 30%. A pacemaker is used only if there is instability of
the escape pacemaker or marked bradycardia which promotes ventricular irritability or hemodynamic derangement (hypotension, congestive failure, or
persisting myocardial ischemia evidenced by continuing or recurring chest
pain).

When complete heart block complicates *anterior* wall myocardial infarction, the infarct is usually large or there has been prior conduction disturbance. The block is below the AV node and both bundle branches are involved. The escape focus is in the distal conduction system. The QRS complexes are wide and the rate is slower (usually less than 40 beats per
minute). The pacemaker focus is frequently unstable leading to sudden and
variable periods of asystole. The onset of complete heart block may be
abrupt, but frequently the development of bifascicular block serves as a
warning. Despite pacemaker therapy, when complete heart block com-

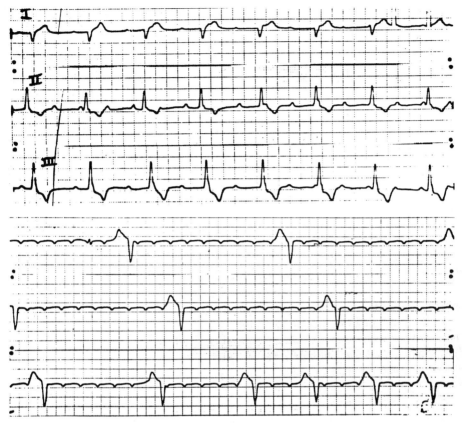

Figure 6 A & B is the electrocardiogram of a 48 year old man with acute anterior myocardial infarction and complete AV block. Panel A shows the complete dissociation of atrial and ventricular events. A complete tracing suggested that the site of origin of the focus responsible for ventricular activation was located in (or near) the left anterior fascicle; its rate stable and adequate at 55 per minute. Panel B provides a dramatic example of the unpredictable nature of such ventricular foci. Without an electrocardiographic (or clinical) alert, the pacemaker focus suddenly slows with a life threatening bradycardia resulting. This potential instability prompts the insertion of a "standby-demand" transvenous electronic pacemaker.

plicates anterior myocardial infarction the mortality approximates 80%, with death primarily related to the size of the infarction. However in many cases, pacing may improve cardiac output and decrease ischemia and ventricular irritability. If the patient survives, the block is apt to be permanent. Even if conduction does return, His bundle recordings are warranted. The finding of a prolonged HV time is ominous and serves to justify the insertion of a permanent pacemaker. It is important to emphasize that the prolongation of HV time can be present despite a normal PR interval in the surface electrocardiogram.

D. *High grade AV block*. High grade AV block includes an assortment of clinical and electrocardiographic pictures. An example might be a patient who has atrial fibrillation with a very slow, but somewhat irregular ventricular response. If he is receiving digitalis the drug should be discontinued. If the rate remains abnormally slow when the digitalis effect has dissipated, there is an inherent defect in AV conduction and pacemaker implantation is indicated. Then, if necessary, digitalis therapy can be reinstituted.

3. *Fascicular blocks*

A. *Acute bifascicular block occurring during myocardial infarction.* This is usually associated with a large anteroseptal myocardial infarction and often heralds complete AV block. If complete block occurs there is significant risk of ventricular asystole or ventricular fibrillation; therefore, as soon as bifascicular block is noted, many physicians would insert a temporary demand type ventricular pacemaker.

B. *Incomplete or intermittent trifascicular block.* This is a foreboding of complete bilateral bundle branch block. The following four conditions should prompt concern:
   1. RBBB and left anterior fascicular block with first degree AV block,
   2. RBBB and left posterior fascicular block with first degree AV block,
   3. LBBB with first degree AV block,
   4. alternating bundle branch block.
Any of these abnormalities is an indication for a temporary pacemaker, if it occurs acutely or if a patient is symptomatic.

If any of the above abnormalities are observed on a routine ECG or if it has been noted previously, the patient may benefit by having a His bundle recording to determine whether the first degree AV block is at the AV node or represents disease in the third fascicle. It would also be important to know whether drugs were responsible. Trifascicular disease has also been observed in some patients who electrocardiographically have only bifascicular block apparent (i.e., the PR interval is normal, but the HV time is prolonged). The prognostic significance of this observation remains to be clarified. Firm prognostic data for bifascicular block with a normal PR interval in a totally asymptomatic patient is being accumulated. At present, prophylactic pacing in the asymptomatic group is not recommended.

4. *Tachyarrhythmias*

A. *Atrial tachycardia and atrial flutter.* Usually DC shock is indicated in preference to pacing for these arrhythmias. However, in the presence of digitalis intoxication, a safer procedure is to pace the right atrium. The artificial pacemaker may be used to stimulate at a rate above the atrial rate (usually about 400/min) and overdrive the atrium. Alternately, the pacemaker discharge may be used to provide single or multiple stimuli intended to depolarize a reentry pathway and thus interrupt it, allowing resumption of normal sinoatrial activity. Atrial pacing successfully converts atrial flutter or paroxysmal atrial tachycardia to sinus rhythm in 50-75% of patients. Not uncommonly atrial fibrillation occurs, but it is found that in the next 24 hours it reverts to sinus rhythm in 50-75% of the patients. It should be noted that one cannot revert atrial fibrillation or an accelerated AV junctional focus (nonparoxysmal AV junctional tachycardia) by overdrive pacing.

B. *Ventricular premature beats and recurrent ventricular tachycardia.* When antiarrhythmic drugs and DC shock have not been successful in controlling these rhythm disturbances, temporary ventricular pacing may be tried, and the rate required to suppress ventricular ectopy established. Often this is only 10-20 beats faster than the patient's spontaneous rate, but on occasion may be higher. Only after careful observation for a period of time can the need for a permanent pacemaker be established.

The bibliography on the subjects covered in this chapter is exhaustive. We have elected to offer suggested reading which covers the contents in a comprehensive manner rather than to document original sources or isolated articles.

SUGGESTED READING

Complications of Pacing — #4, 7, 9, 11, 12, 21
Follow Up of Pacemakers — #6, 20, 21
General Reviews — #4, 12, 14, 20
His Bundle Recordings and Their Application — #2, 13, 16, 17, 18, 19
History of Pacing — #4
Pacemaker Stress Tests — #5
Pacing During Coronary Angiography — #5
Pacing in the Treatment of Tachyarrhythmias — #2, 3, 5
Permanent Atrial Pacing — #15
Prognosis — #10, 19
Temporary Use in Myocardial Infarction — #1, 3, 12, 13, 22
Use in AV Block — #10, 16
Use in Chronic Complete Heart Block — #4, 10
Use in Fascicular Blocks — #5, 10, 12, 17
Use in the "Sick Sinus Node" Syndrome — #3, 5, 8
Use in the Wolff-Parkinson-White Syndrome — #5, 18

READING LIST

1. Atkins, J.M., Leschin, S.J., Blomquist, G., and Mullins, C.B.: Ventricular conduction blocks and sudden death in acute myocardial infarction. *N. Engl. J. Med.*, **288**: 281, 1973.
2. Barold, S.S.: Therapeutic uses of cardiac pacing in tachyarrhythmias. *His Bundle electrocardiography and Clinical Electrophysiology*. F.A. Davis Co., Philadelphia, Pennsylvania, 1975.
3. Batchelder, J.F. and Zipes, D.P.: Treatment of tachyarrhythmias by pacing. *Arch. Intern. Med.*, **135**: 1115, 1975.
4. Chardack, W.M.: Cardiac Pacemakers and Heart Block. 2nd edition. In John H. Gibbon, Jr., David C. Sabiston, Jr., and Frank C. Spencer (Eds.): *Surgery of the Chest*, W.B. Saunders Co., Philadelphia, Pennsylvania, 1969, Chapter 38.

5. Cheng, T.O.: Atrial pacing: Its diagnostic and therapeutic applications. *Prog. in Cardiovascular Dis.*, **14**, (#2): 230, 1971.
6. Escher, D.J.: Follow up of the patient with an implanted cardiac pacemaker. *Mod. Concepts of Cardiovascular Disease*, **43**: 77, 1974.
7. Escher, D.J.: Types of pacemakers and their complications. *Circulation*, **42**: 1119, 1973.
8. Ferrer, M.I.: The Sick Sinus Syndrome. Futura Publishing Co., Mount Kisco, New York, 1974.
9. Grogler, F.M., Frank, G., Greven, G., et al: Complications of permanent transvenous cardiac pacing. *J. Thor. and Cardiovascular Surg.*, **69**: 895, 1975.
10. Kastor, J.A.: Atrioventricular Block. *N. Engl. J. Med.*, **292**: (two parts) 462, 572, 1975.
11. Kitchen, J.G., Ill and Kastor, J.A.: Pacing in acute myocardial infarction. Indications, methods, hazards, and results. *Cardiovascular Clinics*, **7** (2): 219, 1975.
12. Lemberg, L. and Castellanos, A.: Artificial Pacing. In Edward K. Chung, *Cardiac Emergency Care*. Lea and Febiger, Philadelphia, Pennsylvania, 1975, Chapter 10.
13. Lie, K.I., Wellens, H.J., Schuilenburg, R.M., Becker, A.E., and Durrer, D.: Factors influencing prognosis of bundle branch block complicating acute anteroseptal infarction. The value of His bundle recordings. *Circulation*, **50**: 935, 1974.
14. Lown, B. and Kosowsky, B.D.: Artificial cardiac pacemakers. *N. Engl. J. Med.*, **283**: (three parts) 907, 971, 1023, 1970.
15. Moss, A.J.: Therapeutic uses of permanent pervenous atrial pacemakers: A review. *J. Electrocardiology*, **8**: 373, 1975.
16. Narula, O.S.: Current concepts of atrioventricular block. *His Bundle Electrocardiography and Clinical Electrophysiology*. F.A. Davis Co., Philadelphia, Pennsylvania, 1975, Chapter 9.
17. Ibid. Narula, O.S.: Intraventricular conduction defects. Chapter 10.
18. Ibid. Narula, O.S.: Electrophysiologic evaluation of accessory conduction pathways. Chapter 15.
19. Ibid. Narula, O.S., Gann, D., and Samet, P.: Prognostic value of HV intervals. Chapter 20.
20. Parsonnet, V., Furman, S., and Smyth, N.P.: Implantable cardiac pacemakers: Status report and resource guideline. *Am. J. Card.*, **34**: 487, 1974.
21. Parsonnet, V.J., Myers, G.H., Gilbert, L., Zucker, I.R., and Shilling, E.: Follow up of implanted pacemakers. *Am. Heart J.*, **87**: 642, 1974.
22. Scheinman, M. and Brenman, B.: Clinical and anatomic implications of intraventricular conduction blocks in acute myocardial infarction. *Circulation*, **41**: 753, 1972.

CHAPTER 16
Defibrillators

Ward Chambers, M.D.; Robert A. Stratbucker, M.D., Ph.D.;
Barry Dzindzio, M.D.; Alan D. Forker, M.D.

Of the new therapeutic instruments the defibrillator has made the greatest contribution to reduced death toll in acute myocardial infarction. Remarkably it remains superficially understood at the clinical level. This readable Chapter identifies those characteristics of defibrillators that may enlighten its clinical use.

INTRODUCTION

Until the last 15-20 years, very little could be offered to those who fell victim to lethal tachyarrhythmias. With the development of closed chest cardio-pulmonary resucitation and the introduction of defibrillators, routine resuscitation of these patients became possible in the hospital environment. Recent studies have documented the survival rates of those resuscitated and the risk factors for refibrillation[1-3]. Many communities are now making these techniques available to patients with out-of-hospital arrests.

The techniques of both elective and emergency defibrillation have been well described elsewhere[4-6]. This chapter will concentrate on understanding the principles of defibrillation.

HISTORY

The study of fibrillation-defibrillation has its origins in the middle of the nineteenth century. Erickson was probably the first to describe ventricular fibrillation in 1842. Hoffa and Ludwig are credited with the first published report of ventricular fibrillation in 1850[7]. In dogs with open chests, they recorded the movements of the heart during external electrical stimulation. Occasionally, they noted the heart went into a rhythm they called "Flummerin" or fibrillation.

In 1874, Moritz Schiff reported the relationship of chloroform death and ventricular fibrillation in cats[7]. He also discovered that compressing the heart through the closed chest·terminated ventricular fibrillation. The first clinical observation was by MacWilliam in 1888. He opened the chest immediately after death of patients suspected of having heart disease and observed that the hearts were fibrillating[7]. From these observations over 2 centuries ago, much work continues to determine the mechanisms of fibrillation and how to prevent it.

The use of electrical current to defibrillate a heart is also quite old. In 1899, Prevost and Batelli[8,9] reported defibrillating dog hearts using both alternating (AC) current and a capacitor discharge. They were studying the effects of sinusoidal (45 Hz) voltage stimulation upon the heart and occasionally fibrillated it. They describe the events as follows:

> "One can in submitting the animal of which the heart has been put in fibrillary tremulations by a current of low tension, see the heart reestablish ventricular contraction if one submits the animal to a current of high tension."[9]

In addition, they discovered that by applying electrodes directly to the heart and discharging a capacitor directly into the electrodes, the hearts could also be defibrillated. They also observed the decreasing ability to convert hearts that had been fibrillating more than 15 seconds. Only with initial vigorous massage could they successfully defibrillate the heart. This, quite clearly, was a forerunner of present resuscitation techniques.

During the 1920's the power companies were concerned with the frequent accidental deaths of their employees by electrocution. Dr. W.B. Kouwenhover states:

> "In 1926 Dr. L.W. Lieb, Vice-President of Consolidated Edison of New York City, appealed to the Rockefeller Institute for help in reducing the high rate of electric fatalities. As a result of his request five investigations were started. They were conducted by Professor W.H. Howell of the School of Hygiene and Public Health at the Johns Hopkins University, Dr. H.B. Williams of Columbia University, Dr. W.G. MacCallum of the Johns Hopkins Medical School, Dr. Philip Drinker of the Harvard Engineering Committee and Dr. W.J.V. Osterhougt of the Rockefeller Institute Staff."[10]

Work began at Johns Hopkins in 1928. Dr. D.R. Hooker, a physiologist, Dr. O.R. Langworthy, a neurologist, and Dr. W.B. Kouwenhoven, an electrical engineer, were brought together to attack the problem. In 1933 this group published the results of their investigations[11,12]. They were able to defibrillate dogs with both open and closed chests if high voltage alternating current (60 Hz) was applied within 15 seconds.

Only sporadic reports appeared in the literature from the mid 1930's to 1947[13,14]. At that time, Dr. Claude Beck, a Cleveland surgeon, successfully defibrillated a patient by applying 60 Hz current directly on the heart[15]. He had previously successfully defibrillated the human heart, but the patients had not survived. Thereafter, open chest defibrillation became a standard procedure.

This method had the obvious disadvantage of requiring surgical exposure of the heart. Work was intensified to successfully defibrillate the human heart through the closed chest. Several groups were actively working on this problem, including Kouwenhoven and Dr. P.M. Zoll, a cardiologist. Zoll became the first person to externally fibrillate the human heart in 1956[16,17]. He preceded Kouwenhoven by about 6 months.

Although alternating current had been exclusively used clinically for defibrillation, other waveforms were to be extensively studied. Superceding the sinusoidal waveform in efficiency and popularity was the direct current

(DC) or capacitor discharge waveform. In 1962, Dr. B. Lown introduced the DC fibrillator as a new method for converting cardiac arrhythmias[18,19]. Other DC waveforms have been introduced since 1962. The comparative merits of each will be discussed separately. Excellent reviews of the history of defibrillation have been recently published[20,21].

GENERAL PRINCIPLES

Much controversy exists over what constitutes the ideal defibrillator design. In its operation, a defibrillator should (1) be reliable and effective, (2) minimize post-shock myocardial damage, (3) have a low incidence of post-shock arrhythmias, especially for elective cardioversion, and (4) be safe to use. Certain obstacles, such as the inability of the scientific community to agree on which of the several waveform parameters are key factors in determining defibrillator efficency, have delayed the development of the ideal defibrillator. Much of this difficulty centers around the obvious problem of conducting human experiments in numbers adequate to achieve statistical significance.

It must be emphasized, however, that the present defibrillators are effective. The question of optimum performance is yet to be settled. Areas such as waveform analysis, optimal current and energy, electrode size, myocardial damage, and the relative inability to defibrillate heavy subjects provide fields for continuing investigation.

Presently manufactured defibrillators operate more or less as voltage devices; that is, they store a certain voltage on a capacitor and discharge this energy into the thorax and heart. This voltage, impressed across the tissue by means of metallic electrodes, causes a current to flow in the tissue when the operate switch is closed. Ignoring losses within the machine itself, the peak magnitude of this current depends upon two variables: (1) the magnitude of the stored voltage and (2) the chest wall resistance. The current flow is related to the voltage by Ohm's Law: V (voltage) = I (current) x R (resistance). The higher the stored voltage or the lower the chest resistance, the larger the current flow.

Calibration

Defibrillators are not calibrated in voltage or amperes, but in units of total discharge energy. Such units are known as joules or watt-seconds, since the two units are equivalent. For a particular shock, Energy $= \int_{0}^{t} I(t) V(t) \, dt$, that is, the integral of current times voltage. The use of energy as a measure of effectiveness originated with the studies by Mackay and Leeds[22]. Since then, several authors have shown that this probably is not true[23-25]. It appears that a minimum of uniform current flow through the heart for a minimum of time is necessary for successful defibrillation. It is also known that the larger the heart, the greater the current density necessary. This relationship of current magnitude and current duration is similar to the familiar strength-duration stimulation curves for nerve and skeletal muscle (See Figure 1). Below a certain optimum pulse duration, high levels of current are needed for successful defibrillation. Although current density in the region of the heart may be a more important determinant of defibrillator success than is energy, the latter may be more important in myocardial damage or post-shock arrhythmias.

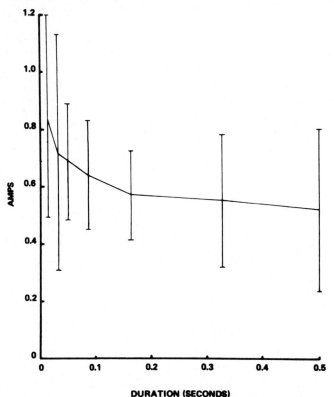

Figure 1 Current-duration relationship for ventricular defibrillation with 60 Hz sinusoidal alternating current applied to the ventricles of 11-24 Kg dogs. (From Witzel, D., Gettes, L.S., McFarlane, J., et al: The influence of cycle frequency on the effectiveness of electrical defibrillation of the canine ventricles. *Cardiovasc. Res. Cent. Bull.*, **5**: 112-118, 1967, with permission.)

Chest Wall Resistance

Another important variable is chest wall resistance. Chest resistance is determined by many variables, not all of which are completely understood. Chest resistance varies with chest size, thoracic configuration[26], voltage level[27], voltage frequency[27], electrode size and position[28], and the nature of the electrode-skin interface[28]. Using standard defibrillator paddles, 9 cm in diameter, placed in either the anterior-anterior or anterior-posterior position, the resistance during a defibrillator shock is most affected by body size and the skin-electrode interface. The resistance using the anterior-posterior configuration is slightly less than with the anterior-anterior position. Stratbucker and Chambers first reported the measurement of thoracic resistance on human subjects during countershock[29]. Their first patient had a measured resistance of approximately 50 ohms. This work has been expanded by others, and now it is known that in most adults, chest resistance falls into the 40-150 ohm range, with the average being nearer the lower figure[26,30].

Also, chest resistance is not constant, but falls significantly with repeated shocks[31,32]. First reported by Stratbucker and Chambers in humans, this phenomenon has recently been well documented in animals by Geddes. Miles and Chambers presented data from humans showing resistance drops of up to 50% between the first and second consecutive shocks during elective cardioversion. This fall appears to level off after the third shock[31].

Geddes el al have recently pointed out a problem in defibrillation of heavy subjects. They noted, in a retrospective study, that successful defibrillation of patients who weigh over 100 kgms is uncommon[33]. They tested this hypothesis in animals and found a linear relationship between animal weight (and thus heart weight) and energy needed for defibrillation[34]. This study was conducted using the Gurvish-Lown type waveform. It would appear that defibrillators currently on the market utilizing the Gurvich-Lown waveform are not adequate to effectively defibrillate patients over 100 kgms. Similar statements concerning the trapezoidal waveform can be made[34], but the exact linear relationship has not been experimentally determined.

Electrodes

As previously noted, it takes a minimum level of uniform current through the heart for a minimum of time for defibrillation. This is a function not only of the current delivered by the defibrillator, but of electrode size, placement and condition of the interface. Rush et al theoretically estimated the current distribution for different electrode positions[35]. In general, the current distribution can be assumed to be fusiform between the paddles. It is estimated that 20-45% of the total current passes through the heart when the paddles are placed in optimum positions[21]. Experimentally, one paddle over the apex and one in the area of the upper sternum results in the highest cardiac current density[36]. If the paddles are placed on the lateral chest wall, the energy needed for defibrillation is doubled[36].

Electrode size and interface have also been found to be important. Recent studies in dogs have shown that an optimal paddle size exists, and deviation from this size decreases effectiveness[37]. The optimum paddle size for humans has not been determined. Electrolytic pastes provide a much better interface for paddles than a metal-skin alone as reflected by lower chest resistance[38]. The effects of the different pastes, creams, and pads on effectiveness for human defibrillation are not known. There have not been any convincing studies published at this time comparing the differences.

Myocardial Damage

A major concern is myocardial damage from excessive energy or repeated countershocks. Several excellent animal studies with microscopic examination of the heart have been reported[38-40]. At levels of one ampere per kilogram there was no histologic damage seen under microscopic examination. At higher levels increasing damage was seen. Ewy et al recently reported that paddle size and time between shocks affected myocardial damage[38]. Small paddles and repeated shocks more often than every three minutes increased myocardial damage. Again, exact recommendations for humans are not possible. Sobel et al[41], have shown that at energy levels used in elective cardioversion, CPK isoenzyme analysis did not indicate myocardial damage. The ideal situation would be to determine chest resistance prior to defibrillation, and then select current levels that would be highly effective and yet minimize myocardial damage. The state of the art has not advanced that far.

Defibrillation Threshold

One of the newer and more exciting areas is the study of the effects of drugs upon the defibrillation threshold. It is well known that hypoxia and acidosis make defibrillation more difficult. Myocardial infarction has also been shown to increase defibrillation threshold. Tacker et al have recently shown that IV ouabain decreases the defibrillation threshold up to 30% in non-toxic doses[42]. If the animals survived toxic doses, the threshold was decreased by 66% at 20 minutes, but rose toward control levels thereafter. Others have shown the danger of elective cardioversion in digitalized patients. The differences may be accounted for by the short term nature of the ouabain experiments. How these relate to chronic digitalis administration is unknown. Nevertheless, these are important observations and should be expanded to other clinically useful cardiac drugs.

Animal Experimental Studies

A final note of caution should be expressed in evaluating experimental defibrillation studies. The extrapolation of the exact results of animal studies to human use should be discouraged. Trends certainly are apparent from animal studies, but numerical results are simply not applicable. Man and experimental animals (particularly dogs) have grossly different body configurations that make great differences in density distribution. In addition, dogs have 2-3 times greater chest wall resistance per kilogram than humans. These and other variables prevent the quantitative application of animal results.

Defibrillator Wave Forms

Many waveforms, as shown in Figure 2, have been used clinically at one time or another.

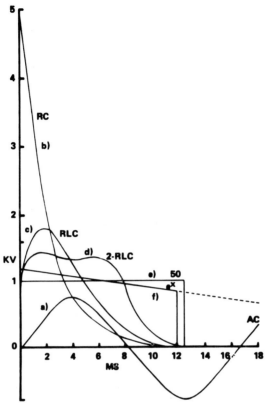

Figure 2 Different waveforms used for ventricular defibrillation. (a) alternating current, (b) capacitor discharge, (c) capacitor-inductor discharge, (d) delay line, (e) square wave, (f) trapazondal or exponential. (From Hagan, W.: Defibrillation techniques. *Medical Electronics and Data*, July/August, 1972, with permission.)

AC Defibrillators

The obvious areas of concern are current level, frequency and duration of the shock. Following the success of Beck in 1947, work was initiated to answer these concerns.

Two studies have been published on the optimal frequency for AC defibrillators[24,43]. One used closed chest animals and the other open chested preparation. Transthoracic electrode application was successful in a frequency range of 60-250 Hz. The open chest range was from 50-400 Hz. The smallest energy requirements occurred at the power line frequency of 60 Hz, a coincidence that is truly remarkable. For this reason, AC defibrillators are powered through a transformer from the regular house current outlets.

Guyton and Satterfield[44] were among the first to investigate the strength-duration relationships of 60 Hz AC current. They found that higher voltage from the defibrillator (and, consequently, higher current) was required if the duration of the shock was less than 0.1 second (6 full sine waves). The voltage remained constant if the duration was between 0.1 and 5 seconds. Guillet et al[45] expanded these findings and constructed a traditional strength-duration curve. (See Figure 1.) Clinical AC defibrillators use shock durations of 0.1 to 0.5 seconds. One hundred volts provided adequate current if the electrodes are placed directly on the heart. For transthoracic application, 300-750 volts are needed. These voltages give a current flow of 3-12 amperes[21].

The evidence for discontinuing AC defibrillation in favor of DC defibrillation was provided by Lown et al in 1962[46]. In well documented experiments, they compared the two waveforms in converting dogs. They found that (1) DC was more effective in converting ventricular fibrillation, (2) more animals died immediately and within one week after conversion with AC current, (3) post-defibrillatory atrial and ventricular arrhythmias were less with DC shocks, and finally, (4) the occurrence of ventricular fibrillation following attempted conversion of atrial fibrillation was much higher with AC. This last point has been noted clinically and commented upon editorially. These results opened the door for the routine use of elective cardioversion, which had been deemed too dangerous to attempt with AC defibrillators. There can be no question that the evidence favoring DC over AC is overwhelming.

Capacitor and Capacitor-Inductor Defibrillators

As previously noted, Prevost and Batelli used capacitor discharge defibrillation. They applied metallic disks to the heart and discharged a condensor directly into them. It has been calculated that the condensors were charged to 18,000 volts[21]. A straight condensor discharge generates a waveform that starts at a maximum and decays exponentially to zero (See Figure 2). The rate of decay depends upon the resistance of the chest wall. This arrangement requires much more energy than the DC units used today and was abandoned[47].

In 1947, Gurvich and Yunivev from Russia discovered the low-energy advantage of placing an inductor in series with the capacitor[48]. This is essentially the same circuit that Lown popularized. The circuit and waveform are seen in Figures 2 and 3. The capacitor discharges its voltage through the inductor and into the chest. The voltage starts at zero, rises to a maximum and decays to zero. This has been called a damped sinusoid. The exact shape of the waveform depends upon the size of the capacitor, inductor, and the amount of chest wall resistance. Since the capacitor and inductor are fixed for a particular defibrillator, the waveform is determined by the chest resistance. Lown has determined by trial and error the values for the capacitor and inductor that appear to be the most effective[46]. The stored energy on the capacitors in most units ranges from 0-400 watt-seconds. Over the range of chest resistances routinely encountered in the adult population, these energies result in peak voltages up to 4,000 volts and peak currents of 50 amps. The pulse width varies from 10-20 milliseconds.

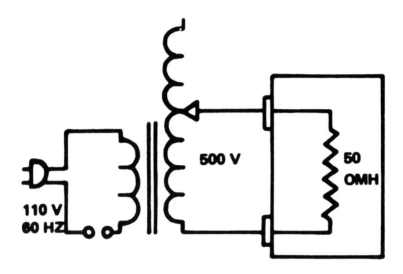

Figure 3a AC

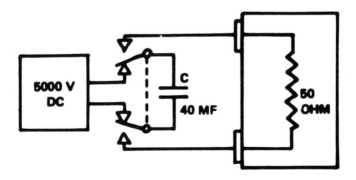

Figure 3b Capacitor Discharge

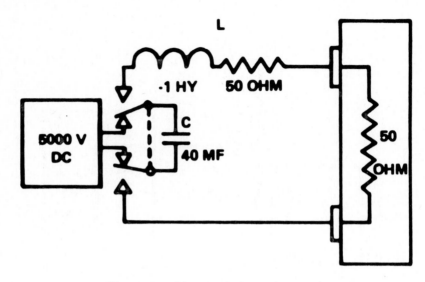

Figure 3c Capacitor-Inductor Discharge

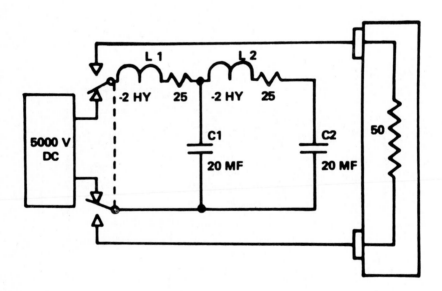

Figure 3d Delay Line

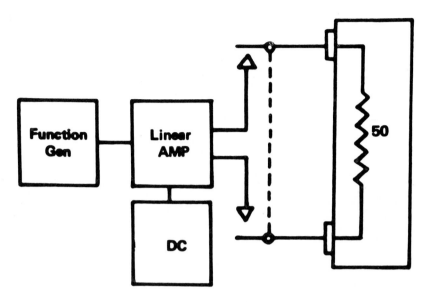

Figure 3e   Square Wave

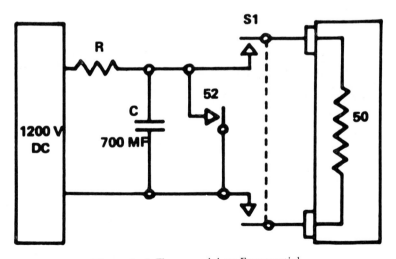

Figure 3e-f Trapazondal or Exponential

Figure 3a-f   Circuit diagrams for creating the different waveforms for ventricular defibrillation. (From Hagan, W.: Defibrillation techniques. *Medical Electronics and Data*, July/August, 1972, with permission.)

Figure 4 shows that the voltage not only falls toward zero, but may actually become negative and become positive again with each oscillation becoming smaller until the voltage becomes zero. This condition is called underdamping. For a particular capacitor and inductor there is a resistance at which this underdamping disappears. The waveform is then said to be critically damped. Below this resistance, the waveform becomes underdamped; and with lower resistances, the excursions become larger and the oscillations greater in number. There has been some concern that these after voltages may cause refibrillation[49]. If the resistance is above the critical value, not only do the oscillations disappear, but the magnitude of the peak voltage and current decreases. During this condition, the waveform is said to be overdamped.

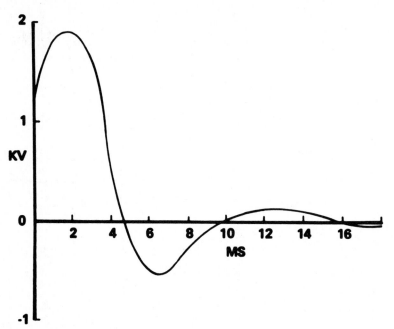

Figure 4 The waveform of an underdamped pulse. The negative portion will increase as electrical resistance due to patient's chest wall decreases. This may result in refibrillation. (From Hagan, W.: Defibrillation techniques. *Medical Electronics and Data*, July/August, 1972, with permission.)

It is readily apparent that the waveform is greatly influenced by the patient's chest resistance. Even if the resistance could be determined for the first shock, subsequent shocks would be into a chest with a different resistance. In addition to the waveform being a function of the chest resistance, the delivered energy is likewise affected.

On earlier models of defibrillators, the indicator meters were calibrated in stored energy. There are some internal energy losses within the defibrillator, and less energy reaches the patient than indicated. Chambers and Stratbucker determined that in some cases this loss amounted to 50%,[29,59] (See Figure 5). Others have reported similar findings[50-52]. A representative graph is shown for eight different commercial defibrillators discharged into a 50 ohm load; however, this is only strictly valid for patients with a chest resistance to 50 ohms.

DEFIBRILLATOR PERFORMANCE CHARACTERISTICS

COMPUTER ANALYSES OF EIGHT POPULAR MODELS

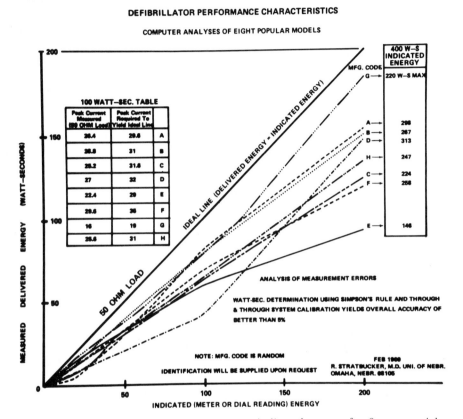

Figure 5 Measured delivery energy versus indicated energy for 8 commercial defibrillators.

The damped sinusoidal waveform presents significant theoretical and practical problems in controlling the amount of current that is injected for any shock. This makes optimizing the waveform for a particular patient rather difficult. In spite of these apparent disadvantages, this waveform is the standard against which all others are measured. It has had 13 years of extensive clinical experience and shown to be effective and safe for both ventricular and supraventricular arrythmias. The problems of maximal efficiency, heavy subject defibrillation, and minimizing myocardial damage remain, but at the present time there is no alternative waveform that has been shown to be clearly superior either experimentally or clinically. Other waveforms have not been as completely evaluated, however, and certain theoretical advantages do exist for some of them. Perhaps future research will answer these problems.

Figure 2 shows the only other capacitor-inductor discharge circuit. The addition of the extra capacitor and inductor lowers the voltage and lengthens the pulse[60]. Maximum voltage is about 1,000 volts, and maximum current is about 25 amperes. The pulse width may be up to 40 plus milliseconds. This circuit has been called the "delay line". It was hoped that the lower voltage and current for the same energy would minimize myocardial damage. This waveform suffers from some of the same problems as the single capacitor-inductor waveform. There are no published reports comparing its performance directly with any of the other waveforms.

Rectangular and Trapezoidal Defibrillators

In the mid 1960's, the evaluation of other waveforms appeared in the literature. The most successful of these were the rectangular and trapezoidal waveforms (See Figure 2). Schuder has had the most extensive experience[49,53-57]. Figure 6 shows a wide range of energies that are successful at a given current. The energy constant is controlled by varying the pulse width, thus the final current is different for different energy levels. He found that a final current of greater than 10 amperes gave higher success rates, and even approached 100%. Decreasing success below 10 amperes is thought to be due to "refibrillation" and may be due to the characteristic trailing edge of any defibrillator pulse that has a long, low amplitude tail. If the waveform does not decay at all (that is, a rectangular waveform), the defibrillative effectiveness is maintained over a wider range of energy levels. From an experimental model, Koning[61] has calculated the strength-duration characteristics for trapezoidal waveforms with different time constants. The time constant is a measure of the rate of fall of the current. The shorter the time constant, the faster the rate of fall. When the duration of the pulse equals the time constant, the current has fallen to about 63% of the initial current. His calculations show that the longer the time constant, the lower the current and energy requirements. This effect is maximal when the waveform is rectangular. This model agrees with the Schuder's experimental results. In addition, if these results are compared to the damped sinusoidal results of Geddes, there appears to be a slight advantage in favor of the rectangular waveform.

In 1972, Hagan introduced a voltage source trapazoidal waveform, portable defibrillator[58]. For ranges of energies used in emergency defibrillation, the initial voltage is about 1,200 volts regardless of the energy setting. The energy varies with the pulse width which in turn is controlled by the chest resistance. Although the current is not controlled, this machine does control the delivered energy. During a shock, an internal computer calculates the energy being delivered at the paddles and interrupts the waveform when the energy level is reached. It also terminates the pulse if the terminal current falls below 10 amps. This is one of the newer innovations in defibrillation.

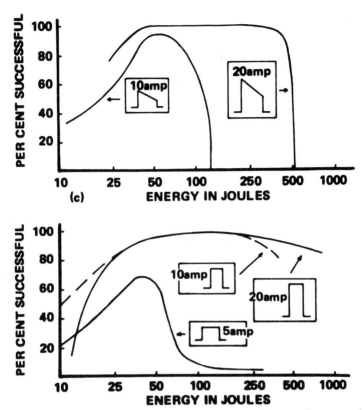

Figure 6 Success rate of defibrillation versus delivered energy for trapezoidal and rectangular pulses. (From Schuder, J.C., Stoeckle, H., West, J.A., Keskar, P.Y.: Transthoracic ventricular defibrillation in the dog with untruncated exponential stimuli. *IEEE Transactions on Biomedical Engineering*, BME **18-6**: 410-415, November 1971, with permission.)

Although current is not directly controlled, the absolute delivered energy is, which is a step in the right direction. Several manufacturers have now marketed this type of defibrillator. Chambers and Miles[31] recently introduced a modification of this design in which the initial voltage on the capacitors is varied. This indirectly controls the initial current depending upon the chest resistance. This could approach the ideal characteristics of a voltage source defibrillator.

Implantable Defibrillators

Another new development is the work being done by Mirowski et al[62-67,73,74] and Schuder[68-71] on implantable defibrillators. Functioning much like a pacemaker, these defibrillators are totally implantable. These devices monitor the electrical and mechanical activities of the heart, and administer defibrillatory shocks automatically. One electrode is in the apex of the right ventricle with the other in the superior vena cava. Schuder's truncated exponential waveform was as efficient as any tested and has significant engineering advantages. They currently have tested it in dogs, and find that energy levels of 5-15 watt-seconds are effective and have had no untoward effects. Human implantation has not been reported, but is anticipated.

References

1. Schagger, W.A. and Cobb, L.A.: Recurrent ventricular fibrillation and modes of death in survivors of out-of-hospital ventricular fibrillation. *N. Engl. J. Med.*, **293**: 259-262, 1975.
2. Baum, R.S., Alvarez, H., and Cob, L.A.: Survival after resuscitation from out-of-hospital ventricular fibrillation. *Circulation*, **50**: 1231-1235, 1974.
3. Liberthson, R.R., Nagel, E.L., Hirschman, J.C., et al: Pre-hospital ventricular fibrillation: prognosis and follow-up. *N. Engl. J. Med.*, **291**: 317-321, 1974.
4. Miscia, V.F. and Pollicina, F.: Emergency pacing and cardioversion. In R.S. Eliot (Ed.): *The Acute Cardiac Emergency*, Futura Publishing, Mt. Kisco, N.Y., 1972.
5. Zipes, D.P.: The clinical application of cardioversion. *Cardiovasc. Clinics*, **2**: 2, 1970.
6. Dreifus, L.S.: Use of DC shock in the treatment of cardiac arrhythmias. *Mod. Treatm.*, **7**: 188, 1970.
7. Benson, D.W.: Historical background and physiology of fibrillation. *J. Assoc. for the Adv. of Med. Instr.*, **3**: 53-57, 1969.
8. Prevost, J.L. and Batelli, F.: Some effects of electric discharge on the hearts of mammals. *CR Acad. Sci. (D) (Paris)*, **129**: 1267-1268, 1899.
9. Prevost, J.L. and Batelli, F.: Death by electric currents (alternating current). *CR Acad. Sci. (D) (Paris)*, **128**: 668-670, 1899.
10. Kouwenhoven, W.B. and Langworthy, O.R.: Cardiopulmonary resuscitation, an account of forty-five years of research. *The Johns Hopkins Medical Journal*, **132**: 186-193, 1973.
11. Hooker, D.R., Kouwenhoven, W.B., and Langworthy, O.R.: The effect of alternating electrical current on the heart. *Am. J. Physiol.*, **103**: 444-454, 1933.
12. Kouwenhoven, W.B. and Hooker, R.D.: Resuscitation by counter-shock. *Elect. Engin.*, **52**: 475-477, 1933.
13. Ferris, L.P., King, B.G., Spence, P.W., et al: Effect of electric shock on the heart. *Elec. Engin.*, **55**: 498-515, 1936.
14. Wiggers, C.J.: The physiologic basis for cardiac resuscitation from ventricular fibrillation—method for serial fibrillation. *Am. Heart J.*, **20**: 413-422, 1940.
15. Beck, C.S., Pritchard, W.H., and Fiel, H.S.: Ventricular fibrillation of long duration abolished by electric shock. *JAMA*, **135**: 985-986, 1947.
16. Zoll, P.M., Linenthal, A.J., Gibson, W., et al: Termination of ventricular fibrillation in man by externally applied electric counter-shock. *N. Engl. J. Med.*, **254**: 727-732, 1956.
17. Zoll, P.M., Paul, M.H., Linenthal, A.J., et al: The effects of external electric currents on the heart. *Circulation*, **14**: 745-756, 1956.
18. Lown, B., Amarasingham, R., Neuman, J., et al: The use of synchronized direct-current countershock in the treatment of cardiac arrhythmias. *J. Clin. Invest.*, **41**: 1381, 1962.
19. Lown, B., Amarasingham, R., and Neuman, J.: New methods for terminating cardiac arrhythmias. *JAMA*, **182**: 458-555, 1962.

20. Zoll, P.M., Linenthal, A.J., and Zarsky, L.R.N.: Ventricular fibrillation treatment and prevention by external electric currents. *N. Engl. J. Med.*, **262**: 105-112, 1960.
21. Geddes, L.A.: Electrical ventricular defibrillation. *Baylor College of Medicine Cardiovascular Research Center*, **10**: 3-42, 1971.
22. Mackay, R.S. and Leeds, S.E.: Physiological effects of condenser discharges with application to tissue stimulation and ventricular defibrillation. *J. Appl. Physiol.*, **6**: 67-75, 1953.
23. Schuder, J.C., Rahmoeller, G.A., and Stoeckle, H.: Transthoracic ventricular defibrillation with triangular and trapezoidal waveforms. *Circ. Res.*, **19**: 689-694, 1966.
24. Ferris, C.D., Moore, T.W., Khazei, A.H., et al: A study of parameters involved in alternating-current defibrillation. *Med. Biol. Engin.*, **7**: 17-29, 1969.
25. Druz, W.S.: The design rationale of defibrillators. *J. Assoc. Advancement Med. Instrumentation*, **3**: 65-69, 1969.
26. Ewy, G.A. and Ewy, M.D.: Chest wall impedance to cardioversion. *Cir. Suppl. III*, **49**: 889, 1974.
27. Geddes, L.A., Tacher, W.A., Cabler, M.S., Kidder, H., and Gothard, R.: The impedance of electrodes used for ventricular fibrillation. *J. Assoc. of Med. Instr.*, **9**: 177-178, 1975.
28. Connell, D.N., Ewy, G.A., et al: Transthoracic impedance to defibrillator discharge—effects of electrode size and electrode-chest wall interface. *J. of Electrocardiology*, **6**: 315-317, 1973.
29. Stratbucker, R.A. and Chambers, W.A.: Defibrillator Performance Characteristics. Scientific Exhibit at American College of Cardiology, Annual Session, 1971.
30. Kugelberg, Jan: The interelectrode electrical resistance at defibrillation. *Scand. J. Thor. Cardiovasc. Surg.*, **6**: 274-277, 1972.
31. Chambers, W.A. and Miles, R.R.: A New Defibrillator Design Employing Dual Compensation for Wide Ranges of Thoracic Resistance and Thoracic Mass. J. Assoc. Advancement Medical Institute Annual Session, 1975.
32. Geddes, L.A., Tacker, W.A., et al: The decrease in transthoracic impedance during successive ventricular defibrillation trials. *J. Assoc. of Med. Instr.*, **9**: 179, 1975.
33. Tacker, W.A., Galioto, F.M., Jr., Giuliani, E., Geddes, L.A., and McNamara, D.G.: Energy dosage for human transchest electrical ventricular defibrillation. *N. Engl. J. Med.*, **290**: 214, 1974.
34. Tacker, W.A., Jr.: Electrical Dose for Defibrillation. Cardiac Defibrillation Conference, Purdue University, West Lafayette, Indiana, Oct. 1-3, 1975.
35. Rush, S., Gregoritsch, A.J., and Lepeschkin, E.: Theoretical and Model Studies of Current Pathways From Defibrillating Electrodes. 20th Annual Conference on Engineering in Medicine and Biology, Boston, Nov. 13-16, 1967 (Publication No. 14-3).
36. Kouwenhoven, W.B., Milnor, W.R., Knickerbocker, G.G., et al: Closed chest defibrillation of the heart. *Surgery*, **42**: 550-561, 1957.
37. Ewy, G.A.: Defibrillation for Paddle Electrodes. Proceedings of Cardiac Defibrillation Conference, Purdue University, West Lafayette, Indiana, 1975.
38. Dahl, C.F., Ewy, G.A., et al: Myocardial necrosis from direct current countershock: effect of paddle electrode size and time interval between discharge. *Circulation*, **50**: 956, 1974.
39. Lepeschkin, E., Jones, J.L., Rush, S., and Jones, R.E.: Analysis of Cardiac Damage Following Elective Cardiac Defibrillation. Cardiac Defibrillation Conference, Purdue University, West Lafayette, Indiana, Oct. 1-3, 1975.
40. Tacker, W.A., Davis, J.S., and Geddes, L.A.: Damage Produced in Canine

Hearts Following Trans-Chest DC Electrical Shock. Proceedings of Cardiac Defibrillation Conference, Purdue University, West Lafayette, Indiana, 1975.

41. Ehsani, A.A., Ewy, G.A., and Sobel, B.E.: CPK isoenzyme elevations after electrical countershock. *Circulation*, Suppl., **4**: 511, 1973.

42. Tacker, W.A., et al: Alteration of Electrical Defibrillation Threshold by the Cardiac Glycoside, Ouaban. Proceedings of Cardiac Defibrillation Conference. Purdue University, West Lafayette, Indiana, 1975.

43. Witzel, D., Geddes, L.A., McFarlane, J., et al: The influence of cycle frequency on the effectiveness of electrical defibrillation of the canine ventricles. *Cardiovasc. Res. Cent. Bull.*, **5**: 112-118, 1967.

44. Guyton, A.C. and Satterfield, J.: Factors concerned in electrical defibrillation of the heart particularly through the unopened chest. *Am. J. Physiol.*, **167**: 81-87, 1951.

45. Guillet, J.R., Havens, W.W., Tacker, W.A., et al: Optimum duration of 60 Hz current for direct ventricular defibrillation in the dog. *Cardiovasc. Res. Cent. Bull.*, **6**: 117-123, 1968.

46. Lown, B., Neuman, J., Amarasingham, R., et al: Comparison of alternating current with direct countershock across the closed chest. *Am. J. Cardiol.*, **10**: 223-233, 1962.

47. Peleska, B.: Optimal parameters of electrical impulses for defibrillation by condenser discharges. *Circ. Res.*, **18**: 10-17, 1966.

48. Gurvich, N.L. and Yuniev, G.S.: Restoration of heart rhythm during fibrillation by a condenser discharge. *Am. Rev. Soviet Med.*, **4**: 252-256, 1947.

49. Schuder, J.C., Stoeckle, H., West, J.A., et al: Transthoracic ventricular defibrillation in the dog with truncated and untruncated exponential stimuli. *IEEE Trans. Biomed. Engin.*, **18**: 410-415, 1971.

50. Ewy, A.: Defibrillator Output. Cardiac Defibrillation Conference, Purdue University, West Lafayette, Indiana, Oct. 1-3, 1975.

51. Balagot, R.C. and Bandelin, V.R.: Comparative evaluation of some DC cardiac defibrillators. *J. Assoc. Advancement Med. Instrumentation*, 1972.

52. Flynn, C., Fox, F., and Bourland, J.: Indicated and delivered energy by defibrillators. *J. Assoc. Advancement Med. Instrumentation*, 1972.

53. Schuder, C., Stoeckle, H., and Gold, J.H.: Effectiveness of Transthoracic Ventricular Defibrillation With Square and Trapezoidal Waveforms. Cardiac Defibrillation Conference, Purdue University, West Lafayette, Indiana, Oct. 1-3, 1975.

54. Schuder, J.C., Rahmoeller, G.A., and Stoeckle, H.: Transthoracic ventricular defibrillation with triangular and trapezoidal waveforms. *Circ. Res.*, **19**: 689, 1966.

55. Schuder, J.C., Rahmoeller, G.A., Nellis, S.H., Stoeckle, H., and Mackenzie, J.W.: Transthoracic ventricular defibrillation with very high amplitude rectangular pulses. *J. Appl. Physiol.*, **22**: 1110, 1967.

56. Schuder, J.C., Stoeckle, H., West, J.A., and Keskar, P.Y.: Transthoracic ventricular defibrillation in the dog with truncated and untruncated exponential stimuli. *IEEE Transactions on Bio-Medical Engineering*, BME-18: 410, 1971.

57. Schuder, J.C., Stoeckle, H., West, J.A., and Dolan, A.M.: A very high power amplifier for experimental external defibrillation. *Proceedings of the 16th Annual Conference on Engineering in Medicine and Biology*, **5**: 40, 1963.

58. Hagan, W.K.: Efficacy of a Small, Solid-State Defibrillation Employing Truncated Exponential Discharges. Ninth Annual Rocky Mountain Engineering Symposium, 1972.

59. Stratbucker, R., Chambers, W., and Hagern, W.: Defibrillator performance characteristics. *J. Assoc. Advancement Medical Instr.*, **5**: 2, 1971.

60. Balagot, R.C., Druz, W.A., Ramadan, M., et al: A monopulse DC current defibrillator for ventricular defibrillation. *J. Thorac. Cardiovasc. Surg.*, **47**: 487-504, 1974.

61. Koning, G.: Strength-Duration Curves For Direct Ventricular Defibrillation With Rectangular Current Pulses. Cardiac Defibrillation Conference, Purdue University, West Lafayette, Indiana, Oct. 1-3, 1975.

61. Mirowski, M., Mower, M.M., Langer, A., and Heilman, M.S.: Implanted Defibrillators. Cardiac Defibrillation Conference, Purdue University, West Lafayette, Indiana, Oct. 1-3, 1975.

63. Mirowski, M., Mower, M.M., Staewen, W.S., Tabatznik, B., and Mendeloff, A.I.: Standby automatic defibrillator. *Arch. Intern. Med.*, **126**: 158-161, 1970.

64. Mirowski, M., Mower, M.M., Staewen, W.S., Denniston, R.H., Tabatznik, B., and Mendeloff, A.I.: Ventricular defibrillation through a single intravascular catheter electrode system. (abstr) *Clin. Res.*, **19**: 328, 1971.

65. Mirowski, M., Mower, M.M., Staewen, W.S., Denniston, R.H., and Mendeloff, A.I.: The development of the transvenous automatic defibrillator. *Arch. Intern. Med.*, **129**: 773-779, 1972.

66. Mirowski, M., Mower, M.M., Gott, V.L., Brawley, R.K., and Denniston, R.H.: Transvenous automatic defibrillator—preliminary clinical tests of its defibrillating subsystem. *Trans. Am. Soc. Artif. Int. Organs*, **16**: 520-524, 1972.

67. Mirowski, M., Mower, M.M., Gott, V.L., and Brawley, R.K.: Feasibility and effectiveness of low-energy catheter defibrillation in man. *Circulation*, **47**: 79-85, 1973.

68. Schuder, J.C., Stoeckle, H., Gold, J.H., West, J.A., and Keskar, P.Y.: Experimental ventricular defibrillation with an automatic and completely implanted system. *Trans. Am. Soc. Artif. Int. Organs*, **16**: 207-212, 1970.

69. Schuder, J.C., Stoeckle, H., West, J.A., Keskar, P.Y., Gold, J.H., and Holland, J.A.: Ventricular defibrillation in the dog using implanted and partically implanted electrode systems. *Am. J. Cardiol.*, **33**: 243-247, 1974.

70. Schuder, J.C., Stoeckle, H., West, J.A., and Keskar, P.Y.: Relationship between electrode geometry and effectiveness of ventricular defibrillation in the dog with catheter having one electrode in right ventricle and other electrode in superior vena cava, or external jugular vein, or both. *Cardiovasc. Res.*, **7**: 629-637, 1973.

71. Schuder, J.C., Stoeckle, H., West, J.A., Keskar, P.Y., Gold, J.H., and Denniston, R.H.: Ventricular defibrillation in the dog with a bi-electrode intravascular catheter. *Arch. Intern. Med.*, **132**: 286-290, 1973.

72. Hagan, W.: Defibrillation techniques. *Medical Electronics and Data*, July/August 1972.

73. Mirowski, M., Mower, M.M., Staewen, W.S., et al: Standby automatic defibrillator. *Arch. Intern. Med.*, **126**: 158-161, 1970.

74. Denniston, R.H., Mower, M., and Mirowski, M.: Automatic standby defibrillator. *J. Assoc. Advancement Med. Instrumentation*, **5**: 110, 1971.

CHAPTER 17

Medical and Surgical Approach to Unstable Angina*

John Stoner, III, M.D.; Donald C. Harrison, M.D.

This Chapter presents a thorough and balanced approach to a variety of clinical conditions resulting in unstable angina pectoris. Throughout the clinical course of this condition, a series of therapeutic options are offered in rational relationship to morbidity and mortality. The advantages of medical vs. surgical approaches are discussed by authors displaying an extensive clinical perspective of both available options.

Myocardial infarction remains highly lethal in spite of recent advances in coronary care, largely due to high pre-hospital mortality[1-5]. A substantial reduction in these deaths is likely to occur only with recognition of warning symptoms and earlier hospitalization. Though infarction can occur as the first expression of underlying disease, in the majority of cases there is a recognizable progression of symptoms[6,7]. This progression frequently takes the form of a syndrome we have termed "unstable angina," in which symptoms worsen abruptly, along with prolonged and intense pain unrelated to exertion, and poorly relieved by nitroglycerin[8-13]. Physiologically, this state represents a precarious balance between myocardial oxygen demands and reduced coronary blood flow, in which any increase in the former, or further compromise of the latter, may lead to infarction. It is essential to recognize this syndrome since, at the very least, early hospitalization can reduce the mortality from a subsequent infarction. More importantly, it can possibly prevent infarction through appropriate care aimed at reducing myocardial oxygen demands and increasing coronary blood flow.

In the discussion which follows, we review the natural history of unstable angina and its medical and surgical treatment. Much of the information presented has been summarized from the numerous reports in the recent literature. However, we have also included an outline of our own approach to the management of unstable angina, in the hope that it will be of practical value to the reader.

*This work was supported in part by NIH Grant No. HL-5866 and Program Project Grant No. 1-PO1-HL-15833.

NATURAL HISTORY

Patients with unstable angina frequently have a history of previous but stable symptoms for months or even years, or may experience the sudden onset of disabling pain as the first manifestation of coronary atherosclerotic heart disease[8-14]. Typically, an individual accustomed to angina on exercise begins having pain of greater intensity at rest or with only minimal exertion. Alternatively, a previously asymptomatic patient develops severe and prolonged anginal pain in the absence of obvious precipitating factors. In either case, a key aspect is the duration of anginal pain. While previous attacks may have lasted a few minutes, they now persist for 30 minutes or longer and are poorly responsive to standard drugs such as nitroglycerin and long acting nitrates.

Clinically, it may be difficult to differentiate unstable angina from actual myocardial infarction (Table I). In unstable angina, the electrocardiogram typically shows changes of myocardial ischemia; straightening and depression of the ST segments, and flattening or inversion of the T waves[13,14]. The appearance of new Q waves obviously indicates that transmural infarction has already occurred. However, their absence does not exclude the possibility of a subendocardial myocardial infarction.

TABLE I
DIFFERENTIAL DIAGNOSIS OF PREINFARCTION ANGINA

	Stable Angina	Impending Infarction	Acute Infarction
Pain pattern	Brief pain episodes, usually of substernal origin and lasting 3-5 min. Onset related to physical effort, emotion, eating, or other stress. Prompt response to rest or nitrates.	Severe pain, usually of substernal origin and lasting 15-30 min. Onset unrelated to effort or other known precipitating factors. Responsive to nitrates, but narcotics may be required for relief.	Crushing pain, usually of substernal origin and lasting 15 min. or more. Onset usually unrelated to effort or other known precipitating factors. Narcotics required for relief.
Physical signs	A 3rd or 4th heart sound may appear, related to pain episode.	Arterial blood pressure usually normal or initially decreased, followed by moderate decline.	May develop shock or heart failure. Cold extremeties, sweating, peripheral cyanosis present.
Serum enzymes	Within normal range.	SGOT and LDH levels within normal range. CPK levels normal or slightly elevated to no more than twice maximal normal level.	SGOT, LDH, and CPK levels elevated and show evolutionary pattern.
ECG changes	S-T segment displacement or T-wave inversion in some cases.	Flattened depression of S-T segment. Deep symmetrical T wave inversion. Elevation of S-T segment in anginal variant syndromes (occasional). Transient changes.	Appearance of Q waves. Elevation of S-T segment T wave inversion. Evolutionary changes over days.

(Table reprinted from Harrison, D.C. and Shumway, N.E.: *Hospital Practice*, HP Publishing Co., New York 1974 with permission.)

Serum enzyme determinations may help in diagnosing this latter possibility. Any increase in SGOT or LDH levels into a clearly abnormal range suggests infarction. CPK and its myocardial isoenzyme (MB) may increase slightly on the basis of severe ischemia alone[15]. However, elevations to twice normal levels or higher should be taken as presumptive evidence of myocardial infarction. Care must be taken to avoid intramuscular injections as they may produce skeletal muscle necrosis and increases in LDH and CPK levels (though not increases of the myocardial isoenzyme for CPK)[16].

Currently, available data on the natural history of unstable angina are inconsistent, largely due to differing definitions of the syndrome, insufficient numbers of cases and inadequate follow-up (Table II)[10,12,17-21]. In one of the larger series of the literature, Vakil found that among 156 patients with unstable angina, 77 (50%) developed subsequent myocardial infarction, while 37 (25%) were dead after a minimum follow-up period of three months[18]. Unfortunately, the study was a retrospective analysis of patients seen in the author's practice over a 14-year period, raising questions about the accuracy of the diagnosis and the extent of follow-up in individual cases. Fulton and co-workers, on the other hand, in an equally large series of 167 cases of unstable angina, found a much lower incidence of infarction (14%) and death (2%) during a 3 to 6 month follow-up period[19]. Their definition of unstable angina, however, was considerably more liberal than that used in other studies, since it included all patients with recent onset or worsening of angina, regardless of severity. However, Krause and co-workers found that among 100 patients with more rigorously defined unstable angina admitted to a coronary care unit, there were only six in-hospital infarctions and one death[20]. Twelve months later, 85% of these patients were still alive, though after 20 months 40% had died, most of these acute infarction or sudden death.

In our own experience at Stanford, we have found it helpful to classify patients with unstable angina into two groups. Those who become asymptomatic or nearly so within 48 hours of hospitalization and institution of appropriate medical treatment are classified as having simple unstable angina.

TABLE II
NATURAL HISTORY OF UNSTABLE ANGINA

Study [Ref. No.]	No. of Patients	Length of Follow-up	Infarction No. Patients (%)	Cardiac Death No. Patients (%)
Levy, 1956[10]	158	2 mo.	37 (23%)	51 (32%)
Wood, 1961[12]	50	2 mo.	22 (44%)	30 (60%)
Vakil, 1964[18]	156	>3 mo.	77 (49%)	37 (23%)
Fulton et al., 1972[19]	167	3-6 mo.	23 (14%)	3 (2%)
Krause et al., 1972[20]	100	20 mo.	23 (23%)	22 (22%)
Gazes et al., 1973[21]	140	3 mo.	29 (21%)	14 (10%)

On the other hand, those patients who have persistant and recurrent pain in spite of such therapy are labelled as having the "intermediate coronary syndrome." Approximately 70% of our patients fall into the former category and follow a relatively benign course (Figure 1). Thirty percent however, develop the intermediate coronary syndrome associated with more rapid clinical changes.

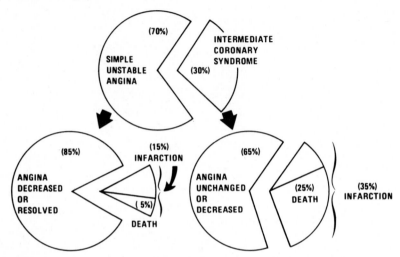

Figure 1 Clinical course of unstable angina.

In a prospective study of 140 patients with unstable angina, Gazes and co-wokers made a similar distinction among their patients[21]. For the group as a whole, they observed a 21% incidence of infarction over a three-month period, with an 82% survival rate at one year. In 74%, the angina became less severe, while in 8% it remained unchanged. However, for a subgroup of high risk patients with persistent unstable angina in spite of intensive medical treatment, the prognosis was much poorer. Thirty-five percent of these patients sustained a myocardial infarction within three months, while 43% died within one year.

MEDICAL APPROACH

General Considerations

The primary aim of therapy in unstable angina is to relieve myocardial ischemia by improving the balance between coronary blood flow and myocardial oxygen demands. This is to prevent acutal myocardial infarction, or at the very least, to minimize the amount of myocardial necrosis. Since a significant proportion of patients with this syndrome do progress to infarction in spite of all efforts, a secondary aim is to provide safeguards against the potential complications of such an outcome, especially fatal arrhythmias.

Accordingly, all patients with unstable angina are hospitalized and observed initially in a Coronary Care Unit with continuous electrocardiogram monitoring. Serial electrocardiograms and serum CPK, SGOT and LDH enzyme determinations are obtained to rule out infarction and document any resolution of ischemic ST segment and T wave abnormalities. Patients are transferred out of the Coronary Care unit only after infarction has been excluded and the patient has had substantial resolution or stabilization of his symptoms.

Environmental stress in the patient's home or business life may play a significant role in the production of unstable angina[13]. Increases in autonomic sympathetic tone and circulating catecholamine levels heighten myocardial oxygen demands by increasing heart rate, blood pressure, and myocardial contractility[22]. This process, to a certain extent, becomes self-reinforcing as the syndrome evolves, with the patient's worsening chest pain creating more and more apprehension. A major effort therefore is made to relieve any anxiety early in the patient's course.

Hospitalization may be helpful in itself, removing the patient from a hostile home or business environment, provided that the Coronary Care Unit to which he has been admitted offers a quiet and restful atmosphere. Clearly some Intensive Care Units, though they may provide electrocardiographic monitoring, are detrimental since they markedly increase the patient's apprehension. Adequate sedation and effective pain relief are also essential. The former can be accomplished with appropriate doses of phenobarbital or diazepam. Chest pain is often unresponsive to nitroglycerin in patients with unstable angina[10-14] and may require morphine or meperidine for relief. Bed rest and limitation of physical activity are important to keep cardiac work and myocardial oxygen consumption to a minimum. Oxygen administration by nasal prongs or facemask is also beneficial, provided that it is well tolerated by the patient. The increase in arterial oxygen content produced is not great, but may be significant in salvaging severely ischemic myocardium.

Contributing Factors

The abrupt onset, or worsening of symptoms, with unstable angina suggests a dramatic change in the balance between coronary blood flow and myocardial oxygen demands. This alteration is primarily due to progressive coronary artery narrowing with reduction of blood flow beyond a critical level. However, there are other contributing factors which are more readily corrected[23].

Poorly controlled arterial hypertension markedly increases cardiac work and, as a result, increases myocardial oxygen consumption[24]. Since coronary blood flow cannot increase appreciably through narrowed atherosclerotic vessels, these new demands cannot be met and myocardial ischemia worsens. Under these circumstances, rapid but accurate lowering of the blood pressure is needed. Often the increase in pressure is secondary to the patient's pain and anxiety, and is easily controlled by sedation and adequate analgesia.

If the hypertension is sustained, a number of agents are available for its control. Methyldopa can be administered orally for mild-to-moderate hypertension, or intravenously when rapid action is needed[25]. In instances of severe hypertension unresponsive to these measures, an intravenous infusion of nitroprusside will invariably succeed in lowering the pressure[26]. However, when using this and other antihypertensive agents, extreme care must be taken to avoid significant hypotension which might further impair coronary perfusion.

Tachycardia worsens myocardial ischemia both by increasing myocardial oxygen requirements and by decreasing the time spent in diastole, when coronary blood flow to the left ventricle is greatest[27]. Rapid control of any increase in heart rate is therefore essential in treating unstable angina. Sinus tachycardia in response to chest pain and anxiety is treated with sedation and appropriate amounts of analgesics. However, sinus tachycardia may also reflect underlying congestive heart failure, in which case appropriate therapy with digoxin and diuretics must be instituted. Supraventricular tachycardia, if persistent and unresponsive to simple maneuvers such as Valsalva and carotid sinus massage, is best treated with intravenous propranolol[28]. This agent has the added advantage of decreasing myocardial oxygen consumption, though it is contraindicated in the presence of overt congestive heart failure[29]. Atrial flutter or fibrillation with a rapid ventricular response can be managed with digoxin to control the rate. If this does not control the ventricular response, then DC cardioversion should be performed.

Patients with advanced coronary artery disease frequently have associated left ventricular dysfunction, either as localized hypokinesis or generalized poor contractility. If severe, these abnormalities may lead to overt congestive heart failure, which in turn may precipitate unstable angina. With left ventricular dilatation, wall tension increases as a function of the chamber radius, according to the LaPlace relationship[30]. This in turn increases myocardial oxygen demands, worsening ischemia. In addition, if pulmonary edema is present there may be significant hypoxemia, which further decreases the amount of oxygen reaching the ischemic myocardium. Accordingly, heart failure is treated aggressively with digoxin, potent diuretics such as furosemide, and oxygen.

Other contributing factors in unstable angina are listed in Table III. Patients with chronic renal failure, a group that frequently develops coronary atherosclerotic heart disease[31], are almost universally anemic. Unstable angina in this setting may require transfusion with packed red blood cells to increase the oxygen-carrying capacity of the blood.

Hyperthyroidism is uncommon among older males, who make up the bulk of the coronary atherosclerotic heart disease population, but is occasionally seen. In addition to endogenous causes, it may be produced by the injudicious use of thyroid supplements of d-thyroxine in the treatment of

TABLE III
CONTRIBUTING FACTORS

A. Increased cardiac work and myocardial oxygen demands
   1. Hypertension
   2. Tachyarrhythmias
   3. Left ventricular failure and dilatation
   4. Physical or emotional stress
   5. Anemia
   6. Hyperthyroidism

B. Decreased coronary blood flow and/or oxygen delivery
   1. Hypotension
   2. Tachyarrhythmias
   3. Hypoxemia (pulmonary edema, lung disease)
   4. Anemia
   5. Increased blood viscosity (polycythemia, hyperlipidemia)

hyperlipidemia. In the presence of unstable angina, such agents should be reduced in dosage or discontinued, if they are not providing physiologic hormonal replacement. Propranolol will block many of the effects on the cardiovascular system, especially, tachycardia[32]. Treatment of an underlying thyroid disorder may require administration of propylthiouracil or methimazole[33].

Anticoagulation

Anticoagulation as a form of therapy for both unstable angina and acute myocardial infarction remains controversial. The obvious rationale for its use is to prevent thrombosis of narrowed atherosclerotic coronary arteries. Recent evidence, however, suggests that antemortem thrombosis occurs in only a minority of patients who die of myocardial infarction[34]. An additional benefit of anticoagulant therapy is the prevention of thrombophlebitis and pulmonary emboli, which occur frequently in bedridden patients with decreased cardiac outputs[35].

Numerous reports have appeared in the literature that ostensibly demonstrate beneficial effects of anticoagulation in unstable angina[18,36-38]. Unfortunately, most of these studies suffer from a lack of adequate controls, insufficient numbers of patients, and inconsistent use of various anticoagulants. As a result, no firm conclusions can be drawn.

In a retrospective analysis of 346 patients with unstable angina, Vakil reported that among 190 patients treated promptly with anti-coagulation, 69 (36%) developed subsequent myocardial infarction[18]. Among 156 patients managed without anticoagulation, 77 (49%) suffered this complication. Because of the retrospective nature of this study, however, patients were not randomly assigned to treatment and control groups, and a consistent anticoagulation regimen was not maintained. In contrast to these results, Master found no significant difference in the frequency of subsequent myocardial infarction or death in a large, controlled series of 172 patients treated with either anticoagulation or bed rest and sedation alone[39].

Given these conflicting and inconclusive results, it is not surprising that current use of anticoagulation in the treatment of unstable angina varies from institution to institution. However, if the decision is made to use anticoagulants, heparin is the agent of choice. Intravenously, it produces prompt prolongation of the clotting parameters. Oral anticoagulants, on the other hand, take several days to produce their maximum effect. In addition, there are theoretical reasons to suspect that heparin may be more effective in preventing coronary artery thrombosis. In contrast to the formation of venous clots, arterial thrombus forms only after an initial nidus of platelets has formed on the vessel wall[40]. Heparin, and other agents such as dipyridamole that inhibit platelet function, can theoretically prevent this initial step.

Hemodynamic Interventions

As previously noted, patients with unstable angina typically experience spontaneous angina at rest without obvious precipitating events. Gorlin has suggested that these episodes may be caused by acute peripheral vasoconstriction, possibly related to catecholamine release[41]. Recent hemodynamic observations in patients with unstable angina tend to support this thesis[42]. Many of these patients develop elevations in heart rate and arterial pressure during episodes of pain. In others, left ventricular filling pressure increases, reflecting either left ventricular dysfunction or decreased compliance[43]. It is unclear whether these changes are the initiating events, as suggested by Gorlin, or the hemodynamic results of chest pain in unstable angina. Regardless of which is the case, they almost certainly increase cardiac work and myocardial oxygen requirements.

Accordingly, control of these hemodynamic changes is an important aim of therapy. Propranolol administered in adequate doses every 6 hours provides continuous beta-adrenergic blockade and effectively prevents significant increases in heart rate and arterial pressure. In addition, by reducing myocardial contractility, this agent more directly lowers myocardial oxygen consumption[44].

A number of well-controlled studies have confirmed propranolol's efficacy in treating stable angina[45-48]. These findings almost certainly apply to unstable angina also, though large scale controlled trials have not been performed. Favorable results have been reported from several uncontrolled series. Master and Jaffe found that among 18 patients with unstable angina who were treated with propranolol, there were no infarctions nor deaths[49].

Because there is substantial individual variation in blood levels achieved with a given dose of propranolol, therapy should be initiated with a low dose, 10 mg every 6 hours, then a gradually increased dosage[50]. Most patients require from 40 to 80 mg every 6 hours to obtain a significant response[51]. As propranolol can depress myocardial contractility, it should not be given to patients who have evidence of significant left ventricular dysfunction and heart failure[52].

Sublingual nitroglycerin and isosorbide dinitrate are well-established agents in the treatment of both stable and unstable angina[23]. Though they are direct vasodilators of the coronary circulation, their beneficial effect is not solely related to this action. In fact, it is unlikely that they can significantly dilate rigid areas of atherosclerotic narrowing. Tissue ischemia itself produces near maximal dilatation of the local coronary vessels, to which these agents probably add very little. Under these circumstances, more important actions are the lowering of systemic arteriolar resistance and venous dilatation[53]. The former provides systolic unloading of the left ventricle, while the latter decreases venous return, thus reducing left ventricular chamber size and wall tension. These effects, in turn, lower myocardial oxygen consumption, bringing it more into balance with existing coronary blood flow.

Although the symptomatic response to nitrates is frequently poor in unstable angina, the use of these agents is beneficial, nonetheless, since systemic resistance is often elevated. Isosorbide dinitrate is administered sublingually in 5 to 10 mg doses every 3 to 4 hours. To obtain a more sustained effect, nitroglycerin may be applied to the skin as a paste for gradual absorption.

It should be emphasized that this therapy carries the potential hazard of dangerously lowering arterial pressure, further impairing coronary blood flow, and actually worsening myocardial ischemia. Recently, intra-aortic balloon counterpulsation has been proposed as a means of avoiding this problem[54]. Counterpulsation provides two beneficial effects: (1) rapid deflation of the balloon at the onset of systole unloads the left ventricle, thus reducing myocardial oxygen requirements; (2) inflation during diastole maintains diastolic pressure at or above its initial level, thus augmenting diastolic coronary blood flow. In a series of 16 patients treated in this manner, all but one had resolution or significant decrease in chest pain and ischemic electrocardiographic changes. All 16 subsequently underwent coronary revascularization with saphenous vein aortocoronary bypass grafts. Though insertion of an intraaortic balloon may seem an overly invasive procedure, it may be the only recourse in patients who continue to have severe angina in spite of more conservative measures. If viewed as a presurgical measure aimed at preserving myocardium until adequate coronary blood flow can be restored by coronary artery bypass grafting, it becomes more reasonable.

In the future, effective counterpulsation may be available through less invasive methods. A purely external device (cardioassist) has recently been developed which augments diastolic pressure by phasic compression of the lower extremities. Its use to date has been limited, but in one report it was found to produce significant hemodynamic improvement after myocardial infarction when used in combination with intravenous nitroprusside[55].

SURGICAL APPROACH

As previously noted, there remains considerable uncertainty about the ultimate outcome of patients with unstable angina. However, based on currently available data, it is probable that 30 to 40% of these patients will progress to actual myocardial infarction within a year. Associated mortality is likely to be 20% or higher, as compared with a 4% yearly mortality for patients with stable angina[56,57]. Knowledge of this rather grim prognosis has led to the current widespread use of surgical revascularization for unstable angina.

Clearly, not all patients are good surgical candidates. Some patients are either too old to be considered (usually those over 70 years of age), or have other life-limiting illness. In others, the coronary artery narrowing may not be extensive enough to warrant the risks of such a procedure, or may be so widespread as to make successful surgery technically impossible. Selective coronary arteriography therefore is essential for identifying those patients who are suitable surgical candidates. Substantial narrowing, equivalent to 70% or more of the vessel lumen, is probably needed before significant reduction of coronary blood flow occurs[58]. Accordingly, surgery is warranted only when narrowing of this degree or greater involves major vessels—the left main coronary artery or its anterior descending branch, the left circumflex coronary artery or one of its large marginal branches, or the right coronary artery. Obstructive lesions of less than 70% probably do not carry a significant risk of subsequent infarction.

Likewise, narrowing of non-dominant vessels that supply only small portions of myocardium, even if they are the source of severe angina, are best treated medically. Infarction, if it does occur, is unlikely to be massive or have a fatal outcome if the patient is appropriately cared for in the Coronary Care Unit.

Diffuse disease with extensive narrowing of the distal coronary arteries generally is not amenable to surgery. The small caliber of the vessels creates technical difficulties, and the associated poor run-off makes significant increases in coronary blood flow unlikely[59]. If, as a result, flow through the bypass is low, it may well thrombose postoperatively[60,61].

Coronary arteriography reveals severe multi-vessel disease in most patients with unstable angina. Based upon data from several larger series[62-65], 44% of patients will have three or more major coronary arteries involved. Thirty-one percent will have two-vessel disease, while only 25% will have significant narrowing limited to one major coronary artery. The anterior descending branch of the left coronary artery is most frequently involved, though the circumflex branch and the right coronary artery are also commonly affected[65].

The timing of coronary arteriography and subsequent surgery is controversial at present. In the past at Stanford Medical Center, and currently at many institutions, patients have been studied on an emergency basis shortly after their admission to the hospital. However, such an approach, with hurried angiography on acutely ill subjects, probably runs the risk of increased complications. In addition, sufficient time is not allowed to exclude the possibility of acute infarction, which markedly increases the angiographic and surgical risks.

Our current approach is to observe all patients for 48 hours in the Coronary Care Unit, where they are managed with bed rest, sedation, nitrates and propranolol, as outlined earlier. Those patients with simple unstable angina who respond to such therapy with resolution or marked reduction of their symptoms are then continued on medical management, with transfer out of the Coronary Care Unit and progressive ambulation after 4 to 5 days.

Those patients with the intermediate coronary syndrome and continued angina at rest are approached more aggressively. After ruling out infarction during the initial 48 hours of observation, coronary arteriography is subsequently performed. If two or more major coronary arteries, or the left main coronary artery, are involved by significant stenosis (greater than 70%), then coronary artery bypass surgery is recommended. Patients with single-vessel disease limited to the right coronary artery or the circumflex branch of the left coronary artery are managed medically. We do, however, recommend surgery for isolated stenosis of the proximal left anterior descending artery when proximal to the first diagonal branch, since the area of myocardium supplied is large and more likely to cause left ventricular failure or death if infarcted.

Propranolol, if previously administered to help control angina, should be discontinued prior to surgery, since it may contribute to postoperative myocardial depression. However, this should not be done abruptly, as angina frequently worsens and the risk of infarction increases[66]. When possible, rapid tapering is preferable, with one-half of the maintenance dose given at 72 hours before surgery, one-quarter at 48 hours before, and discontinuance of the drug at 24 hours before surgery. Since propranolol and its active metabolities are completely cleared within 24 hours, this schedule allows for maximum benefit from the use of beta-blockade, and avoids more severe ischemia or postoperative myocardial depression[67]. In instances where propranolol cannot be discontinued 24 hours ahead of time, isoproterenol can be used postoperatively to reverse the depressant effects, since the beta-receptor blockage produced by propranolol is a competitive one[52].

The risks associated with coronary arteriography are reasonably low when compared with the natural history of unstable angina. Mortality associated with the procedure is approximately 0.1%, and serious complications occur in 1 to 2% of these patients[68]. These figures conceivably could be higher in patients with unstable angina, but as yet we have seen no evidence to suggest this when the procedure described below is used. Anxiety is controlled by adequate premedication (usually with barbiturates), accompanied by additional doses during the procedure if the desired level of sedation is not obtained. The arterial pressure is continuously monitored to avoid significant hypotension that might impair coronary blood flow. Contrast injection is withheld during periods of acute ischemia, which can be detected by monitoring the electrocardiogram for ischemic ST segment of T wave changes.

The surgical procedure is the standard saphenous vein coronary artery bypass, which is currently in widespread use for the treatment of stable angina. This technique involves anastomosis of a reversed segment of the patient's saphenous vein to the aorta and to the distal end of the coronary artery beyond the obstructive lesion, leaving the proximal portion of the artery intact. As might be expected, the risks associated with surgery are considerably higher in patients with unstable angina[63-65,69-73]. Operative mortality rates reported for most large series have ranged from 5 to 22%. More recently, these have been considerably reduced, largely due to refinements in technique and shorter operating times. In addition, initial experience has shown that surgery after progression to acute infarction has already occurred, or in the presence of severe congestive failure, carries a much higher risk[74-76]. The current trend towards longer preoperative observation allows for better identification and exclusion of these patients. In addition, medical treatment during this period may produce considerable improvement in myocardial ischemia, making subsequent surgery less hazardous.

The late results of coronary artery bypass surgery for unstable angina appear quite promising (Table IV). Cheanvechai et al, reporting on 63 patients, found that 55 were free of symptoms postoperatively, and only four continued to have angina[77]. Four patients died and six suffered postoperative infarctions. Bonchek and his colleagues found that among 55 patients undergoing bypass surgery for unstable angina, 23 were free of symptoms, and 19 had angina only with strenous exertion[63]. Eight continued to have angina with daily activities. There were four deaths and nine myocardial infarctions over an average two-year follow-up period. Among the first 81 patients undergoing coronary artery bypass surgery for unstable angina at Stanford Medical Center, the overall mortality was 11% over an average 18-month follow-up period[65]. Complete relief or significant improvement of angina was achieved in 94% of the survivors. However, there was a 16% peri-operative and a 15% late incidence of myocardial infarction. Similar results have been reported by others[78,79], and when compared with existing data on the natural history of unstable angina these results appear encouraging.

However, confirmation of the beneficial effects of coronary bypass surgery must await the results of randomized controlled trials, several of which are currently underway. Bertolasi et al have reported preliminary results from their prospective randomized study of the surgical treatment of unstable angina[80]. Among 44 patients with the intermediate coronary syndrome and severe angina unresponsive to medical management, 24 underwent coronary artery bypass surgery, and 20 were treated conservatively. Over an average follow-up period of 8.3 months, there were two deaths among those treated surgically, (or a mortality rate of 8.5%). Among those treated medically, however, there were seven deaths (35%), suggesting that surgery in these severely ill patients may prolong life, in addition to relieving symptoms.

TABLE IV

CORONARY ARTERY BYPASS GRAFT SURGERY RESULTS

Study [Ref. No.]	No. of Patients	Length of Follow-up	Infarction No. (%)	Cardiac Death No. (%)	Symptoms Improved No. (%)
Lambert et al., 1971[64]	52	*	2 (4%)	3 (6%)	47 (90%)
Scanlon et al., 1973[62]	39	*	10 (25%)	4 (10%)	36 (92%)
Cheanvechai et al., 1973[77]	63	*	6 (9%)	4 (6%)	55 (93%)**
Bonchek et al., 1974[63]	55	12-52 mo.	9 (16%)	4 (7%)	42 (82%)**
Berndt et al., 1975[65]	81	5-34 mo.	25 (30%)	9 (11%)	62 (86%)**

*Length of follow-up not stated
*% of survivors with symptoms improved

Patients with less severe but progressive angina were also randomized to surgical or medical treatment in this study, but there was no difference in mortality.

FOLLOW-UP CARE

Patients with simple unstable angina, whose symptoms are controlled by medical treatment, can be transferred out of the Coronary Care Unit after 4 to 5 days observation. Thereafter, they should gradually increase their physical activity while continuing antianginal therapy with nitrates and propranolol. A treadmill exercise test is helpful after one to two weeks, to establish safe levels of activity, as well as to provide objective evidence of ischemic heart disease. These patients can then be safely studied with coronary arteriography at 6 weeks, and surgery can be performed on an elective basis if significant obstructive lesions are found.

Patients who have undergone surgery, as well as those who are managed conservatively, must be followed closely. In spite of the dramatic symptomatic improvement that is usually produced by coronary artery bypass grafting, evidence of severe ischemia persists in many cases. Berndt and coworkers found a 50% incidence of positive treadmill exercise tests postoperatively, though 95% of their patients had experienced partial or complete relief of angina[65]. This discrepancy suggests that the mechanism of pain relief following surgery may vary. In addition to improved coronary blood flow, relief of symptoms may be due to perioperative infarction of the ischemic area or denervation during the operative dissection[81]. In addition, there is undoubtedly considerable placebo effect associated with the procedure.

Clearly, objective methods of assessing the patient's cardiac status are needed during the postoperative period. Serial treadmill exercise tests are currently the best means of determining safe levels of exertion. The appearance of ischemic electrocardiographic changes or arrhythmias sets the upper limits of physical activity. Initially, such tests may be performed every one to two months, as the patient's activity is gradually increased. Later they may be scheduled every 6 to 12 months, as part of routine followup examinations, to detect any worsening of ischemia. Ambulatory electrocardiographic monitoring is also helpful during the follow-up period. By identifying those patients with arrhythmias and instituting appropriate antiarrhythmic therapy, it is hoped that late sudden deaths can be prevented[82,83].

A carefully graded program of exercise training may be beneficial. Although there is no convincing evidence to suggest that exercise actually increases coronary blood flow, it does improve the patient's functional capacity[83]. Such a program can usually be safely started 3 to 4 months after recovery from the acute episode, providing severe angina does not persist. The initial level of exercise should be low, then gradually increased. The safety of each new level of activity can be determined by serial treadmill exercise tests.

Control of major coronary risk factors is also important in the follow-up period. Patients in general should eat foods low in calories, cholesterol and saturated fats. Serum cholesterol and triglyceride levels are determined and, if elevated, treated with appropriate dietary restrictions and drugs. If the patient if overweight, a low calorie, weight-reducing diet is instituted. Hypertension must be carefully controlled and cigarette smoking discontinued.

SUMMARY

Individuals with coronary atherosclerotic heart disease may experience abrupt worsening of their symptoms, with severe and prolonged episodes of angina in the absence of known precipitating factors, a syndrome we have termed "unstable angina." The ultimate prognosis, though not clearly defined, appears quite grim, with a 30 to 40% risk of myocardial infarction within a year, and a yearly mortality rate of approximately 20%. Medical therapy is directed at decreasing myocardial oxygen demands with bed rest, sedation, nitrates and propranolol, while treating potentially fatal complications such as arrhythmias (Figure 2). Approximately 70% of such patients will respond to this therapy with resolution or marked reduction of their symptoms. They may then be safely managed by continued medical treatment, with elective coronary arteriography and coronary artery bypass surgery, if indicated, six weeks following the acute episode. Thirty percent of patients with unstable angina, however, will develop the intermediate coronary syndrome characterized by persistent, severe angina, in spite of intensive medical therapy. These patients have a much poorer prognosis and may benefit from a more aggressive therapeutic approach, with early performance of coronary arteriography and coronary artery bypass surgery, if appropriate lesions are found. Subsequent management of both medically and

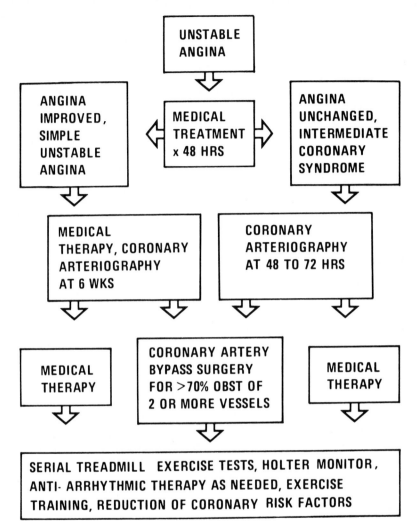

Figure 2 Medical and surgical management of unstable angina. Abbreviation: obst. = obstruction

surgically treated patients is directed towards determining safe levels of physical activity, identifying and treating potentially fatal arrhythmias, and reducing major coronary risk factors.

References

1. Kuller, L., Lilienfeld, A., and Fisher, R.: Epidemiological study of sudden and unexpected deaths due to arteriosclerotic heart disease. *Circulation*, **34**: 1056, 1966.

2. McNeilly, R.H. and Pemberton, J.: Duration of last attack in 998 fatal cases of coronary artery disease and its relation to possible cardiac resuscitation. *Brit. Med. J.*, **3**: 139, 1968.

3. Fulton, M., Julian, D.G., and Oliver, M.F.: Sudden death and myocardial infarction. *Circulation*, **40** Suppl IV: IV-182, 1968 (Abstract).

4. Armstrong, A., Duncan, B., Oliver, M.F., Julian, D.G., Donald, K.W., Fulton, M., Lutz, W., and Morrison, S.L.: Natural history of acute coronary heart attacks. *Brit. Heart J.*, **34**: 67, 1972.

5. Bainton, C.R. and Peterson, D.R.: Deaths from coronary heart disease in persons fifty years of age and younger. *N. Engl. J. Med.*, **268**: 569, 1963.

6. Solomon, H.A., Edwards, A.L., and Killip, T.: Prodromata in acute myocardial infarction. *Circulation*, **40**: 463, 1969.

7. Stowers, M. and Short, D.: Warning symptoms before major myocardial infarction. *Brit. Heart J.*, **32**: 833, 1970.

8. Graybiel, A.: The intermediate coronary syndrome. *U.S. Armed Forces Med. J.*, **6**: 1, 1955.

9. Master, A.M., Jaffe, H.L., Field, L.E., and Donoso, E.: Acute coronary insufficiency: its differential diagnosis and treatment. *Ann. Intern. Med.*, **45**: 561, 1956.

10. Levy, H.: The natural history of changing patterns of angina pectoris. *Ann. Intern. Med.*, **44**: 1123, 1956.

11. Papp, C. and Smith, K.S.: Status anginosus. *Brit. Heart J.*, **22**: 259, 1966.

12. Wood, P.: Acute and subacute coronary insufficiency. *Brit. Med. J.*, **1**: 1779, 1961.

13. Vakil, R.J.: Intermediate coronary syndrome. *Circulation*, **24**: 557, 961.

14. Harrison, D.C. and Shumway. N.E.: Evaluation and surgery for impending myocardial infarction. In E. Braunwald (Ed.): *The Myocardium: Failure and Infarction.* H.P. Publishing Co., New York, 1974, p. 353.

15. Chiong, M.A., West, R., and Parker, J.O.: Myocardial balance of inorganic phosphate and enzymes in man, effects of tachycardia and ischemia. *Circulation*, **49**: 283, 1974.

16. Meltzer, H.Y., Mrozak, S., and Boyer, M.: Effect of intramuscular injections on serum creatine phosphokinase activity. *Am. J. Med. Sci.*, **259**: 42, 1970.

17. Master, A.M.: The treatment of impending infarction. *Dis. Chest*, **43**: 302, 1963.

18. Vakil, J.V.: Preinfarction syndrome. Management and follow-up. *Am. J. Cardiol.*, **14**: 55, 1964.

19. Fulton, M., Lutz, W., Donald, F.W., Kirby, B.J., Duncan, B., Morrison, S.L., Kerr, F., and Julian, D.G.: Natural history of unstable angina. *Lancet*, **1**: 860, 1972.

20. Krause, K.R., Hutter, A.M., Jr., and DeSanctis, R.W.: Acute coronary insufficiency. *Arch. Intern. Med.*, **129**: 808, 1972.

21. Gazes, P.C., Mobley, E.M., Jr., Faris, H.M., Jr., Duncan, R.C., and Humphries, G.B.: Preinfarction angina—a prospective study. Ten year follow-up. *Circulation*, **48**: 331, 1973.

22. Sonnenblick, E.H., Ross, J., Jr., and Braunwald, E.: Oxygen consumption of the heart: newer concepts of its multifactorial determination. *Am. J. Cardiol.*, **22**: 238, 1968.

23. Harrison, T.R. and Reeves, J.J.: Management of preinfarctional angina. In *Principles and Problems of Ischemic Heart Disease.* Yearbook Publishers, Chicago, 1968, p. 261.

24. Braunwald, E.: Control of myocardial oxygen consumption: physiologic and clinical considerations. *Am. J. Cardiol.*, **27**: 416, 1971.

25. Nickerson, M. and Rvedy, J.: Antihypertensive agents and the drug therapy of hypertension. In L.S. Goodman and A. Gilman (Eds.): *The Pharmacologic Basis of Therapeutics.* MacMillan Publishing Co., New York, 1973, p. 707.

26. Gifford, R.W., Jr. and Richards, N.G.: Hypertensive encephalopathy. Differential diagnosis and treatment. *Curr. Concepts Cerebrovasc. Dis. Stroke*, **5**: 43, 1970.

27. Schlant, R.C.: Altered cardiovascular physiology of coronary atherosclerotic heart disease. In J.W. Hurst (Ed.): *The Heart*. McGraw Hill Book Co., New York, 1974, p. 1020.

28. Irons, G.V., Ginn, W.N., and Orgain, E.S.: Use of a beta-adrenergic receptor blocking agent (propranolol) in the treatment of cardiac arrhythmias. *Am. J. Med.*, **43**: 1967.

29. Robin, E., Cowan, C., Puri, P., Ganguly, S., DeBoyrie, M.M., Stock, T., and Bing, R.J.: A comparative study of nitroglycerin and propranolol. *Circulation*, **36**: 175, 1967.

30. Badeer, H.S.: Contractile tension in the myocardium. *Am. Heart J.*, **66**: 432, 1963.

31. Lindner, A., Charra, B., Sheppard, O.J., and Scribner, B.H.: Accelerated atherosclerosis in prolonged maintenance hemodialysis. *N. Engl. J. Med.*, **290**: 697, 1974.

32. Riddle, M.C. and Schwartz, T.B.: New tactics for hyperthyroidism: Sympathetic blockade. *Ann. Intern. Med.*, **72**: 749, 1970.

33. Ingbar, S.H. and Woeber, K.A.: The thyroid gland. In R.H. Williams (Ed.): *Textbook of Endocrinology*. W.B. Saunders Co., Philadelphia, 1974, p. 175.

34. Roberts, W.C.: Coronary thrombosis and fatal myocardial ischemia. *Circulation*, **49**: 1, 1974.

35. Wray, R., Maurer, B., and Shillingford, J.: Prophylactic anticoagulant therapy in prevention of calf vein thrombosis after myocardial infarction. *N. Engl. J. Med.*, **288**: 815, 1973.

36. Nichol, E.S., Phillips, W.C., and Casten, G.G.: Virtue of prompt anticoagulant therapy in acute coronary insufficiency or impending myocardial infarction. *Ann. Intern. Med.*, **50**: 1158, 1959.

37. Maurice, P., Beaumont, J.L., Leupin, A., and Lenegre, J.: La periode premonitaire de l'infarctus du myocarde. *Arch. Mal Coeur*, **48**: 551, 1955.

38. Beamish, R.E. and Storrie, V.M.: Impending myocardial infarction. Recognition and management. *Circulation*, **21**: 1107, 1960.

39. Master, A.M.: Impending myocardial infarction. the value of anticoagulant therapy. *Gen. Practice*, **32**: 122, 1965.

40. Mustard, J.F., Murphy, E.A., Rowsell, H.C., and Downie, H.G.: Factors influencing thrombus formation in vivo. *Am. J. Med.*, **33**: 621, 1962.

41. Gorlin, R.: Pathophysiology of cardiac pain. *Circulation*, **32**: 138, 1965.

42. Cannom, D.S., Harrison, D.C., and Schroeder, J.S.: Hemodynamic observations in patients with unstable angina pectoris. *Am. J. Cardiol.*, **33**: 17, 1974.

43. Roughgarden, J.W.: Circulatory changes associated with spontaneous angina pectoris. *Am. J. Med.*, **41**: 947, 1966.

44. Aronow, W.S.: The medical treatment of angina pectoris. Propranolol as an antianginal drug. *Am. Heart J.*, **84**: 706, 1972.

45. Alderman, E.L. and Harrison, D.C.: Beta adrenergic blockade in the management of angina pectoris. In D.C. Harrison (Ed.): *Circulatory Effects and Uses of Beta-Adrenergic Blocking Drugs*. Excerpta Medica, Amsterdam, 1971, p. 67.

46. Sharma, B. and Taylor, S.H.: A critical review of the symptomatic electrocardiographic and circulatory effects of adrenergic beta receptor antagonists in angina pectoris. In D.M. Burlye, J.H. Frier, R.K. Randel, and S.H. Taylor (Eds.: *New Perspectives in Beta-Blockade*. Horsham, England: CIBA, 1973.

47. Gianelly, R.E., Goldman, R.H., Treister, B., and Harrison, D.C.: Propranolol in patients with angina pectoris. *Ann. Intern. Med.*, **67**: 1216, 1967.

48. Grant, R.H.E., Keelan, P., Kernohan, R.J., Leonard, J.C., Nancekievill, L., and Sinclair, K.: Multicenter trial of propranolol in angina pectoris. *Am. J. Cardiol.*, **18**: 361, 1966.

354 / Cardiac Emergencies

49. Master, A.M. and Jaffe, H.L.: Propranolol vs. saphenous vein graft bypass for impending infarction (preinfarction syndrome). *Am. Heart J.*, **97**: 321, 1974.
50. Nies, A.S. and Shand, J.D.: Clinical pharmacology of propranolol. *Circulation*, **52**: 6, 1973.
51. Alderman, E.L., Davies, R.O., Crowley, J.J., Lopes, M.G., Brooker, J.Z., Friedman, J.P., Graham, A.F., Matlof, H.J., and Harrison, D.C.: Dose response effectiveness of propranolol for the treatment of angina pectoris. *Circulation*, **51**: 964, 1975.
52. Greenblatt, O.J. and Koch-Weser, J.: Adverse reactions to propranolol in hospitalized medical patients: a report from the Boston Collaborative Drug Surveillance Program. *Am. Heart J.*, **86**: 478, 1973.
53. Cohn, P.F. and Gorlin, R.: Physiologic and clinical actions of nitroglycerine. *Med. Clin. North Am.*, **58**: 407, 1974.
54. Weintraub, R.M., Voukydis, P.C., Aroesty, J.M., Cohen, S.I., Ford, P., Kurland, G.S., Laraia, P.J., Morkin, E., and Paulin, S.: Treatment of preinfarction angina with intra-aortic balloon counterpulsation and surgery. *Am. J. Cardiol.*, **34**: 809, 1974.
55. Parmley, W.W., Chatterjee, K., Charuzi, Y., and Swan, H.J.C.: Hemodynamic effects of non-invasive systolic unloading (nitroprusside) and diastolic augmentation (external counterpulsation) in patients with acute myocardial infarction. *Am. J. Cardiol.*, **33**: 619, 1974.
56. Block, W.J., Jr., Crumpacker, E.L., and Dry, T.J.: Prognosis of angina pectoris. Observations in 6,882 cases. *JAMA*, **150**: 259, 1952.
57. Kannel, W.B. and Feinleib, M.: Natural history of angina pectoris in the Framingham study. Prognosis and survival. *Am. J. Cardiol.*, **29**: 154, 1972.
58. Roberts, W.C.: Coronary arteries in fatal acute myocardial infarction. *Circulation*, **45**: 215, 1972.
59. Swan, H.J., Chatterjee, K., Corday, E., Ganz, W., Marcus, H., Matloff, J., and Parmely, W.: Myocardial revascularization for acute and chronic coronary heart disease. *Ann. Intern. Med.*, **79**: 851, 1973.
60. Grondin, C.M., LePage, G., Castonguay, Y.R., Meere, C., and Grondin, P.: Aortocoronary bypass graft, initial bloodflow through the graft and early postoperative patency. *Circulation*, **44**: 815, 1971.
61. Walker, J.A., Friedberg, H.O., Flemma, R.J., and Johnson, D.: Determinants of angiographic patency of aortocoronary vein bypass grafts. *Circulation*, **45** Suppl I: I-86, 1972.
62. Scanlon, P.J., Rimguadas, N., Moran, J.F., Talano, J.V., Pirouz, A., and Pifarra, R.: Accelerated angina pectoris. *Circulation*, **47**: 19, 1973.
63. Bonchek, L.I., Rahimtoola, S.H., Anderson, R.P., McAnulty, J.A., Rosch, J., Bristow, J.O., and Starr, A.: Late results following emergency saphenous vein bypass grafting for unstable angina. *Circulation*, **50**: 972, 1974.
64. Lambert, C.J., Adam, M., Geisler, G.F., Verzosa, E., Nazarian, M., and Mitchell, B.F.: Emergency myocardial revascularization for impending infarctions and arrhythmias. *J. Thorac. Cardiovasc. Surg.*, **62**: 522, 1971.
65. Berndt, T.B., Miller, D., Silverman, J.F., Stinson, E.B., Harrison, D.C., and Schroeder, J.S.: Coronary bypass surgery for unstable angina pectoris. Clinical follow-up and results of postoperative treadmill electrocardiograms. *Am. J. Med.*, **58**: 171, 1975.
66. Alderman, E.L., Coltart, D.J., Wettach, G.E., and Harrison, D.C.: Coronary artery syndromes after sudden propranolol withdrawal. *Ann. Intern. Med.*, **81**: 625, 1975.
67. Coltart, D.J., Cayen, M.N., Stinson, E.B., Goldman, R.H., Davies, R.O., and Harrison, D.C.: Investigation of the safe withdrawal period for propranolol in patients scheduled for open-heart surgery. *Brit. Heart J.*, In press.

68. Ross, R.S. and Gorlin, R.: Coronary arteriography. In E. Braunwald and H.J.C. Swan (Eds.): *Cooperative Study on Cardiac Catheterization.* American Heart Association, New York, 1968, pp. III-67.
69. Miller, D.C., Cannom, D.S., Fogarty, T.J., Schroeder, J.S., Daily, P.O., and Harrison, D.C.: Saphenous vein coronary artery bypass in patients with "preinfarction angina." *Circulation,* **47**: 234, 1973.
70. Favaloro, R.G., Effler, D.B., Cheanvechai, C., Quint, R.A., and Sones, F.M.: Acute coronary insufficiency: impending myocardial infarction and myocardial infarction. *Am. J. Cardiol.,* **28**: 598, 1971.
71. Conti, C.R., Greene, B., Pitt, B., Griffith, L., Humphries, O., Brawley, R., Taylor, D., Bender, H., Gott, U., and Ross, R.: Coronary surgery in unstable angina pectoris. *Circulation,* **44** Suppl II: II-154, 1971.
72. Conti, C.R., Greene, B., Pitt, B., Griffith, L., Humphries, O., Brawley, R., Taylor, D., Bender, H., Gott, U., and Ross, R.: Coronary surgery in unstable angina pectoris. *Circulation,* **49** Suppl II: II-154, 1971 (Abstract).
73. Segal, B.L., Likoff, W., Van Den Broef, H., Adam, A., Blanco, S., Kimbris, D., and Najmi, H.: Saphenous vein bypass for impending myocardial infarction. *Am. J. Cardiol.,* **29**: 290, 1972.
74. Dawson, J.T., Hall, R.J., Hallman, G.L., and Cooley, D.A.: Mortality in patients undergoing coronary artery bypass surgery after myocardial infarction. *Am. J. Cardiol.,* **33**: 483, 1974.
75. Lea, R.E., Tector, A.J., Flemma, R.J., Johnson, W.D., Beddingfield, G.W., and Lepley, D., Jr.: Prognostic significance of reduced left ventricular ejection fraction in coronary artery surgery. *Circulation,* **46** Suppl II: II-49, 1972 (Abstract).
76. Hill, D.J., Kerth, W.J., DeLeval, M.R., Yokota, M., and Gerbode, F.: Myocardial infarction and preinfarction: results of emergency myocardial revascularization. *J. Cardiovasc. Surg.,* **15**: 205, 1974.
77. Cheanvechai, C., Effler, D.B., Loop, F.D., Groves, L.K., Sheldon, W.C., Razavi, M., and Sones, F.M., Jr.: Emergency myocardial revascularization. *Am. J. Cardiol.,* **32**: 901, 1973.
78. Motlagh, F.A., Pansegran, D.G., and Wilson, H.E.: Direct myocardial revascularization for preinfarction syndrome. *Circulation,* **45** and **46** Suppl II: II-195, 1972 (Abstract).
79. Flemma, R.J., Johnson, D., Tector, A.J., Lepley, D., and Blitz, J.: Surgical treatment of preinfarction angina. *Arch. Intern. Med.,* **129**: 828, 1972.
80. Bertolasi, C.A., Tronge, J.E., Carreno, C.A., Jalon, J., and Vega, M.R.: Unstable angina—prospective and randomized study of its evolution, with and without surgery. Preliminary report. *Am. J. Cardiol.,* **33**: 201, 1974.
81. Griffith, L.S.C., Achuff, S.C., Conti, C.R., Humphries, J., Brawley, R.K., Gott, U.L., and Ross, R.S.: Changes in coronary circulation and ventricular motion after bypass surgery. *N. Engl. J. Med.,* **288**: 589, 1973.
82. Tominaga, S., Blackburn, H.: Prognostic importance of premature beats following myocardial infarction: experience in the Coronary Drug Project. *JAMA,* **223**: 1116, 1973.
83. Redwood, D.R., Rosing, D.R., and Epstein, S.E.: Circulatory and symptomatic effects of physical training in patients with coronary artery disease and angina pectoris. *N. Engl. J. Med.,* **286**: 959, 1972.

CHAPTER 18
Drug Management of
Hypertensive Emergencies

Gerald L. Wolf, Ph.D., M.D.; Frederick Dalske, Ph.D.;
Hope Sass, M.D.

Few physicians see hypertensive crises frequently. In this Chapter, the authors present a concise and practical discussion of current drugs most useful in lowering blood pressure safely and quickly. Intravenous agents have replaced those given by intramuscular routes. The pharmacologic characteristics of each agent importantly influence which one to select for specific crises. Tables provide ready future reference.

The essence of a hypertensive emergency is the need for rapid reduction of blood pressure. The actual blood pressure does not define an emergency—more relevant are the clinical signs and symptoms associated with a particular pressure elevation. When the function of such vital organs as the brain, heart, or kidney is acutely impaired by an elevated blood pressure, it is mandatory to safely institute effective antihypertensive therapy. This therapeutic goal should be achieved within a period of several minutes to a few hours.

Fortunately, parenteral drugs have become available that can permit selection of the proper pharmacophysiologic intervention for nearly all hypertensive emergencies. These agents include diazoxide (Hyperstat®), trimethaphan (Arfonad®) and nitroprusside (Nipride®). The pharmacologic effects of these agents differ importantly and this influences the drug of choice for a particular crisis.

In this chapter, we will review the relation between drug characteristics and different pathophysiologic states that may cause hypertensive emergencies. We will first consider the pharmacologic basis for the treatment of hypertensive encephalopathy. Next, the emergency treatment of functional impairment in other organ systems will be contrasted with that for hypertensive encephalopathy to define the changes in therapeutic strategy that are required. However, the same pharmacologic principles may be used to quickly lower severely elevated blood pressure that is not associated with imminent functional loss or to lower a mildly elevated blood pressure in situations that are aggravated by hypertension such as dissecting aneurysm, intracranial hemorrhage, or postoperative bleeding.

357

TREATMENT OF HYPERTENSIVE ENCEPHALOPATHY

Hypertensive encephalopathy presents as an elevated blood pressure, usually greater than 120 mm Hg diastolic, *and* clinical evidence for recent impairment of brain function. The clinical portrait may include severe headache, nausea, vomiting, mental confusion, seizures, nystagmus, papilledema, Babinski's sign, localized weakness, reflex asymmetries, coma or stupor. The cerebral symptoms and signs may wax and wane and frequently appear at night. They can be caused by almost any acute increase in blood pressure, but are usually associated with values close to 220/130 mm Hg. This is a true medical emergency for these patients may expire within a few hours.

The brain faces several mechanical disadvantages when blood pressure is acutely raised because the cerebral circulation is unique. First, there are actually three functional intracranial volume compartments as shown in Figure 1. Nervous tissue is, in effect, suspended between the vascular compartment and the cerebral spinal fluid compartment, and all three are encased in a rigid container, the skull. One compartment cannot expand without reductions in the volume of another. The vascular endothelium has unusually small pores (blood brain barrier) while the functional interstitial space is small and nearly protein free. During cerebral edema the barrier is disrupted, allowing protein and fluid to be pushed into the interstitial fluid space by perfusion pressure. This volume expansion impairs nervous function.

The regulation of the vascular compartment is accomplished without significant direct control by the sympathetic nervous system. Brain arterioles possess few α-receptors for vasoconstriction; local sympathetic nerves and circulating hormonal factors are equally unimpressive in changing cerebral blood flow. In fact, interstitial hydrogen ion seems to be the only physiologic vasodilator within the cerebral circulation. For the most part, matching of cerebral flow to physiologic requirements is accomplished by very strong local regulation of flow. As shown in Figure 2, when blood pressure rises this autoregulatory mechanism constricts the arterioles just enough to maintain constant flow; the opposite response is induced when pressure falls. It is now recognized that there is an upper limit as well as a lower limit for autoregulation of cerebral blood flow[1].

There are two theories about what happens to the brain when the blood pressure goes up acutely. One dates from 1859 and holds that segmental narrowing or vasospasm develops, leading to cerebral ischemia and thence to hypertensive encephalopathy (Figure 3). These observations are probably at least partly true, and certainly vasospasm in the retinal circulation is prominent in this condition.

Currently, the more popular theory is inappropriate arteriolar dilatation. Under the stress of acute hypertension, some vessels do not maintain adequate tone and may, in fact, dilate. This forces too much pressure into more

PECULIARITIES OF CEREBRAL CIRCULATION

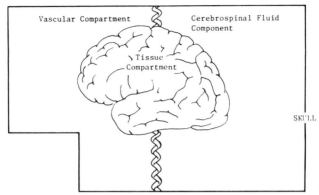

1. Tight vascular endothelium
   (Blood Brain Barrier)

2. Small Interstitial Fluid Space
   with little protein

3. Few sympathetic vasoconstrictor
   receptors

4. Interstitial H^+ is physiologic
   vasodilator

5. Very strong local flow control
   (Autoregulation)

Figure 1 Schematic representation of the peculiarities of cerebral circulation. Functional nervous tissue is, in effect, suspended between the vascular and cerebrospinal fluid compartments. The vascular compartment differs from other circulatory beds in its anatomy and function as enumerated.

distal vessels, overcoming the physical processes which maintain the blood brain barrier. Local ultrafiltration occurs, causing cerebral edema which may physically restrict the vessels and lead to cerebral ischemia (Figure 3).

The pathophysiologic process is therefore an autoregulatory breakthrough, and initially blood flow goes up markedly. No matter what the pressure, as long as the arteriolar vessel can constrict, the pressure is not transmitted downstream into smaller vessels where untrafiltration would occur.

Each patient has his own characteristic autoregulatory curve and its associated breakthrough point. The curve is importantly influenced by several variables. Acidosis shifts the curve as shown in Figure 2 and allows breakthrough at lower absolute pressures. This may be one reason that patients frequently develop their symptoms at night when the arterial CO_2 increases. For similar reasons, tranquilizing and sedative drugs that decrease ventilation are potential precipitating agents.

Chronic hypertension shifts the whole curve toward the right, so that the hypertensive patient tolerates higher pressures even better than the normotensive one. It usually takes an additional acute increase in pressure to in-

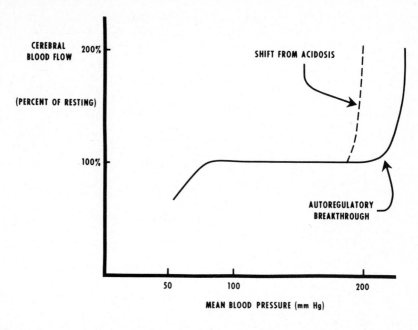

Figure 2 Autoregulation of cerebral circulation. The autoregulatory plateau is a zone in which cerebral flow is kept constant despite increases or decreases in blood pressure. The breakthrough point represents failure of autoregulation, and blood flow climbs steeply leading to encephalopathy. With acidosis, the breakthrough point shifts to the left. The adaptation to chronic hypertension shifts the entire curve to the right.

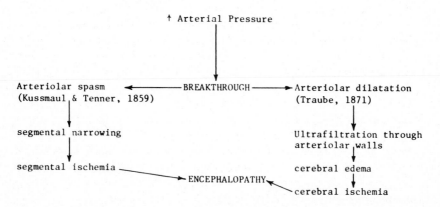

Figure 3 Theories of the etiology of cerebral ischemia with hypertension. The vasoconstrictive and vasodilator theories both lead to ischemia and may, in fact, coexist.

duce symptoms in hypertensive patients. However, the entire curve is shifted so that it also takes more pressure to keep flow from falling on the lower part of the plateau. This is an extremely important therapeutic consideration; one can lower the pressure too far in these patients and induce cerebral ischemia iatrogenically.

The treatment of hypertensive encephalopathy consists of judicious lowering of blood pressure. The desire to reverse cerebral ischemia as quickly as possible makes parenteral therapy the best. The therapeutic goal for the first few days is a blood pressure near 140/100 mm Hg with suitable allowances for the usual pressure prior to the onset of encephalopathy. We must now consider the pharmacology of parenteral drugs that are recommended for managing hypertensive encephalopathy.

Diazoxide

There are three drugs preferred for the treatment of hypertensive crisis-diazoxide (Hyperstat®), sodium nitroprusside (Nipride®), and trimethaphan camsylate (Arfonad®). All are fast and effective when administered intravenously, but probably the easiest to handle in terms of specialized equipment needed or attention to the patient's response is diazoxide.

Diazoxide is chemically related to the thiazide diuretics, but, paradoxically, causes salt and water retention. The anithypertensive response to diazoxide depends on the drug's ability to directly relax arteriolar, but not venular, smooth muscle in all vascular beds. Since diazoxide does not interfere with sympathetic neurotransmission, the distinction between vascular sites of action is an important one. Venous return to the heart is maintained during diazoxide-induced arteriolar dilation; this, when coupled with the reflex tachycardia that diazoxide produces, leads to an increased stroke volume and left ventricular ejection rate that combine to augment cardiac output (Figure 4). The drop in peripheral resistance is much greater with diazoxide than with either nitroprusside or trimethaphan, since the rise in cardiac output must be offset in order to maintain a lowered arterial pressure. Diazoxide has no direct stimulatory effect on the heart; all cardiac actions are mediated by reflex. Blood flow to all vascular beds, including renal, is usually maintained; postural hypotension does not occur, due to the intact autonomic reflexes.

Diazoxide is given in a bolus intravenous dose of 300 mg or 5 mg/kg (Table I). The drug is rapidly bound to serum albumin and must be given within 10-15 seconds to allow sufficient free drug to reach vasodilatory receptor sites at the arteriolar wall. Diazoxide solutions are very alkaline and should be administered via an IV line. Extravasation must be avoided if the drug is given directly into a vein. Maximum reduction in blood pressure occurs within 3-5 minutes, but often as quickly as 1 minute. The hypotensive response may last as little as 30 minutes, but generally lasts 6-12 hours. A se-

	Diazoxide (300 mg iv in 9 patients)		Trimetaphan (1 mg/ml iv infusion in 6 patients)		Sodium Nitroprusside (60 μg/ml iv infusion in 7 patients)	
	C	D	C	D	C	D
Mean Arterial Pressure (mm Hg)	142	111	142	108	152	112
Heart Rate (beats/min)	74	97	85	100	83	98
Cardiac Output (litres/min/M²)	3.1	4.2	3.3	3.0	3.0	2.7
Left Ventricular Ejection Rate (ml/sec/M²)	158	177	149	132	157	135
Total Peripheral Resistance (mm Hg/ml/min)	0.024	0.014	0.023	0.019	0.027	0.023

C = Control.
D = Active drug.

Figure 4 Comparison of the hemodynamic responses in patients with hypertensive crisis treated with the three recommended drugs. The effects upon arterial pressure, heart rate, and peripheral resistance are similar. However, important differences are noted in the response of cardiac output and ejection rate. (From Bhatia, S.K. and Frohlich, E.D.: Hemodynamic comparison of agents useful in hypertensive emergencies. *Am. Heart J.*, **85**: 367-373, 1973, with permission.)

cond dose may be given after 30 minutes if the initial response is not sufficient. Patients should remain recumbent and be closely monitored for the first 15 minutes after each dose, with hourly pressure checks thereafter. Subsequent doses may be given at intervals determined by the hypotensive response, although oral antihypertensive medication should be initiated with the first dose to minimize the need for continued intravenous injections. Although blood pressure rarely falls to below normotensive levels, pressor amines may be used to counter any undue hypotensive response. Signs of cerebral or myocardial ischemia may occur during the initial response to diazoxide, especially in patients with previously compromised cerebral or coronary circulations. Patients with a history of chronic hypertension usually require a diastolic pressure of about 100 mm Hg to maintain cerebral flow, due to the autoregulatory shift described above.

Diazoxide causes hyperglycemia and hyperuricemia, but neither is serious during the usual brief course of therapy unless diabetes or renal insufficiency are present, in which case insulin dosage adjustments or allopurinol, respectively, are indicated. Marked salt and water retention are a normal conse-

TABLE I
SUMMARY OF CLINICAL PHARMACOLOGY
FOR THE PREFERRED DRUGS

Drug	Mode of Action	Onset	Peak	Duration	Dosage
Diazoxide (Hyperstat®)	Direct dilation of arterioles	1-2 min	3-5 min	3-14 hr.	300 mg IV bolus
Sodium nitroprusside (Nipride®)	Direct dilation of arterioles and venules	½-1 min	1-2 min	3-5 min	30-500 micrograms per min IV infusion
Trimethaphan camsylate (Arfonad®)	Ganglionic blockade	1-2 min	2-5 min	10 min	1-15 mg per min IV infusion ± postural change

quence of diazoxide use, but can be effectively countered with diuretics. The more potent loop diuretics, furosemide or ethacrynic acid, are usually needed; when given prior to diazoxide, either agent will not only offset the deleterious effects of volume retention but also help maintain function which may be compromised in a hypertensive crisis (Figure 5). Diazoxide crosses the placenta, and may also interrupt labor if given during hypertensive crisis due to eclampsia. Uterine contractions can be reestablished with oxytocin. Renin levels may rise during diazoxide therapy, but this is a minor consideration in an emergency situation.

Diazoxide's effect may be potentiated in a patient already receiving propranolol or guanethidine, since the reflex rise in cardiac output will be diminished or blocked by these agents. The dosage of coumarin anticoagulants or other drugs which bind to plasma albumin should be reduced, since diazoxide displaces these drugs from their binding sites.

In comparison with nitroprusside and trimethaphan, diazoxide has the advantage of requiring only a single dose with a minimum of patient monitoring thereafter. Disadvantages include the reflex cardiac stimulation that attends its use, as well as the inability to make minute-to-minute adjustments in blood pressure. The consistency of diazoxide's effect runs a close second to that of nitroprusside.

Nitroprusside

Sodium nitroprusside is the most rapidly acting and consistently effective agent presently available for managing acute hypertensive crises. Unfortunately, unfounded fears of cyanide toxicity and the time-consuming process necessary to prepare the drug immediately before use have worked against its acceptance as a valuable hypotensive agent. Recently, however, a

	DIAZOXIDE	FUROSEMIDE	DIAZOXIDE + FUROSEMIDE
MAP	↓↓	↓	↓↓↓
CO	↑↑	↓↑	↑↑
SODIUM BALANCE	(+)(+)	(−)(−)	(−)
URINARY OUTPUT	↓↓	↑↑	↑

Figure 5 The advantages of combined therapy with diazoxide and furosemide. The adverse effects of diazoxide upon urinary excretion are countered by furosemide. Both drugs are additive in decreasing mean arterial pressure (MAP) and maintaining cardiac output (CO). (From Russek, H.I., and Zohman, B.: *Cardiovascular Therapy: The Art and the Science*. Williams and Wilkins, Baltimore, 1971, with permission.)

commercial lyophilized form requiring much less preparation time has been introduced (Nipride®).

Nitroprusside does release cyanide ions in the body as a consequence of its action on vascular smooth muscle. However, the release of cyanide is a relatively slow process, and the enzymatic action of rhodanase mitigates against any buildup of this ion. Rhodanase rapidly converts cyanide into thiocyanate, which is then excreted by the kidney in the same manner as chloride.

Unlike diazoxide, nitroprusside relaxes both arteriolar and venular smooth muscle in all vascular beds. The consequence of this nonspecific vascular action is to diminish venous return as well as to decrease total peripheral resistance. As is the case with diazoxide, nitroprusside has no effect on adrenergic function, and sympathetic cardiovascular reflexes are maintained. Thus, tachycardia occurs, but cardiac output rarely rises and usually falls, since the increased heart rate cannot compensate for the decreased stroke volume and reduced left ventricular ejection rate that results from venous pooling. Nitroprusside has no direct cardiac action. Blood flow is usually maintained to all vascular beds, but the combination of arterial dilation and reduced cardiac output may lead to signs of insufficiency in an already compromised cerebral or coronary circulation when pressure is lowered too far.

Nitroprusside should be prepared fresh by dilution in 5% dextrose solution just prior to use. Solutions are normally stable for about four hours, but if protected from light by wrapping in aluminum foil the effective life of solutions may be extended up to 24 hours. The drug must be given intravenously using a micro-drip regulator or, preferably, an infusion pump, because small changes in administration rate can cause large changes in blood pressure. Nitroprusside's onset of action is almost instantaneous; blood pressure can be maintained at almost any level by appropriate adjustment of the infusion rate. However, arterial pressure returns to pretreatment level within minutes after stopping the infusion. Thus, constant supervision and observation of the patient is mandatory, with pressure checks every 4-5 minutes. Virtually no one is refractory to nitroprusside's action, but sensitivity varies tremendously—effective doses range from 0.3-8 μg/kg/min. Nitroprusside therapy may be continued for days, if necessary, since tolerance rarely occurs. As with diazoxide, oral antihypertensive medication should be started concomitant with nitroprusside use, and the patient weaned from IV therapy as soon as practicable.

Most of the side effects that occur during nitroprusside therapy are due to an excessive fall in blood pressure; careful supervision of the infusion rate generally results in asymptomatic treatment. The thiocyanate end product is normally excreted harmlessly by the kidney. However, if nitroprusside is infused at high rates or for longer than 48 hours, serum thiocyanate levels should be monitored and the infusion stopped if levels exceed 10 mg%. Patients with renal insufficiency are especially prone to thiocyanate accumulation and must be carefully monitored. In addition, nitroprusside should be used with caution in patients with hypothyroidism, since thiocyanate inhibits the uptake and binding of iodine in the thyroid. Plasma renin levels increase during nitroprusside therapy, but the duration of treatment is usually short enough to preclude any untoward effects of increased renin.

Nitroprusside thus offers the advantages of immediate onset, high potency, and ability to minutely adjust blood pressure. However, use of the drug requires constant patient monitoring and precise regulation of infusion rates.

Trimethaphan

Prior to the development of diazoxide and the resurrection of nitroprusside, trimethaphan (Arfonad®) was a mainstay in the treatment of hypertensive emergencies. Now, however, trimethaphan is relegated to only occasional use, except for those physicians who "grew up" with this agent and are sufficiently experienced in its use.

Although the hemodynamic consequences of trimethaphan administration are similar to those of nitroprusside (Figure 4), the former drug has no direct effect on vascular smooth muscle. Trimethaphan is a ganglionic blocking agent, acting to prevent impulse transmission at all autonomic ganglia. This results in impaired parasympathetic and, more importantly, sympathetic transmission. Thus, tonic adrenergic stimulation is reduced in both arteriolar and venular beds, leading to a fall in peripheral resistance and venous pooling of blood. In addition, cardiovascular reflex mechanisms are also impaired, resulting in greatly reduced myocardial reflex stimulation. Cardiac output is diminished as a result of venous pooling, and this contributes to the fall in arterial pressure. This effect is magnified in the upright position as a result of the orthostatic hypotension produced. In spite of the ganglionic blockade, some tachycardia usually results, but this has little effect on the hypotensive response. Blood flow to most vascular beds is reduced, but renal flow is most affected.

Like nitroprusside, trimethaphan has a very rapid onset and offset of action. It is best administered by a slow IV infusion, preferably by an infusion pump. Again, oral antihypertensive medication should be started concomitant with trimethaphan therapy. Careful patient monitoring is necessary to control fluctuations in blood pressure. The hypotensive action can be enhanced by mechanical measures (raising the head of the bed) that take advantage of the orthostatic effect. Similarly, larger doses will be needed in a completely supine patient. Although tachyphylaxis has been claimed to occur after several days therapy with trimethaphan, the more likely explanation is that the patient appears refractory because intravascular volume has expanded; diuretic therapy will markedly improve the hypotensive response. It should also be remembered that ganglionic blockade produces a form of denervation supersensitivity; this supersensitivity to sympathomimetic drugs dictates extreme caution in any attempt to raise arterial pressure with these agents.

Most of the side effects associated with trimethaphan's use are related to inhibition of the parasympathetic system. The most important are the development of paralytic ileus or atony of the bladder, first noticeable at 24 hours. An indwelling catheter is indicated to prevent urinary retention in patients treated for more than 48 hours. Another complication of ganglionic blockade is the inactivation of pupillary reflexes which may interfere with the neurologic evaluation in hypertensive encephalopathy. Finally, trimethaphan crosses the placenta and should not be used during pregnancy.

Figure 4 presents a comparison of the hemodynamic responses seen when each of the drugs were given to patients with hypertensive crises. The clinical pharmacology of the drugs is summarized in Table I.

For the treatment of hypertensive encephalopathy, nitroprusside is the preferred agent if intensive monitoring is readily available. The minute-to-minute control of pressure makes it the ideal drug under these circumstances. Under less optimum conditions, diazoxide becomes the drug of choice because of its safety for use when intensive monitoring is unavailable. Trimethaphan is inferior to both of the above drugs, but much preferred to other drugs such as reserpine, methyldopa, guanethidine, or clonidine.

CHOOSING A DRUG FOR OTHER HYPERTENSIVE CRISES

Coronary ischemia

If the patient with a hypertensive emergency has evidence of coronary artery disease, drugs that increase myocardial oxygen demand are contra-indicated (Table II). Of course, lowering blood pressure and afterload will usually reduce myocardial oxygen requirements. However, drugs such as hydralazine and diazoxide may cause increased cardiac output and aggravate ischemia because their action is limited to arterioles. On the other hand, nitroprusside will diminish both afterload and preload through its action upon arteries and veins. Severe diastolic hypotension must be avoided since myocardial perfusion, especially with coronary artery disease, depends upon diastolic pressure. When one knows the usual diastolic pressure before the crisis occurred, this level can be safely set as the therapeutic goal. Otherwise, aim for a diastolic pressure of 100 mm Hg.

TABLE II
SPECIAL THERAPEUTIC PROBLEMS

	Preferred Drugs	Drugs To Avoid
1. Patients with coronary ischemia	Nitroprusside	Hydralazine Diazoxide
2. Intracranial Hemorrhage or ischemia	Nitroprusside Trimethaphan Hydralazine	Diazoxide Reserpine Methyldopa
3. Acute left ventricular failure	Nitroprusside Trimethaphan	Hydralazine Diazoxide
4. Diminished renal function	Diazoxide Nitroprusside Hydralazine Loop Diuretics	Trimethaphan
5. Dissecting aneurysm or post-operative bleeding	Nitroprusside Trimethaphan Reserpine Propranolol	Diazoxide Hydralazine

Intracranial Hemorrhage

When a patient in hypertensive crisis also has intracranial hemorrhage, reserpine and methyldopa are not recommended. These drugs may interfere with accurate evaluation of the patient's CNS function and may even shift the autoregulatory curve further to the left by reducing ventilation. The drug of choice is nitroprusside because accurate blood pressure control is required. Diazoxide's effects are not as quickly modified. Trimethaphan is an excellent drug for this clinical situation.

Dissecting Aneurysm

The ingenious experiments of Palmer et al in turkeys, dogs, and patients have shown that management of this condition demands special anti-hypertensive therapy. In this situation both the absolute pressure and the rate of pressure change must be controlled, for each influences the forces in the arterial wall that promote further dissection. Both diazoxide and hydralazine unload the heart and allow more rapid ejection of ventricular volume. Both are contraindicated for use in dissecting aneurysm. Nitroprusside is better, but agents like trimethaphan and propranolol best combine effective antihypertensive actions along with diminished cardiac contractility. Reserpine and guanethidine have also proven clinically excellent in this condition although they do not act as rapidly as trimethaphan and propranolol.

Cathecholamine Crisis

Several clinical conditions may create a hypertensive emergency due to excessive catechol action. Pheochromocytoma is the classic example, but drugs are more frequently responsible for the emergency. The patient may have used excessive sympathomimetic drugs such as bronchodilators or appetite suppressants or may be unduly sensitive to small amounts of these drugs or even food products because he is taking MAO inhibitors. Whatever the etiology, emergency management begins with the alpha blocker, phentolamine (Table III). In some patients an excessive beta receptor stimulation may also be seen and must be blocked with propranolol.

TABLE III

MANAGEMENT OF CATECHOLAMINE CRISIS

Drug	Mode of Action	Onset	Peak	Duration	Dosage
Phentolamine (Regitine®)	α-receptor blockade	½-1 min.	1-2 min.	10-15 min.	5-15 mg IV bolus, sustain with infusion
Propranolol (Inderal®)	β-receptor blockade	1-2 min.	2-5 min.	3-6 hr.	1 mg/min IV 1-3 mg total dose

THE TRANSITION TO ORAL THERAPY

The necessity to start oral antihypertensive medication as soon as practicable has been noted for each of the parenteral agents discussed above. The specific oral drug to use is, of course, dependent upon the severity of the patient's hypertension; but generally the choice will be among alphamethyl dopa, clonidine and/or guanethidine. All are effective in moderate to severe hypertension. Clonidine can produce a significant fall in arterial pressure within 2-4 hours after oral administration; the time course for alphamethyl dopa's effect is slightly longer, about 4-6 hours. Guanethidine is the most potent oral agent available, but the usual course of therapy may require up to 7 days to achieve adequate pressure control. However, a recent study[2] has shown favorable results utilizing a loading-maintenance dose regimen, achieving satisfactory results after 1-3 days. Nearly every patient will require a diuretic agent in addition. When renal function is nearly normal, the thiazide diuretics are preferred. If renal function is less than one-third of normal, the thiazide diuretics are contraindicated and titration with loop diuretics is necessary.

References

1. Strangaard, S., Jones, J.V., Mackenzie, E.T., et al: Upper limit of cerebral blood flow autoregulation in experimental renovascular hypertension in the baboon. *Circ. Res.*, **37**: 164-167, 1975.
2. Shand, D.G., Nies, A.S., McAllister, R.G., et al: A loading-maintenance program for more rapid initiation of the effect of guanethidine. *Clin. Pharm. Ther.*, **18**: 139-144, 1975.

Suggested for Additional Reading

Bhatia, S.K. and Frohlich, E.D.: Hemodynamic comparison of agents useful in hypertensive emergencies. *Am. Heart J.*, **85**: 367-373, 1973.

Diazoxide: A review of its pharmacological properties and therapeutic use in hypertensive crises. *Drugs*, **2**: 78-137, 1971.

Drug Commentary: Evaluation of diazoxide (Hyperstat IV). *JAMA*, **224**: 1422-1423, 1973.

Koch-Weser, J.: Hypertensive emergencies. *N. Engl. J. Med.*, **290**: 211-214, 1974.

Palmer, R.F. and Lasseter, K.C.: Sodium nitroprusside. *N. Engl. J. Med.*, **292**: 294-297, 1975.

Tuzel, I.H.: Sodium nitroprusside: a review of its clinical effectiveness as a hypotensive agent. *J. Clin. Pharmacol.*, **14**: 494-503, 1974.

Index

Tables are indicated with page numbers followed by t